LIFESTYLE COUNSELING FOR ADJUSTMENT TO DISABILITY

Edited by

Warren R. Rule, Ph.D.

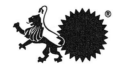

AN ASPEN PUBLICATION®
Aspen Systems Corporation
Rockville, Maryland
Royal Tunbridge Wells
1984

Library of Congress Cataloging in Publication Data
Main entry under title:

Lifestyle counseling for adjustment to disability.

Bibliography: p. 329
Includes index.
1. Handicapped—Counseling of. 2. Rehabilitation. 3. Adler, Alfred,
1870-1937. 4. Choice (Psychology)
I. Rule, Warren R.
HV1568.L53   1983   362.4'045323   83-15777
ISBN: 0-89443-895-6

Publisher: John Marozsan
Editorial Director: Margaret Quinlin
Executive Managing Editor: Margot Raphael
Editorial Services: Ruth Judy
Printing and Manufacturing: Debbie Collins

Poem by E.E. Cummings reprinted from *Complete Poems 1913-1962*
by permission of Harcourt Brace Jovanovich, Inc., and Granada
Publishing Limited. Copyright 1947 by E.E. Cummings

Library of Congress Catalog Card Number: 83-15777
ISBN: 0-89443-895-6

Printed in the United States of America

1 2 3 4 5

This book
is
dedicated
with love
to
my parents,
Richard William and Iris Geraldine Rule
of
Glassboro, New Jersey

Your
caring and sacrifice,
savvy and teaching,
earthiness and balance,
are gratefully appreciated

i thank You God for most this amazing
day: for the leaping greenly spirits of trees
and a blue true dream of sky; and for everything
which is natural which is infinite which is yes
                                        E.E. Cummings

Table of Contents

Preface

Disabled individuals make up a sizable portion of our population. Therefore, the inference could logically be drawn that many different and creative counseling approaches have been developed for assisting people to adjust to their disabilities. However, this has not been entirely so. For instance, surprisingly few books have appeared that explore adjustment to disability within the framework of a specific counseling perspective. This book is such an effort.

Lifestyle Counseling for Adjustment to Disability was designed so that much of the material discussed would be broadly consistent with several of the major premises of the founder of the lifestyle concept, Alfred Adler. The term "lifestyle" has come to have many meanings to different people and is being increasingly heard in everyday living as well as within the ranks of the helping professions. As will be discussed in the introductory chapter, however, most contemporary meanings of the term do not reflect the depth of the concept as it was originally intended or as it is used in this book.

This cannot be properly called an Adlerian book, in a pure and total sense. Rather, it is a practitioner's adaptation of many of Adler's ideas to adjustment to disability. Accordingly, the contributors, who have each had training at Virginia Commonwealth University in the fundamentals of the Adlerian lifestyle approach, were asked to be, broadly speaking, Adlerian eclectics. They were requested to include in their chapters whatever Adlerian lifestyle concepts and techniques that *worked for them,* as long as their overall approach was consistent with the Adlerian theoretical underpinnings of the holistic and goal-directed lifestyle. Because this is intended as a practitioner-oriented book, the use itself of these practical variations is largely consistent with the spirit of Adler's approach as a "psychology of use."

Lifestyle Counseling for Adjustment to Disability is intended for the variety of helping professionals who strive to facilitate the adjustment of the disabled. This includes practitioners in institutional and field settings as well as students in educational settings. The scope of the definition of disability in this book is decidedly broad, including the mental and emotional realms as well as the physical.

The book is divided into five parts. The first part is designed to provide background information, particularly a perspective on Adlerian lifestyle fundamentals. The second section explores family and lifespan considerations. The third includes chapters that discuss practical considerations relating to disabilities in general. Each chapter in the fourth part applies lifestyle concepts to specific types of disabilities. Finally, in the fifth section, attention is given to the counselor as a person.

In my editorial capacity, I respected whichever manner each contributor chose to express unidentified pronouns (e.g., "he" only, "he or she"). Whichever the choice, I doubt that inherent superiority—either male or female—is intended or implied by these contributors. My own personal belief is that the usage of dual personal and possessive pronouns is unjustifiably unwieldy in communication and that a more acceptable alternative is the selection of pronouns that are in keeping with one's own gender.

A host of individuals deserve acknowledgment for their contributions or support. Special appreciation is extended to my wife, Jane, for her understanding and patience, particularly while I was working on this manuscript. I am also very grateful to my daughter, Lauren, and son, Brian, for being themselves, for the warm sense of connectedness, and for frequently keeping me in touch with the realization that I was once an expert on children—until I had children of my own.

Heartfelt thanks are due my parents, to whom this book is dedicated. I would indeed be remiss in a book that focuses on some of Adler's concepts if I did not gratefully acknowledge the developmental contributions of my brother, Dick, and my sister, Cindy. In addition, the Brady family has been a supportive influence in many ways.

Sincere gratitude is extended to my original Adlerian mentor, Francis X. Walton, encourager par excellence and friend. Special thanks are offered to Harold and Birdie Mosak for their spirit of social interest as well as for their other contributions. Very significantly, the magic of the late Don McKenzie, doctoral advisor and teacher, continues to be gentle on my mind.

I am indebted to the Virginia Commonwealth University students who explored with me Adlerian ideas and variations of the lifestyle approach. This group, spanning ten years of classes, is affectionately and mischievously referred to as the "Adlerian Incorrigibles" and has taught me a great deal.

Deep gratitude is acknowledged to the many clients who directly and indirectly influenced the ideas offered in this book. Often, these persons are the ultimate—and unheralded—teachers.

Appreciation is expressed to my departmental chairman of rehabilitation counseling at Virginia Commonwealth University, Richard Hardy, for his ongoing support. Warm thanks are due my colleagues Bob Lassiter and "Mr. Rehab,"

Keith Wright, for their initial encouragement and sage advice regarding the undertaking of this manuscript. George Jarrell and Dr. Gerald Gandy also contributed very human qualities to a supportive academic environment.

Special thanks are due Allison Gosney for her typing assistance as well as for her consistently cheerful attitude and watchful eye.

I would like to express appreciation to John Marozsan of Aspen for his timely encouragement and to Anne M. Gousha, also of Aspen, for her eager and reliable assistance. In addition, a respectful and well-deserved tip of the hat goes to Adele Gorelick, copy editor, for her thoroughness and insightful suggestions.

Warren Rule
Richmond, Virginia

Part I

Fundamentals of Lifestyle Counseling

Chapter 1

Introduction

Warren R. Rule

In contemporary living, the term "lifestyle" has a broad range of meanings to different individuals and is used in an expanding variety of contexts:

> The television advertisement shows an attractive young woman, her long, blond hair flowing with the wind as she rides along the sunlit beach in her convertible sportscar. The TV announcer pleads with the viewers to use Goldendust Shampoo "so your lifestyle, too, will be golden and glamorous!"

> The middle-aged banker sits behind a neatly organized desk. He is alone and in a wistful mood. This melancholy person reflects on the past, assesses the present, projects into the future, and hears himself declare aloud, "I need a change in lifestyles."

> The panting jogger runs up the hill and, despite his physical discomfort, creates in his mind the shopping list of items he will use this evening: various vitamins, selected vegetables, juices, etc. He then prides himself for making the right decision "to live a healthy lifestyle."

> The couple, while dining in an exclusive restaurant, raise glasses of wine in a toast to each other. One glowingly says, "Our lifestyle is really filled with fun, isn't it?"

> The teenager gazes in despair out of her hospital window. Recently she has been told that she will never walk again. She quietly cries and thinks over and over, "My lifestyle is ruined forever."

These examples reflect an array of meanings attributed to the term "lifestyle." The connotations suggest that one's lifestyle is basically one's appearance, which can be embellished by discreet selection of consumer products; that one's lifestyle can be readily and radically changed by doing something different in one's life, such as switching jobs; that one's lifestyle is essentially one's commitment to managing a healthy body; that lifestyle is a joint enterprise that also can be measured by the number of fun activities it entails; and that one's lifestyle can be ruined by a major occurrence such as a severe injury. Many other examples abound in the spoken and written language.

However, the term "lifestyle," coined by Alfred Adler more than 50 years ago, meant something considerably more fundamental than is reflected in the above contemporary examples. Adler, a pioneer in the helping professions, conceptualized the lifestyle as being more basic and unique to the individual as a person and, as such, would be the mental pattern itself that influenced the individual choices made in each of the above examples. This concept would seem to be a much more useful approach to understanding the individual than the various implications of the term currently in vogue. Adler's view of lifestyle—one that can be very valuable to the helping practitioner—constitutes one of the broad underpinnings of this book.

LIFESTYLE

Adler believed that each individual develops a "lifestyle" during his early years that exerts a major influence on one's thoughts, feelings, and behavior throughout life. These childhood years certainly do not totally determine how an individual will develop in later life; however, they probably have a large bearing on the thought patterns on which the person will take a sensitive position. Adler's definition of lifestyle focuses heavily on the core of personality, especially on the individual's unique mental map. Lifestyle is seen as the pattern of dimly conscious beliefs and goals that the person uses for interacting with others and for measuring self-worth. Expressed another way, the emphasis is on the individual's long-standing holistic pattern of dimly conscious expectations.

In general, we are not aware of how pervasively the lifestyle pattern is at work in our daily lives: the way we relate to others, our choice of clothes, our choice of mate, our successes, our failures, the situations we avoid, the viewpoint we take toward the limitations of a disability, etc. Each individual lifestyle has a bearing on the choices already made and on the ones to be made.

The overriding mental pattern is regarded as the bottom line: this subjective pattern reflects those key cognitive dimensions on which a person takes a sensitive position. This mental pattern, in turn, influences the individual's feelings and behaviors in response to life's circumstances. Therefore, as the person moves through life, this overriding pattern is usually more difficult to alter than are feelings and behaviors.

Because of the consistency of the cognitive nature of the lifestyle, it is often very useful to the individual to have an awareness of his unique lifestyle pattern when he is facing problems or making decisions. This is particularly so because the life-style—the time-tested pattern of fundamental expectations—becomes most apparent (especially to the skilled observer) when the individual is experiencing stress.

The lifestyle concept and methods of lifestyle assessment will be discussed extensively in the next two chapters. Now let us direct our attention to an overview of important historical considerations.

BACKGROUND

"It is the personal meaning of the disability to the individual that is crucial in rehabilitation counseling practice" (Wright, 1980, p. 73). This perspective is certainly in keeping with the lifestyle counseling approach illustrated in this book. However, traditionally the personal meaning of disability was not always accepted by helping practitioners as the most beneficial consideration in adjustment to disability. Even today, acceptance of this concept is not universal, although it may be seen as a professional milestone, which values the dignity of the individual as ultimately significant.

Historical Perspective

According to Shontz's (1975) historical review, contemporary health practices evolved from two contrasting traditions: animism and mechanism. *Animism* assumes that "a special substance or force gives life or magic powers to otherwise non-living objects. The substance or force is usually called soul or spirit, and it usually has mental powers" (p. 4). Animistic thinking has expressed itself, especially in the early stages of health care, in practices to release evil influences (e.g., skull boring, torture, purgatives, bleeding), as well as in the more humane practices of prayer, incantation, rest, and recreation. *Mechanism* focuses on the orderly materialism that served as the foundation for early science and technology. The ancient Greeks (e.g., Democritus, Hippocrates) provided the intellectual orientation for the mechanistic approach. This method of thinking received a rebirth after the thirteenth century, particularly in the form of naturalistic observation, as demonstrated by the anatomist Vesalius and the biologist Harvey.

Centuries later, much controversy stemmed from variations and refinements of the viewpoints of animism and mechanism. Some further developed their ideas in accordance with one or the other framework, particularly the mechanistic, e.g., Darwin, Freud, Skinner; some attempted resolution, e.g., Descartes for religion and science, Kant for mind and body, and Smuts for unity of mind and body, which launched the holistic perspective (Shontz, 1975).

The holistic viewpoint, a very significant concept in lifestyle understanding, was developed, as Shontz explains,

> to decompartmentalize the study and treatment of the human being. According to this view, the person is an indivisible totality and must be understood as such. Holism is responsible for the team approach to patient care, and it has provoked a return to concern for all aspects of the patient's condition. Because of its influence, medical specialists have become more willing to respect the opinions of nurses, social workers, vocational counselors, psychologists, and others whose professional concern is with less obviously somatic aspects of patients' problems. (p. 26)

Shontz further concluded that while holism is not yet a science, its doctrines have evolved in several directions. One direction is the variations of humanistic psychology that recognize the limitations of the mechanistic view of human nature and focus on the uniqueness of each person. Such concepts as identity, way of life, integrity, self-direction have been developed by Maslow, Rogers, some existentialists, and gestaltists. Another direction of holism is general systems theory, as developed by von Bertalanffy, which asserts that "systems exhibit lawful uniformities and must be studied intact if these uniformities are to appear; at present, however, systems theorists admit that their ability to deal with structures as complex as living organisms is limited" (Shontz, 1975, p. 27).

Adler, along with his lifestyle approach, would primarily be aligned with the humanistic psychology movement (Ansbacher & Ansbacher, 1956), although he has, as well, been described as being "[t]he psychological theorist who most closely approximated an application of systems concepts to the individual level" (Amerikaner, 1981, p. 33). We need to know a bit more about this creative and most influential man.

Adler and His Influence

Alfred Adler was born in Vienna in 1870. As a child he suffered from rickets and his decision to pursue a medical career resulted in part from a near fatal bout with pneumonia at age five. After several years as a general medical practitioner, Adler became associated with Sigmund Freud and turned his attention to psychoanalytic explorations. However, Adler's developing concepts were at odds with Freud's (Adler was especially dissatisfied with Freud's view of the sexual instinct as omnipotent) and they parted ways. Thereafter he continued to develop his own approach, being influenced as well by other viewpoints (e.g., Vaihinger's philosophy of "As If," Smut's approach to holism and evolution) and by his experiences as a physician in World War I. Before coming to the United States he established a network of child guidance clinics and societies. He continued to have an impact in this country through his teaching, lecturing, and writing. While on a lecture tour in Scotland in 1937, he died at the age of 67.

For many years, Adler's thinking was overshadowed by that of Freud. Some have even naively regarded the two as similar. However, as Ford and Urban (1963) noted in their comparative review of systems of psychotherapy:

> In contrast to Sigmund Freud, Adler developed a point of view that sought to study behavior from the vantage point of the subjective rather than the objective observer; emphasized the goal-directed rather than the drive-impelled causation of behavior; stressed the unity and integration of behavior rather than the conflict of disparate elements; proposed the use of molar and holistic concepts rather than restricted units of analysis; held an idiographic rather than a nomothetic purpose in studying behavior; and in short, differed from Freud in the most fundamental and basic fashions possible. (p. 303)

Adler's ideas are receiving increasing attention, as evidenced by increasing Adlerian practitioners, research, writings, educational opportunities, and societies (Allen, 1971; Ansbacher & Ansbacher, 1970). In addition, many theorists who studied under Adler have developed eminence in their own right (e.g., Eric Berne, Rollo May, Victor Frankl). Adler's approach, which he termed ''Individual Psychology'' to stress the indivisible nature of the individual, has achieved widespread influence. Sometimes only the barest acknowledgment is given by others, as discussed in O'Connell's ''The 'Friends of Adler' Phenomenon'' (1976), and sometimes forthright declarations are rendered, such as Albert Ellis' conclusion (1973) regarding Adler's contribution: ''It is highly probable that without his pioneering work, the main elements of rational-emotive therapy might never have been developed'' (p. 112). Ellenberger (1970), in his comprehensive review of the history and evolution of psychiatry, observed that:

> Any attempt to assess the influences of Adler's work brings about a paradox. The impact of Individual Psychology stands beyond any doubt. . . . It would not be easy to find another author from which so much has been borrowed from all sides without acknowledgment than Alfred Adler. (p 645)

Thus, Adler's influence has been receiving justified recognition; however, misunderstandings regarding many of Adler's concepts continue to persist.

Misunderstandings of Adler

Unfortunately, a number of writers in the field of rehabilitation and adjustment to disability have contributed to a misrepresentation or an oversimplification of some of Adler's ideas. This seems to be the result of either a superficial understanding of Adler's concepts or an overemphasis on his earlier writings.

Early in his career (1907) Adler developed a theory of behavior based upon organ inferiority. This concept, as well as related ones, such as compensation and inferiority, have received particular attention in the field of rehabilitation. Often overlooked is the fact, however, that in the subsequent quarter century, Adler continued to develop and to refine his approach, especially the central concept, the lifestyle. A number of those attempting to apply Adler's ideas to the field of rehabilitation have focused on the original, less-developed concepts, which seem, because of their labels at the time, to be the most related to rehabilitation. In so doing, unfortunately, some critics have been tempted to generalize from the shortcomings of this limited perspective to the overall worth of the Adlerian approach to rehabilitation.

Adler's refined concept of the lifestyle is a more complete approach to understanding human nature. His later thinking reflects a shift from an organic to a sociopsychological explanation of behavior, a refinement of inferiority and compensation, an increased emphasis on the creativity of the individual, and an even sharper focus on the personal attitude toward disability and the goals to which a disability can be directed. Indeed, as we shall note frequently, the lifestyle approach developed by Adler is essentially *educational* in nature.

DISABILITY

The concept of disability used in this book is intentionally broad. The description by Goldenson (1978) is generally appropriate:

> As used today, it denotes any relatively severe chronic impairment of function resulting from disease, accident or congenital defect. The impairment, or limitation, may be in one or more of the following spheres: (a) physical, affecting ambulation, coordination, speech production, vision, etc.; (b) mental, affecting ability to think, remember, and comprehend, or general learning ability; (c) social, affecting ability to communicate and establish relationships with other people; (d) emotional, affecting self-image, self-acceptance, mental health; (e) occupational, affecting vocational or homemaking ability. (p. 7)

Concepts related to disability, such as handicap and limitation, are frequently used interchangeably. In fact, Wright (1980), in referring to the terms "disability," "limitation," and "handicap," concluded that "no other area of the rehabilitation nomenclature produces such semantic confusion as these three words" (p. 67). As an example, he noted that "It is particularly confusing that the words *disability* and *handicap* in rehabilitation are comparable to *impairment* and *disability,* respectively in American medicine" (p. 69). Various distinctions regarding the difference between "disability" and "handicap" (e.g., Bitter, 1979; Dunham & Dunham, 1978; Wright, 1980) suggest that "disability" is essentially the physical, mental, or emotional impairment that becomes a "handicap" if the condition contributes to lowered self-assessment, reduced function, or limited opportunities. Thus, in this sense, a disability may not be a handicap. However, Dunham and Dunham (1978) note that "Differentiating between 'disability' and 'handicap' becomes more controversial with the mentally ill. . . . The concept gets even more blurred when applied to the criminal, the obese, the drug addict, or the alcoholic" (p. 13).

Another relevant issue is the role that others' attitudes and actions have in contributing to an individual handicap. This influence will be discussed in this book only to the extent that such discrimination becomes a part of the individual's awareness; exploration of the broad societal implications of discrimination against the disabled is outside the scope of this book.

In order to avoid semantic dilemmas, the term "disability" will be consistently used throughout this book. This use of "disability" is intended to incorporate individually determined implications of the term "handicap" because, as noted previously, the personal meaning of the disability to the individual *is* the important issue in lifestyle counseling for adjustment to disability.

ADJUSTMENT

In view of the estimate that there are at least 25 million disabled individuals in the United States (Goldenson, R.M., Dunham, J.R., & Dunham, C.S., 1978) the issue of adjustment to disabilities is one of no small consequence. The ideal is for health services to regard the disabled individual in a holistic manner, not simply to "dissect the patient, distribute portions of him to appropriate repair shops, and reassemble him when all parts are in working order" (Shontz, 1975, p. vi).

The concept of general adjustment can be viewed from many perspectives (Sechrest & Wallace, 1967): the survival model focuses on adjustment to the basic levels, such as keeping alive, maintaining health, reproductiveness; the medical model emphasizes treatment of underlying causes, often to the neglect of environmental influences; the positive striving model is directed at the process of fulfilling one's self-potential, yet, paradoxically, may entail conflicts with idealism and pragmatism; and there are other, less notable, models, such as the drive reduction model, the engineering model, the social conformity model.

From the perspective of adjustment to disability, however, most of the above models, with the possible exception of the positive striving model, do not seem to be entirely satisfactory. Roessler and Bolton (1978) noted that talking abstractly about the effects of disability is important from an analytic or scientific perspective but the overriding focus in helping should be on an empathic awareness of the significance of the disability to a person's life. Moreover, Shontz (1977) concluded, after reviewing numerous studies related to the treatment of various disabilities, that:

> What has been uniformly regarded as crucial is the personal meaning of his disability to each individual client. . . . Virtually all of these authors have cautioned that psychological treatment must be directed toward individual situations and reactions rather than toward psychological processes that can be assumed to be constant from patient to patient. (p. 324)

At least two fundamental issues are involved in defining adjustment; they have to do with achievement versus process (Lazarus, 1969) and with frame of reference (Sechrest & Wallace, 1967). In discussing these key concepts, Roessler and Bolton (1978) noted that the achievement or final state conception of adjustment implies a final, trouble-free state, may foster unrealistically high expectations, and presumes that all problems are solvable; however, the process orientation to adjustment emphasizes how to adapt to a succession of situations and the expectation that life will not be trouble free. Also important is the frame of reference of the person assessing the level of adjustment. Essentially two frames of reference exist: the disabled person himself or an external person, such as a helping practitioner. The convergence of both frames of reference is crucial to the individual's process of adjustment.

The lifestyle approach to adjustment to disability incorporates the key factors discussed in the foregoing paragraphs. The lifestyle approach certainly respects the personalized meaning of the disability to the individual because lifestyle assessment attempts to identify the individual's general expectations of self, others, and life. Regarding the achievement versus process issue, lifestyle understanding focuses on goal-directedness, or fixed consequences to be achieved, within the context of the individual's overall pattern of movement through life. Thus, short-term goals are viewed within the perspective of overriding long-term goals.

As for internal versus external frames of reference, there is a shift, with the lifestyle approach, as the counselor assists the client in getting, psychologically speaking (Carkhuff, 1980), from where he is to where he wants to be. This entails focusing primarily on the client's frame of reference in the earlier phases with an increased blending of the counselor's frame of reference (which sometimes includes occasional nudging of the client) in the later stages. Throughout the process of lifestyle counseling for adjustment to disability, however, the counselor does not lose sight of the client's subjective, or internal, frame of reference. Because individuals are regarded, within the lifestyle framework, as being the product of both general laws and individually created laws (to be discussed more fully in the next chapter), the counselor is essentially more of an artist than a scientist in his role of attempting to understand and replicate the client's mental map.

THE HELPING PROCESS: A PERSPECTIVE

Many who apply psychological concepts to the broad field of rehabilitation perceive helping the disabled as an art. As Stubbins (1977) concluded: "Partly as a consequence of self-understanding and partly through trained judgment, they practice the helping role as an art—something difficult to define but which most practitioners agree is important in applied psychology" (p. 295).

Should those who regard the helping process, at least in its present state, as primarily a subjective art and secondarily as an objective science feel compelled to make apologies? Probably not. Lewis Thomas, regarded by some as the world's foremost scientific essayist, concluded that "The only solid piece of scientific truth about which I feel totally confident is that we are profoundly ignorant about nature" (1979, p. 73). Speaking also in terms of scientific limitations, Merleau-Ponty (1962) expressed well the importance of respecting the subjective perspective:

> I cannot shut myself up within the realm of science. All my knowledge of the world, even my scientific knowledge, is gained from my own particular point of view, or from some experience of the world without which the symbols of science would be meaningless. The whole universe of science is built upon the world as directly experienced, and if we want to subject science itself to rigorous scrutiny and arrive at a precise assessment of its meaning and scope, we must begin by reawakening the basic experience of the world of which science is the second order of expression. (p. viii)

Thus, a heightened respect for the subjective experience, which is perhaps both the means and the end of an artistic approach, may be a key factor in the overall helping process. This respect for the subjective experience is especially important in lifestyle counseling, wherein the counselor's subjective expression attempts to illuminate the patterns of the client's subjective experience.

Can lifestyle practitioners afford to lose sight of scientific research, especially the increasing number of reliability and validity studies on lifestyle assessment and outcome? Again, probably not. These contributions decrease the likelihood of deluding ourselves and our clients. Yet, we may similarly delude ourselves if we believe that, in counseling, objective influences can be the total masters of subjective ones. A complete awareness on the counselor's part of all the scientific studies ever done in counseling process and outcome will not prevent the counselor's own subjective lifestyle from oozing through the mask of objectivity into the counseling experience.

REFERENCES

Allen, T.W. The individual psychology of Alfred Adler: An item of history and a promise of a revolution. *The Counseling Psychologist,* 1971, *3*(1), 3–24.

Amerikaner, M.J. Continuing theoretical convergence: A general systems theory perspective on personal growth and development. *Journal of Individual Psychology,* 1981, *37,* 31–53.

Ansbacher, H.L., & Ansbacher, R.R. (Eds.). *The individual psychology of Alfred Adler.* New York: Basic Books, 1956.

Ansbacher, H.L., & Ansbacher, R.R. (Eds.). *Superiority and social interest* (2nd ed.). Evanston, Ill.: Northwestern University Press, 1970.

Bitter, J.A. *Introduction to rehabilitation.* St. Louis: C.V. Mosby, 1979.

Carkhuff, R. *The art of helping IV.* Amherst, Mass.: Human Resources Development Press, 1980.

Dunham, J.R., & Dunham, C.S. Psychological aspects of disability. In R.M. Goldensen, J.R. Dunham, & C.S. Dunham (Eds.), *Disability and rehabilitation handbook.* New York: McGraw-Hill, 1978.

Ellenberger, H. *The discovery of the unconscious: The history and evaluation of dynamic psychiatry.* New York: Basic Books, 1970.

Ellis, A. *Humanistic psychotherapy.* New York: McGraw-Hill, 1973.

Ford, D.H., & Urban, H.B. *Systems of psychotherapy.* New York: Wiley, 1963.

Goldensen, R.M. Dimensions of the field. In R.M. Goldensen, J.R. Dunham, & C.S. Dunham (Eds.), *Disability and rehabilitation handbook.* New York: McGraw-Hill, 1978.

Goldensen, R.M., Dunham, J.R., & Dunham, C.S. A word to the reader. In R.M. Goldensen, J.R. Dunham, & C.S. Dunham (Eds.), *Disability and rehabilitation handbook.* New York: McGraw-Hill, 1978.

Lazarus, R. *Patterns of adjustment in human effectiveness.* New York: McGraw-Hill, 1969.

Merleau-Ponty, M. *Phenomenology of perception* (C. Smith, Trans.) London: Routledge & Kegan Paul, 1962.

O'Connell, W.E. The "friends of Adler" phenomenon. *Journal of Individual Psychology,* 1976, *32,* 5–18.

Roessler, R., & Bolton, B. *Psychosocial adjustment to disability.* Baltimore: University Park Press, 1978.

Sechrest, L., & Wallace, J. *Psychology and human problems.* Columbus, Ohio: Charles E. Merrill, 1967.

Shontz, F.C. *The psychological aspects of physical illness and disability.* New York: Macmillan, 1975.

Shontz, F.C. Physical disability and personality: Theory and recent research. In J.E. Stubbins (Ed.), *Social and psychological aspects of disability*. Baltimore: University Park Press, 1977.

Stubbins, J. Editorial introduction (Part III). In J. Stubbins (Ed.), *Social and psychological aspects of disability*. Baltimore: University Park Press, 1977.

Thomas, Lewis. *The medusa and the snail*. New York: Viking Press, 1979.

Wright, G.N. *Total rehabilitation*. Boston: Little, Brown, 1980.

Chapter 2

Lifestyle and Adjustment to Disability

Warren R. Rule

Many assumptions and issues are involved in the relationship between lifestyle and adjustment to disability. First of all, it is very likely that the practitioner cannot avoid being influenced by his assumptions regarding the nature of man. The conscious and dimly conscious beliefs that the helper holds about man's personality development and nature will influence his method of intervention. Moreover, this will be subtly in operation regardless of whether the disability is congenital or acquired. The practitioner's beliefs as to whether man is determined by his past or freely chooses from moment to moment, whether he is basically driven by instincts or is shaped by his environment, whether an individual creates his feelings or is possessed by his feelings, and so on, all unavoidably influence how one goes about helping others. Getting in touch with the dimensions of one's personal "personality theory" can be a worthwhile first step. Subsequently, the individual who has made this self-inventory is in a better position to supplement or even change his beliefs as a result of considering more formalized personality theories.

An approach to understanding personality based on the concept of the Adlerian lifestyle provides a holistic framework for viewing disability. It is both substantial and broad based enough that it could have appeal to practitioners with an eclectic orientation. This approach, along with variations, may be helpful to the practitioner because an increased awareness of the individual lifestyle may be a key to understanding his own perception of and reaction to disability.

ADLERIAN LIFESTYLE

As we noted in Chapter 1, Adler believed that each individual develops a "lifestyle" during his childhood years that exerts a major influence on his thoughts, feelings, and behavior throughout life. Adler coined this term more than 50 years ago and he developed this concept over a span of a quarter of a century. Shulman (1973) summarized the lifestyle as:

> a superordinate organizational pattern that directs behavior. By means of selective perception, cognition, memory, etc., it codifies rules for characteristic attitudinal positions. It becomes the intervening variable between efficient cause and effect, between stimulation of the outside world and the responsive behaviors of the person. It is formed early in childhood and is self-reinforcing through selectivity. It is self-consistent, coherent, and unified. It is constant; it does not change from time to time or situation to situation, though it is not necessarily rigid. It can be recognized by its repeated appearance as a theme in the life history of even everyday behavior of an individual. It develops through trial and error and is influenced by physical, developmental, cultural, and familial factors. It is a necessary rule for coping behavior, to bring order into one's relationship with the challenging and confronting world. It is therefore of critical significance to the clinician who wishes to understand the "whys?" of human behavior. (p. 44)

The focus is not on the feelings or behavior that a person uses as he moves through life; rather, the emphasis is on the pattern of goal-directed thinking. Let us examine further some of the important assumptions upon which the lifestyle concept rests.

The Holistic Nature of Man

A basic assumption that fits securely into the perspective of the psychosocial adjustment of the individual is Adler's belief about the wholeness of the individual. A person's wholeness, or "holistic" nature, is irreducible; to break up the personality or fragment it into parts is to destroy the wholeness and thereby undermine the understanding of the individual. A person cannot be dissected without losing some understanding of the pattern or theme that runs through his life. Adler used an analogy from music: music cannot be fully appreciated by studying each note itself—one needs to have the context of the other notes in order to experience the melody.

Adler chose the term "lifestyle" to depict this holistic pattern that is greater than the sum of the parts. The assumption that the unit (the individual) is indivisible is important, particularly for understanding the relationship of an individual to disability. This is so because the way in which individuals organize themselves as whole people influences their perceptions of themselves and others and has a large bearing on their goals and behavioral interactions with others.

Heredity and Environment

Adler was strongly convinced of the creative power of the individual, believing in "soft determinism" as opposed to "hard determinism" (Ansbacher & Ansbacher, 1956). He stated:

> Do not forget the most important fact that not heredity and not environment are determining factors.—Both are giving only the frame and the influences which are answered by the individual in regard to his styled creative power. (p. xxiv)

Dreikurs, who was probably Adler's foremost student in the United States, observed that:

> The genetic emphasis on heredity factors is equally mechanistic as the behavioristic analysis of environmental influences. Even the efforts to describe the interrelationships between heredity and environmental influences on the development of the personality structure result in a mechanistic picture of a struggle between antagonistic or supplementary forces. (1967, p. 168)

A closely related issue is that of lifestyle as a cause of behavior or a determiner of behavior. Shulman (1973) noted that the lifestyle is a "cause" of behavior in the sense that Aristotle discussed the *causa formalis*, the "ordering or patterning of relationships that leads to specific results" (p. 18). Shulman further concluded that the lifestyle acts as a "determiner" in the sense that it limits, as does any law, and it governs in terms of directing overall line of movement and providing feedback that serves to reinforce or inhibit the movement.

Cause-and-effect thinking can sometimes work to the practitioner's disadvantage when applied to life issues other than the validity of the lifestyle concept. The following passage, although not written from an Adlerian perspective, richly illustrates the limitations of mechanistic cause-and-effect thinking when used as a framework for understanding the complexity of life's flow:

> "What is fate?" Nasrudin was asked by a scholar.
> "An endless succession of intertwined events, each influencing the other."
> "That is hardly a satisfactory answer. I believe in cause and effect."
> "Very well," said the Mulla, "look at that." He pointed to a procession passing in the street.
> "That man is being taken to be hanged. Is that because someone gave him a silver piece and enabled him to buy the knife with which he

committed the murder; or because someone saw him do it; or because nobody stopped him?'' (Ornstein, 1972, p. 75)

Social Context

Adler believed that man is a social being and that behavior can only be fully understood in a social context. Ansbacher & Ansbacher (1956) noted that Adler's approach could properly be referred to as a "context" psychology. He regarded personal problems basically as social problems. Related to this assumption about man's social nature is the idea that in each of us there exists the desire to belong. Expressed in another way, each of us strives to have a place of significance in the eyes of others. The goal of obtaining a "place of somebodyness" is handled differently by different people. Correspondingly, a congenital or acquired disability would be handled differently by different lifestyles because both the perceived "place of somebodyness" and the social context would vary from person to person.

Broadly speaking, the goals a person pursues and the behaviors an individual learns can be indirectly related to the innate desire to enhance oneself within a social context. Thus, in attempting to understand another person, a workable framework would be: "How is this person seeking to be known by others?" The answer has obvious implications for the psychosocial adjustment of an individual with a disability. Another Adlerian assumption, the goal-directed nature of behavior, further increases our understanding of the social implications of disability.

Goal-Directedness

Adler believed that all behavior, including emotions, is goal directed. Stated another way, everything we do has a purpose and is a function of our ideas—both conscious and dimly conscious—about consequences to be obtained in the future. Behaviors that seemingly cannot be explained become more understood as the goal or purpose comes to light. So, even though at times we are consciously aware of the purpose of thinking, feeling, or acting in a certain fashion, most of the time we are unaware of our unique self-concerned goals that are in operation at a dimly conscious level. We are not aware of how pervasively lifestyle goals are at work in our daily life: in the way we interact with others, in our choice of friends or consumer products, in our sense of accomplishment or vulnerability, in the viewpoint we take toward the implications of disability, etc.

Thus, the individual seems to operate from a subjective mental framework and is not always fully conscious of his goals. In understanding someone, the focus must be on the person's subjective or internal frame of reference. This seems necessary because the individual's perceptions, including his inner biases influencing his perceptions, determine his behavior more than "reality" does. Furthermore, the individual organizes his perceptions into expectations that influence his personal goals.

It is noteworthy that a wide range of behavioral patterns is usually available to the individual for any given lifestyle conclusion or "characteristic attitudinal position" (Shulman, 1973). The lifestyle approach asserts that people can, in fact, change in major ways; however, the sensitive position on a lifestyle notion may be the common thread that runs through the "changes" a person regards himself as having made throughout the span of his life. These behavioral changes, even seemingly major ones, may actually be variations of the same theme. Or, expressed another way, these changes could be different creative behavioral implementations—in response to changing environmental situations—of the same lifestyle conclusions that the person continues to take a sensitive position on. Mosak (1958) illustrates some of the different behavioral implementations a person could use who has taken a sensitive position on the lifestyle conclusion "Life is dangerous":

> Such a person, behaviorally, may see danger where none exists. He may exaggerate the dangers of life. He may retreat from these perceived dangers with anxious or phobic behavior. Or he may call upon certain defense mechanisms to cope with the omnipotent threat. In the compulsive individual, for example, one observes reliance upon ritual and feelings of omnipotence and the necessity to control as response to danger. Many compulsives are preoccupied with death because this is the greatest threat—the one force which cannot be controlled. Hypochondriacs may exaggerate each body symptom as expressing their conviction that life is fraught with danger. Other individuals may develop into towers of strength or become dependent upon or identify with "strong" people or groups in order to minimize the dangers of life. Still others may actually court or provoke personal disaster in order to confirm their basic attitude. Some flirt with danger in order to prove that they possess a charmed life. While these reactions do not exhaust the repertoire available to people who feel that life is dangerous, they do serve to exemplify the variety of reactions which are possible within a single dimension of an individual's perceptual frame of reference. (p. 306)

Thus, the individual creativity is ever present as the person moves through life. In terms of bringing together the relationships of these different concepts, the following broad generalizations may be useful: from a sensitive position on lifestyle conclusions (e.g., I am . . . , others are . . . , life is . . .) the individual creates both dimly conscious goals and conscious goals to guide him through life; emotions are the energizers that transform the goals into behavior.

Subjectively Striving to Overcome

Adler believed that this pattern of lifestyle goals is organized around the subjectively determined concept of the ideal self, much of which the individual created during childhood years. The person, in his private logic, continually moves through life with this self ideal as a general reference point. Almost as if the individual is wearing blinders, he strives—at a dimly conscious level—to become like the imagined ideal self. Subsequently, the person seems to treat himself at a vague level of awareness as if he will only be truly OK or have a total sense of significance in the eyes of others and have a real feeling of security when he lives up to the ideal self. Thus, this network of lifestyle goals is patterned after an ideal concept of self. It provides the main thrust for the lifestyle that enables each of us to move, on a daily basis and throughout our lives, from a position of dimly felt inferiority or noncoping to a position of overcoming or coping.

Adler believed that this pattern of goals is organized around a single "fictional final goal." This concept has been criticized for its simplicity (e.g., Ford & Urban, 1963), but from the practitioner's vantage point adopted in this book, the significance lies in the concept that a pattern of complementing major goals flows in a unified direction; the issue of whether or not one goal slightly edges out the rest is somewhat academic.

Commensurate with the goal-directed nature of behavior, the individual is able, by his own standards, to move from the felt minus state of non-enoughness to the felt plus state of enoughness. As the individual moves through life, it seems that he never quite gets "there" or is absolutely and totally satisfied.

Adler believed that early conclusions drawn before approximately age six or seven go a long way toward determining the dimly conscious goals that comprise the lifestyle. These conclusions appear to be drawn from experiences related to the person's first social group, the family. Approximately age six or seven can be chosen as a general cutoff primarily because at that period the child is beginning to become enmeshed in a school setting; i.e., the individual has begun to broaden the range of influences received from his first social group, the family, to those of the next social group, the school. Adlerians assert that the childhood conclusions drawn about self, others, and life approximately before age six or seven largely contribute to the internalized guidelines that the person uses in his present striving. The child creatively uses heredity and environment as tools from which he molds a lifestyle.

The early conclusions that become goals of the lifestyle are drawn from a host of childhood impressions and experiences. Exceedingly important is the family constellation, including siblings' development, age differences, ordering of sexes, alliance groups, etc. Moreover, parental influences and expectations, family values and atmosphere, peers, neighbors, all contribute to the biased slice of life that is the *only* slice of life the child has available to generalize from.

Considerable emphasis is placed, in attempting to understand a person's lifestyle, on the psychological "territory" the individual chose to stake out as his own in an attempt to feel "others take notice of me when I am like this." This sense of self-significance or belonging can be manifested in a variety of outlets, e.g., being the best, the worst, the charmer, the tough one, etc. Each sibling, Adlerians hypothesize, will move in a different overall direction in these areas or may even try to overtake a sibling in a chosen area.

Individuals learn at an early age, through trial and error, not only what goals will be most apt to help them move toward a place of significance, but they also begin to experiment with which kinds of behavior are most useful in implementing the goals. Not surprisingly, individuals also learn behaviors, including emotions, in keeping with the dimly conscious goals of the lifestyle that safeguard their vulnerabilities and sense of self-esteem. Generally speaking, then, the chosen lifestyle allows individuals to evaluate, to understand, to predict, and to control experience (Mosak, 1979a).

Adler's approach to understanding the nature of man can be used, either in whole or in part, as a basis for a broadly eclectic approach to counseling. His concepts have influenced many in the helping professions, as discussed in the previous chapter, and his ideas have been of interest to some from other professional disciplines. The anecdote below is one such example:

> I remember this incident mostly because I used to think to myself, "It must be wonderful to be someone like Adler. You'd never have to worry about whether you were intelligent or not." This incident opened my eyes to the fact that everyone, no matter who you are, questions their intelligence and needs reassurance from time to time.
>
> Adler was coming to dinner at my father's house one night. He rang the doorbell. We opened the door. He walked in, and without any greeting, stood there with the most beaming smile and said in his slow speaking way, "I have a new (long, drawn out and softly accented) follower. Guess who?" Of course none of us could guess. And he said, very slowly, and beaming all the time, "Albert Einstein."
>
> He had received a letter from Einstein, who had attended one or more of his lectures, stating that he (Einstein) considered Adler's Individual Psychology to be the most scientific and closest to the truth for today. (Matteson, 1977, p. 48)

LIFESTYLE ASSESSMENT

The lifestyle assessment technique has traditionally been used with adolescents and adults. Some Adlerians, however, have experimented with lifestyle techniques for children; some variations will be discussed in Chapters 4 and 5.

Sources of Lifestyle Information

There are a number of ways by which the practitioner can learn more about an individual's lifestyle. Some of these sources of information are very broad and some are relatively narrow; others draw from readily available data and others require the gathering of additional information. Lombardi (1973) discusses eight different avenues that yield information about the consistent and patterned lifestyle:

1. Case history data—knowing about subject
2. Psychological interviewing—talking to subject
3. Expressive behavior—observing subject
4. Psychological testing—measuring subject
5. Family constellation—social influence on subject
6. Early recollections—subject's meaning of life
7. Grouping—interacting with subject
8. Symptomatic behavior—subject's tell tale signs. (p. 6)

While the most ideal approach is to obtain information from all of the above avenues, oftentimes the practitioner must expediently settle for less. Perhaps one of the most widely used procedures for learning about an individual's lifestyle entails using a lifestyle assessment form. Several versions exist; one of the most popular being the form originally developed by Dreikurs (1967). This form, which has since been modified by other practitioners to suit individual preferences, has incorporated several of the above-listed avenues for obtaining lifestyle information. The section below will expand on the nature of this somewhat structured approach to obtaining lifestyle information. Two variations of the Dreikurs form, a long and an abbreviated form, are included in the Appendix.

Significance of Early Memory

Memory is selective. As Dreikurs (1967) observed, people operate on an economy principle by selectively using their memories in accordance with their individual purposes. Thus our memories from early childhood serve as anchoring orientation points, reflecting the most important conclusions, expectations, and goals that crystallized during this formative period. Adlerians believe that these early impressions and memories reflect those firm ideas that are embedded in the individual's *present* outlook. So, in utilizing the selectivity of memory phenomenon, the helping practitioner is able to gather lifestyle information by asking the client significant questions and, as a result, is able tentatively to reconstruct important aspects of the client's early environment. Once this is accomplished, the helper can look for themes in the remembered early environment that reflect the dimly conscious notions and goals the client is presently using.

Based on the client's memories (both real and sometimes imagined) before approximately age six or seven, areas of lifestyle information include descriptions of self and siblings, sibling rankings on possible areas of competition (e.g., intelligence, pleasing, having own way, athletics, appearance, temper, etc.), sibling interrelationships, parents and parental influence, family values and atmosphere, relationship to peers, and specific early recollections and dreams.

Family Constellation

Particular emphasis is given in the Adlerian lifestyle approach to family constellation from a psychosocial perspective. Accordingly, attention is directed to sibling age differences, ordering of sexes, favoritism, uniquenesses, alliance groups, development of patterns of siblings, how client felt about his position, etc. Only-born children are often compared with playmates.

Shulman (1973) listed five basic positions: only, eldest, second, middle, and youngest child. Different variations and combinations for these basic positions exist. Each basic position has several very modest probabilities of stereotyped characteristics attached to it. The helper considers and refines these tentative hypotheses in line with the direction of movement reflected by the other lifestyle variables. For example, sometimes first-born children (both oldest and only-born) have taken a sensitive position in their early lives on mandates, e.g., "shoulds," "musts," and "ought to's." This heightened sensitivity may have been the result of strong parental expectations. Or, it might have been influenced by the conclusion that one is only OK when one "achieves" in life (hence the usefulness of mandates as stimulators). A host of possible influences may have contributed to this sensitivity to "shoulds." For the purpose of illustration, we will assume below that a consistent pattern of this characteristic has emerged from the rest of the lifestyle information, including the early recollections.

How is an awareness of this pattern or any other pattern helpful to the practitioner? The practitioner can explore how this particular sensitivity is useful to the client in his own unique lifestyle as he moves through life. Does he use it to align himself with authority or established values? Does he strive to be Number One by setting lofty—perhaps unreasonable—"shoulds" for himself? Does he passive-aggressively resist most of life's mandates? The emphasis for the practitioner would be on relating patterns of lifestyle movement, which are grounded in childhood conclusions, to difficulties that the client is presently experiencing. Expressed another way, the practitioner is interested in helping the client get in touch with how his lifestyle is contributing—however consciously—to his problems.

This same flexible process of lifestyle analysis would be used to validate or reject tentative hypotheses the helping practitioner would have in mind about an individual with respect to position in the family constellation. For instance, some youngest borns sometimes strive to be charmers, others choose a pattern of irresponsibility with the expectation that others should step in and help them, some are eager to be the boss, others—particularly from big families—seek to outdo the preceding siblings and become top-notch achievers, and so on. In working with a youngest-born client, the Adlerian practitioner might look for these and/or related patterns, fully keeping in mind that while very modest stereotypes of family constellations exist, the individual is unique in his lifestyle development. Since early influences on the child can be so varied, the modest probabilities of family constellation may or may not be confirmed. The lifestyle interview is designed to pinpoint many of these other early influences so that the practitioner can digest and refine them in the process of bringing the client's lifestyle into sharper focus.

Specific Early Recollections

In rounding out the lifestyle understanding, much importance is given to the client's early recollections, memories, and dreams. Adlerians believe that there are no chance memories. That is to say, from the thousands and thousands of experiences to which an individual has been exposed in early childhood, only those recollections are remembered that coincide with one's present outlook on self, others, or life. Thus, the person's early recollections reflect the same patterns; they are reminders the individual carries around regarding personal limits and the meaning of circumstances (Ansbacher & Ansbacher, 1956).

Generally speaking, individuals can remember, when asked, at least six specific incidents that occurred during their early childhood. Each early recollection, when considered in the context of the accompanying feeling about the remembered incident, reflects a current expectation. Adlerians focus on the manifest content of the early memory, not on hidden, symbolic meanings. Moreover, each recollection supplements and rounds out the outlook reflected by the other early recollections.

Adlerian practitioners generally believe that the individual is the product of both individual "laws" and general "laws." In other words, a person is the result of individual laws that he created for himself and the result of general laws that apply to all people or specified groups of individuals. So, in seeking to understand more fully another person, the practitioner keeps an eye on both individual (idiographic) and general (nomothetic) understanding.

The Lifestyle Interview

The lifestyle interview can take several hours to complete or a shorter interview can be conducted. Several variables are involved here, such as time availability and the purpose for performing a lifestyle analysis. If a greater amount of information is gathered, the likelihood is increased of obtaining more accurate and well-rounded results.

Some examples of different lifestyle themes are cited by Mosak (1971), who cautioned that predictions cannot be made as to what behavior will coincide with a given lifestyle. In addition, Mosak (1976b) emphasized that the uniqueness of the individual is violated by typologies, which should be viewed as strictly didactic contributions. Examples of these themes are controlling, getting, driving, always being right, pleasing, being the center or the best, being admired for moral superiority, being against, being the baby or a charmer, being victimized, being intellectually superior, being an excitement seeker, being a martyr, etc.

If these examples appear to have a distinct self-serving flavor, several points might be kept in mind. First, individuals want to move from a position of dimly felt inferiority to a position of significance. The labels given to the themes reflect the powerful determination to enhance the self. Second, the lifestyle works to one's advantage as well as one's disadvantage. These themes can be channeled on the socially useful side of life and truly enhance others as well as the self. Third, the creativity of the individual is ever present in choosing the subtle as well as the more obvious ways the lifestyle is implemented.

The question of the reliability and validity of the lifestyle approach is not to be taken lightly. Discussion of studies related to these issues may be found in sources such as Allen (1971), Kern, Matheny, and Patterson (1978), and Mosak (1979a). Birth-order research has generated over 500 studies and the bulk of the significant results have been discussed by Forer (1976) and Sutton-Smith and Rosenberg (1970). Early recollections have been the subject of increasing research studies; many of those having Adlerian application are discussed by Mosak (1958, 1977), Olson (1979), and Taylor (1975). A comprehensive bibliography by Mosak and Mosak (1975) is a useful reference for most of these studies. Statistical research can make a contribution in the study of nomothetic, or general, laws as related to the lifestyle approach; however, the idiographic laws, which the individual created for himself as dimly conscious guidelines for moving through life, are more difficult to study with statistical methods.

Experience and familiarity with lifestyle variables and assessment are understandably significant factors in determining how helpful the approach is to the practitioner. Further reading, in addition to supervision, would provide a solid start. Suggested readings and resources for training opportunities are provided in the Appendix.

LIFESTYLE FACTORS AND DISABILITY

In considering the utility of the Adlerian lifestyle approach as a means to better understand adjustment to disability, it is important to keep in mind that "lifestyle" awareness is just as applicable to disabled groups as to "normal" groups. Reviews (e.g., Dunham and Dunham, 1978; English, 1974) of relevant investigations have concluded that few, if any, personality differences exist between the disabled and the normal population. The lifestyle analysis would seem to have as much merit for understanding the "personality" of a disabled individual as a nondisabled person. In addition, once a measure of lifestyle understanding is achieved between the practitioner and the client, exploration can be devoted to the extremely important issue of the relationship between the client's lifestyle and his disability. The focus would be on how the client's lifestyle notions and goals are contributing to—or undermining—adjustment to the disability.

Other Theoretical Perspectives

In comparison to some of the other major theories that attempt to explain psychological reaction to disability, the lifestyle approach seems to have some distinct advantages. The psychoanalytic theory is so grounded in the total determinism of early childhood that it does not appear to have the flexibility of the "soft determinism" of the Adlerian approach. Though definitely emphasizing the importance of early childhood, Adler strongly believed that the individual creatively molds, while exercising a measure of free choice, his lifestyle from environment and heredity. Correspondingly, one's reaction to disability was viewed by Adler as being less deterministic than the psychoanalytic position.

Proponents of the "Body Image" theory or the "Social Role" theory, as discussed by English (1974), would perhaps find their method of assessing reaction to disability enhanced by the lifestyle technique. Briefly stated, the "body image" theorists place much importance on those attitudes individuals have toward themselves and others with regard to physical characteristics. The "social role" theorists emphasize that people interact according to learned role expectations, including how to behave in a sick or disabled role. A heightened awareness of the more broadly based basic lifestyle notions and goals, which have a psychosocial foundation, would enhance or supplement the results obtained by focusing on either the individual's perceptions of body image or his disability role expectations.

Shontz (1977) regarded the "interpersonal" theoretical ideas as probably being the best developed (e.g., Barker and Wright, 1953; Wright, 1960). These ideas, which overlap with the "Social Role" theory discussed above, emphasize the values assigned to the disability and body by self and others and use descriptive concepts such as spread, value loss, containment of disability effects, etc. Shontz also noted other perspectives: motivation theories, e.g., Maslow (1954), who emphasized level of needs; crises theory, involving stages or cycles of the crisis experience; comparison level theory, which focuses on level of payoff or reinforcement; stress theory, which attempts to relate physiological and psychological processes; and attitudes toward disability.

Attitudes Toward Disability

Negative attitudes toward the disabled often contribute to the difficulties faced by them. Although the emphasis in this book is on the personal meaning of the disability to the individual, the following conclusions drawn by Roessler and Bolton (1978), based on reviews by Barker, Wright, Meyerson, and Gonick (1953) and Siller (1976), are worth noting:

> First, attitudes toward disabled persons are typically unfavorable, despite what most people say when asked. Second, negative attitudes toward the disabled result in real barriers and restricted opportunities; again, prejudice produces discrimination against disabled persons. Third, the unfavorable attitudes held by nondisabled persons may influence disabled persons' views of their worth. . . . Fourth, disabled persons often live with unfavorable attitudes from a very early age because even their parents may have difficulty treating them normally. (p. 11)

Adlerian Implications

A heightened awareness of the more broadly based basic lifestyle notions and goals, which act as a psychosocial filter for the individual, may enhance or supplement whatever results are obtained using the theoretical perspective discussed in the preceding two sections.

As we noted in Chapter 1, several of Adler's concepts have sometimes been inconsistently and/or superficially discussed in the disability literature. Adler's student, Rudolf Dreikurs (1967), was aware of the increasing misunderstanding of Adler's concepts in the health field and he published a paper, originally appearing in 1948, in which he attempted to qualify Adler's ideas, especially as they relate to disability.

The concept of organ inferiority, developed very early in Adler's career, is a main source of confusion in the rehabilitation field, especially as it is related to the concept of compensation. Since originally developing the idea of organ inferiority ("organ" meaning any physically identifiable part of the body) and compensation, Adler considerably modified and expanded his ideas during the next 25 years. In this evolutionary process, the concept moved toward and contributed to the sociopsychological orientation of the lifestyle approach as the basis of behavior and away from the earlier emphasis on the physical realm as being the basis of behavior. Unfortunately, many reviewers focused on the earlier emphases, thus missing Adler's refined—and more useful—concepts.

Regarding those individuals with a disability, Adler believed that the creativity of the individual is foremost and that concepts predicting rigid, deterministic reactions to disability were useless. For instance, he believed that a number of possible responses exist, depending on lifestyle variables of the individual: courageous compensation; despair leading to retreat; a protective, hesitating attitude. Dreikurs (1967) observed that the courageous response converts the difficulty into a blessing, the despairing response can mean retreat into disability, and the neurotic response says, "How much better could I do if I had not this disability!" (p. 174).

In regard to the aforementioned evolutionary stages of Adler's thinking, Rychlak (1973) noted that:

> It was this belief in the multiplicity of response to organic inferiority which gave Adler his first inkling that the patient as an interactional person contributed something subjectively to the situation in which he found himself. Illness was not a simple cause-effect business. (p. 99)

Dreikurs further attempted to clarify the confusion related to the uses of the term "inferiority." The words "inferiority," "inferiority feelings," and "inferiority complex" are often not differentiated in the literature. The following passage (Dreikurs, 1967) distinguishes the usages of these terms, which have an important bearing on psychosocial adjustment and lifestyle:

> Inferiority can refer to any objective inadequacy in function or in status. But it does not necessarily produce an inferiority feeling. A person may be weak, deficient or of low status without any realization of inferiority. On the other hand, an inferiority feeling may exist without any real inferiority. The decisive factor in the dynamics of inferiority feelings is the person's assumption of being inferior, either physically, socially, or in comparison to his own goals and standards. This assumption may not always be expressed on a conscious or verbal level as the individual may not be fully aware of it. . . . Only the inferiority feeling can stimulate a compensation on the part of the individual. The situation is different in regard to biological inferiorities and organ deficiencies, because the whole organism takes them into consideration and may, therefore, prompt biological compensations and over compensations, without any necessary awareness by the individual. The term "Inferiority Complex" applies to an entirely different psychological mechanism. A discouraged individual may use a real or assumed deficiency for the purpose of special benefit, generally as an excuse or an alibi for nonparticipation and withdrawal, or as a means to get special services or consideration. This is the only type of inferiority of which the individual is fully aware, as he tries to impress others and his own conscience with the magnitude of his defects. The "Inferiority Complex" does not lead

to any compensation. It is a deadlock for any further development. (pp. 175–176)

In terms of purposes served within various lifestyles, "inferiority" is a somewhat objective assessment or comparison, "inferiority feelings" have been present in everyone at various times and influence future development, and "inferiority complex" is a fatalistic reaction to a very difficult situation without attempting to correct or improve it.

ADJUSTMENT TO DISABILITY

The concept of disability brings a variety of thoughts to the minds of individuals in both the general public and the helping professions. Some of these thoughts are based on reality, others are grounded in stereotypes, and more than a few are fallacies. Let us first note several misconceptions related to personality and disability (primarily physical).

The first widely held belief is that specific disabilities are associated with specific types of personality. Another frequently held viewpoint is that different types of disability cause specific personality reactions. A third common assumption is that severity of disability is directly related to degree of psychological impairment. Extensive reviews of the literature by Shontz (1977) and Roessler and Bolton (1978) indicated that all of the above-stated beliefs are misconceptions that have virtually no solid research support. Shontz (1977) observed that:

> No authority claims that disability never affects personality; individual reactions frequently are profound and intense. What is denied is the systematic and universal correlation of type or degree of disability with type or degree of personality adjustment. (p. 334)

Thus there is a broad scope of reactions to disability. Persons with the same disabilities may have entirely different responses. This phenomenon as well as Shontz's conclusions, based on a review of the literature, that "basic personality structure appears to be remarkably stable even in the face of serious somatic change" (p. 345) are both consistent with the lifestyle approach to disability, which focuses on the individual meaning of the disability to the person.

In terms of this important issue of individual versus general approaches, Roessler and Bolton (1978) concluded that:

> Hence, an individual-by-individual approach to adjustment to disability is important. However, generalizations, if they are not binding, help in providing both an explanation for what one is observing and a frame-

work for a theoretical understanding of adjustment and disability that leads to hypotheses about new ways to serve the disabled. (p. 18)

Brief summaries are listed below of various generalizations related to adjustment to disability. These generalizations should be viewed as tentative considerations that may or may not apply to an individual lifestyle:

• Wright (1977) asserted that basically four issues exist in overcoming emotional barriers to adjustment: (1) enlarging the scope of values, which entails extending one's horizons beyond the disability and the self; (2) subordinating physique, involving the elevation of other values than physique; (3) containing disability effects, which entails preventing the spread of the disability limitations into nondisability-related areas; and (4) upholding asset evaluation, involving a focus on the positive or basic requirements, and on nonjudgmental standards of comparison.

• Kubler-Ross (1973) developed a five-stage theory that relates to adjustment to death, yet has a direct parallel to adjustment to disability: denial ("No, not me"), rage and anger ("Why me?"), bargaining ("Yes, me, but . . ."), depression ("Yes, me"), acceptance.

• Gunther (1969) observed that the somewhat orderly process of adjustment to disability generally involves the following stages, which may vary in duration: shock, partial recognition, initial stabilization, regression, and resolution of the regression phase.

• Eisenberg (1977) noted that, in addition to the use of defense mechanisms, which are employed by everyone (the common ones used by individuals with disabilities being withdrawal, denial and repression, projection, displacement, regression, rationalization), misconceptions about disability and adjustment should be considered. These include such misconceptions as the expectation of excellence in compensatory efforts, obtaining inner peace through suffering, adjustment by disowning a defective body part, and waiting for a miracle cure.

• Siller (1976) observed that noteworthy long-term reactions to traumatization, particularly as related to spinal cord injured persons, could be: passivity; dependency, including pseudoindependent phenomena (e.g., obstinacy, inappropriate confidence, inability to accept appropriate offers of help, and unrealistic goal setting); aggression; and compensation.

• Thompson (1982) has drawn parallels between Erikson's life continuum of eight distinct stages and adjustment to severe disability, such as spinal cord injury.

The stages are infancy, autonomy, initiative, industry, adolescence, identity, generativity, and integrity. In each stage it is assumed that there is a danger— unsuccessful development pushes the person toward the opposite, or negative, pole.

• Cohn (1961) isolated stages that she regards as somewhat fluid points on a continuum rather than as discrete categories. These stages of adjustment refer to permanently disabled persons whose physical conditions are not likely to improve appreciably: shock ("This isn't me"), expectancy of recovery ("I'm sick, but I'll get well"), mourning ("All is lost"), defense (healthy: "I'll go on in spite of it," neurotic: marked use of defense mechanisms to deny the effects of the disability), adjustment ("It's different, but not 'bad.' ").

• Falek and Britton (1974), in a review of studies on human reaction to stress, isolated a sequence of responses that enable a person to regain a "psychological steady state": denial (behavioral focus including being stunned or dazed, refusing to accept information, insisting there has been a mistake, not understanding what has been said); anxiety and fear (possibly expressed in the form of generalized nervousness, overactivity, irritability, headaches, fatigue, insomnia, loss of appetite, somatic complaints); anger and hostility; depression; equilibrium.

• Roessler and Bolton (1978) listed variables affecting rehabilitation outcome, which is very closely related to reaction to disability: person variables (organismic variables, behavioral competencies, self-regulatory systems and plans, expectancies, encoding and personal constructs, subjective stimulus values); environmental variables; nature of disability; cultural factors in rehabilitation; and interaction position.

The above generalizations may be useful when considered within a lifestyle perspective. In terms of generalizing about generalities, Shontz's (1975) observation, although specifically directed toward physical illness, has implications for the broad range of disabilities:

> The broadest view recognizes that suffering in physical illness is the resultant of physiological, subjective (cognitive, emotional), and environmental influences, all operating together. The relative importance of each, and the relations among them, differs among persons and conditions and may be understood only by close study of each individual and his situation. (p. 271)

SUMMARY

The lifestyle often provides an increased understanding of an individual's dimly conscious cognitive map regarding self, others, and life. This information, when viewed in the context of the goal-directed nature of thinking, feeling, and behaving, can provide a useful perspective on the individual's adjustment to disability.

Lifestyle factors were discussed as they relate to disability, other theoretical perspectives, and Adlerian implications. In addition, generalizations were considered that relate to the broad area of adjustment to disability.

REFERENCES

Allen, T.W. The individual psychology of Alfred Adler: An item of history and a promise of a revolution. *The Counseling Psychologist*, 1971, *3*(1), 3–24.

Ansbacher, H.L., & Ansbacher, R.R. (Eds.). *The individual psychology of Alfred Adler*. New York: Basic Books, 1956.

Barker, R.G., & Wright, B.A. The social psychology of adjustment to physical disability. In J.F. Garrett (Ed.), *Psychological aspects of physical disability* (Rehabilitation Services Series No. 310). Washington, D.C.: Office of Vocational Rehabilitation, Department of Health, Education, and Welfare, 1953, pp. 18–22.

Barker, R.G., Wright, B.A., Meyerson, L., & Gonick, M.R. *Adjustment to physical handicap and illness: A survey of the social psychology of physique and disability* (Rev. Ed.). New York: Social Science Research Council, 1953.

Cohn, N.K. Understanding the process of adjustment to disability. *Journal of Rehabilitation*, 1961, *27*(6), 16–18.

Dreikurs, R. *Psychodynamics, psychotherapy, and counseling*. Chicago: Alfred Adler Institute, 1967.

Dunham, J.R., & Dunham, C.S. Psychosocial aspects of disability. In R. Goldenson, J. Dunham, C. Dunham (Eds.), *Disability and Rehabilitation Handbook*. New York: McGraw–Hill, 1978.

Eisenberg, M. *Psychological aspects of physical disability: A guide for the health care worker*. New York: National League of Nursing, 1977.

English, R.W. The application of personality theory to explain psychological reactions to physical disability. In J. Cull & R. Hardy (Eds.), *Rehabilitation techniques in severe disability*. Springfield, Ill.: Charles C Thomas, 1974.

Falek, A., & Britton, S. Phases in coping. *Social Biology*, 1974, *21*(1), 1–7.

Ford, D.H., & Urban, H.B. *Systems of Psychotherapy*. New York: Wiley, 1963.

Forer, L. *The birth order factor*. New York: McKay, 1976.

Gunther, M. Emotional aspects of spinal cord injury. In D. Ruge (Ed.), *Spinal cord injuries*. Springfield, Ill.: Charles C Thomas, 1969.

Kern, R.M., Matheny, K.B., & Patterson, D. *A case for Adlerian counseling: Theory, techniques, and research evidence*. Chicago: Alfred Adler Institute, 1978.

Kubler-Ross, E. On death and dying. In E. Wyschogrod (Ed.), *The phenomenon of death*. New York: Harper & Row, 1973.

Lombardi, D.N. Eight avenues of life style consistency. *The Individual Psychologist*, 1973, *10*(2), 5–9.

Maslow, A.H. *Motivation and personality*. New York: Harper & Row, 1954.

Matteson, P. Excerpt on "Friends and Community." In G.J. Manaster, G. Painter, D. Deutsch, & B.J. Overholt (Eds.), *Alfred Adler: As we remember him*. Austin, Tex.: North American Society of Adlerian Psychology, 1977.

Mosak, H.H. Early recollections as a projective technique. *Journal of Projective Techniques*, 1958, 22(3), 302–311.

Mosak, H.H. Lifestyle. In A. Nikelly (Ed.), *Techniques for behavior change*. Springfield, Ill.: Charles C Thomas, 1971.

Mosak, H.H. *On purpose*. Chicago: Alfred Adler Institute, 1977.

Mosak, H.H. Adlerian psychotherapy. In R. Corsini (Ed.), *Current psychotherapies* (2nd ed.). Itasca, Ill.: Peacock, 1979. (a)

Mosak, H.H. Mosak's typology: An update. *Journal of Individual Psychology*, 1979, 35(2), 192–195. (b)

Mosak, H.H., & Mosak, B. *A bibliography for Adlerian psychology*. Washington, D.C.: Hemisphere, 1975.

Olson, G. *Early recollections: Their use in diagnosis and psychotherapy*. Springfield, Ill.: Charles C Thomas, 1979.

Ornstein, R.E. *The psychology of consciousness*. San Francisco: Freeman, 1972.

Roessler, R., & Bolton, R. *Psychosocial adjustment to disability*. Baltimore: University Park Press, 1978.

Rychlak, J.E. *Introduction to personality and psychotherapy: A theory-construction approach*. Boston: Houghton Mifflin, 1973.

Shontz, F.C. *The psychological aspects of physical illness and disability*. New York: Macmillan, 1975.

Shontz, F.C. Physical disability and personality: Theory and recent research. In J. Stubbins (Ed.), *Social and psychological aspects of disability*. Baltimore: University Park Press, 1977.

Shulman, B.H. *Contributions to individual psychology*. Chicago: Alfred Adler Institute, 1973.

Siller, J.R. Psychological situation of the disabled with spinal cord injuries. *Rehabilitation Literature*, 1969, 30, 290–296.

Siller, J.R. Attitudes toward disability. In H. Rusalem & D. Malikin (Eds.), *Contemporary vocational rehabilitation*. New York: New York University Press, 1976.

Sutton-Smith, B., & Rosenberg, B.G. *The sibling*. New York: Holt, Rinehart & Winston, 1970.

Taylor, J. Early recollections as a projective technique: A review of some recent validation studies. *Journal of Individual Psychology*, 1975, 31(2), 213–218.

Thompson, D.D. In psychosocial redevelopment: Erikson's model. In J. Lott, J. Owens, & W. Wilson (Eds.), *A holistic approach to employment for persons with spinal cord injury*. Fishersville, Va.: Virginia Spinal Cord Injury System, 1982.

Wright, B.A. *Physical disability—A psychological approach*. New York: Harper & Row, 1960.

Wright, B.A. Issues in overcoming emotional barriers to adjustment in the handicapped. In R.P. Marinelli & A.E. Dell Orto (Eds.), *The psychological and social impact of physical disability*. New York: Springer, 1977.

Chapter 3

Structured Processes and Techniques of Lifestyle Counseling

Warren R. Rule

Whereas the preceding chapter focused primarily on the concepts of lifestyle understanding and adjustment to disability, this chapter presents a somewhat structured approach to implementing these concepts. This counseling process for adjustment to disability can be viewed as having four phases. These phases, an adaptation of the Adlerian process (Dreikurs, 1967), are Relationship, Lifestyle Investigation, Lifestyle Interpretation, and Reorientation. The initial discussion will focus primarily on procedures in an individual setting with subsequent brief discussion on adapting these procedures to a group approach.

RELATIONSHIP

The relationship phase is not actually a ''phase'' in the sense that it has a distinct ending. The practitioner begins the helping process by building a relationship of trust, respect, genuineness, and empathy. These and other relationship factors presumably continue to operate and provide the basis for the development of the subsequent phases.

In addition to fostering those qualities upon which a solid counseling relationship is built, the relationship phase also serves other purposes. In this phase the client (1) has the opportunity to explore himself in relationship to the disability; (2) the practitioner learns more about the client's internal frame of reference; and (3) the opportunity is provided for an exchange of specific information (e.g., medical, case history, procedural, etc.) between the practitioner and the client.

Subjective Exploration

The overriding function of client exploration, according to Carkhuff (1980), is for the individual to begin to understand where he is in relationship to where he wants to be. As part of this process of self-exploration, which is skillfully guided by the practitioner, the client is better able to clarify his inner experiencing so that he can understand himself more fully. The future oriented goal-directed framework of this exploration process is crucial: the here and now in relationship to the ideal future. This goal-oriented framework not only is consistent with the Adlerian view of all of man's behavior, but also is an extremely helpful approach to specificity in the counseling process itself. The client's subjectively identifying the perceived present in relation to the perceived ideal future gives the practitioner a valuable perspective as well as serves to give direction to the counseling process. At a later phase in the counseling process, these ideas can be discussed within the context of the client's overall lifestyle.

Carkhuff (1980) has developed a number of considerations that are helpful in the exploration and understanding process. These points are useful in general, yet seem to be especially applicable to practitioners who emphasize the importance of increasing awareness of another's internal frame of reference. A summary of these ideas follows:

Attending

Very basic to facilitating the exploration process is attending or giving undivided attention. Attending personally involves posturing oneself as a helper in order to communicate interest and attentiveness. Attending contextually refers to arranging the practitioner's helping environment so that it conveys open communication and support, rather than power or elevated authority.

A major component of attending is observing, because the client, often unknowingly, reveals many clues to his inner experiences through his physical behavior and appearance. Actually, the client's physical behavior is often the most fertile source of information, especially when the client's remarks are inconsistent or confusing. Energy level, posture, grooming, nonverbal behavior are all important indices of the client's experience and level of functioning. Particularly noteworthy are discrepancies in the client's nonverbal behavior and verbal behavior. Listening is another attending skill that is extremely important. What the client says (who, what, when, where, why, and how) and how he says it (e.g., tone of voice) are keys to facilitation. The more the practitioner is able to suspend personal judgment and resist distractions, the greater will be his ability to listen for the recurrent, important themes in what the client is expressing.

Responding

The manner in which the practitioner verbally responds to the client's experiences is extremely crucial. As a result of the attending skills of accurate observing and listening, the helping person attempts to respond in a manner that expresses empathy, not sympathy. Empathy conveys the idea that the practitioner has an understanding or awareness of the client's experience and it is accomplished by responding initially at an interchangeable level with the client in terms of both feeling and content. By communicating to the client what the client has expressed, at the level of exploration the client expressed it, the practitioner is able to obtain a more accurate picture of the client's inner world. Moreover, the client is able to respond to the helper's empathic responses and this can result in further exploration or a clarification of the helper's understanding.

Interchangeable responding by the practitioner does not mean simply parroting back what the client has expressed; rather, it entails concisely expressing in a sentence the feeling state, which the client might or might not be aware of, along with a fresh understanding of the content of what the client has said. Initially, this counseling base of interchangeable responses would exist for whatever range of emotional states (e.g., anger, sadness, happiness, etc.) the client is experiencing. A working vocabulary of words and phrases that pinpoint various feeling states is essential for the practitioner.

Personalizing

After the client has explored the many dimensions of the problem, the client may be ready to move beyond interchangeable communication with the helper into deeper levels of self-understanding. Carkhuff (1980) views understanding as the next step after exploration. The readiness to do this may be signaled by sustaining self-exploratory responses without the practitioner's help or perhaps the client may make interchangeable responses with earlier remarks. At this point the helper may want to draw from the dominant theme the client has been expressing as well as from the helper's own experiences. In doing this, the practitioner will attempt to personalize the problem by helping the client understand what the client cannot do for himself that is contributing to his difficulty. (As will be discussed later, the lifestyle approach also helps the client see from a different and broader perspective what he is doing or not doing to contribute to his own difficulty.)

Thus, the issue focuses on what the individual presently is lacking or is unable to do for himself that prevents him from resolving the unwanted situation. In discussing such a deficit, the helper must be especially sensitive to the client's feeling about the deficit. In addition, the practitioner should be responsive to inconsistencies in what the client says, feels, or does as a source of useful information about what the client is unable to do for himself.

Upon reaching an awareness of this exceedingly important variable—what the client is unable to do that is contributing to the problem—the practitioner and the client are in a much better position to continue the counseling process.

As the practitioner attempts to grasp the personal meaning of the client's disability, it may be helpful to keep Shontz's (1975) broad principles in mind for viewing clients as whole, living people. These principles, while written for health professionals and not from a lifestyle perspective per se, appear generally consistent with the overall framework:

1. There are often multiple causes in life, rather than simple cause and effect relationships.
2. The person functions or attempts to function as an integrated unit.
3. The person responds to reality as he interprets it.
4. Behavior is determined by the context of the situation at the current moment.
5. Behavior maximizes construed consistency between past, present, and anticipated future experience.
6. Behavior is a function of relationships within an integrated organism-environment totality. (pp. 191–198)

Information Sharing

In addition to subjective exploration, another important component of the relationship phase is information sharing. Information sharing takes place as needed throughout the relationship phase and relates to primarily content-oriented material that has minimal emotional overtones. Information sharing would, in most cases, supplement the subjective exploration, rather than the reverse. However, it is far too easy to deal with exchanges between the helper and the client in terms of simply content; one must be prepared to respond to the emotions behind the content, even to client statements as seemingly innocuous as "information" sharing. In general, "information sharing" material might be questions and responses regarding strictly medical information, misconceptions about disability, procedural details, miscellaneous clarification, and the like. The information sharing components, which are intertwined with the subjective exploration dimension, can yield information for both the practitioner and the client.

LIFESTYLE INVESTIGATION

Prior to conducting the lifestyle investigation, Adlerian practitioners often obtain from the client information that may have a significant bearing on the subsequent lifestyle discussion. The helper explores with the client how he is functioning in the three areas of social living, sometimes referred to as the three tasks of life. Adlerians believe that everyone takes a position—with varying degrees of success or failure—on these three areas of social living: work (or school), love, and friendship. As Dreikurs (1953) notes, if one of the tasks is evaded, difficulties may ultimately unfold in the other tasks as well. The Adlerian belief is that the individual's lifestyle, including its unique strengths, weaknesses, and blind spots, functions as a coping device in all areas of life. Therefore, an increased awareness of how things are going for the client in the three main areas of life provides a fuller picture of how the client's chosen lifestyle is presently contributing to his problems or his happiness. Generally, Adlerians believe that the lifestyle becomes most apparent when the individual is experiencing stress. It is then that what has proven most useful, i.e., the lifestyle, is relied on with greater intensity.

Another procedure that some practitioners use is that of asking ''The Question.'' This is simply asking the client what would be different if he were well or if the problem did not exist. Sometimes the answer to this question indicates for what purpose the individual is experiencing unusual difficulties, against whom or what the symptoms are directed, or against what demand or threat he is defending himself by having such a difficult adjustment.

The exploration of the three tasks of life and ''The Question'' normally would precede the gathering of the lifestyle information. This pre-lifestyle material might sometimes be discussed in the relationship phase, depending on appropriateness and the flow of the interaction. The demarcation points between the various stages, especially between relationship and lifestyle investigation, are not rigid; rather, one stage overlaps another until the later stage clearly emerges from the former.

The procedure for one type of formal lifestyle investigation (Dreikurs, 1967) was highlighted in the previous chapter, which also discussed other avenues for obtaining lifestyle information. The rationale for conducting the lifestyle investigation should be introduced to the client in a concise, respectful manner. An example might go something like this:

> John, sometimes it is helpful to be in touch with some pretty broad attitudes and goals that are at work in major areas of a person's life. We are talking here about important beliefs an individual has learned about himself, other people, and life that he probably is not completely aware of. One way I have found very useful in trying to help someone identify them is by taking a look at what impressions from early childhood a person is choosing to continue to believe. You and I could discuss for a while some of your early impressions and then talk about how these are operating right now, in your everyday life. Want to give it a try?

In the overwhelming majority of cases, clients are intrigued by the prospect of learning what relationship exists between early childhood and the present. This seems hold for individuals who experienced relatively unpleasant childhoods as well as for those who experienced pleasant ones. The counselor's introductory remarks, as well as his subsequent comments, should not depict the lifestyle exploration as a mystical, murky endeavor. Rather, the emphasis ought to reflect a sharing, educational process in which relationships between the early past and present are discussed. As we have noted, Adlerians rely on the selectivity of memory as providing information that is currently useful to the individual's chosen lifestyle; accordingly, emphasis is placed on the manifest content of memory, not on symbolic meanings.

LIFESTYLE INTERPRETATION

The process itself of gathering the lifestyle information helps to cement the counseling relationship. This step, in addition to the ongoing efforts initiated during the relationship phase, provides a foundation for the practitioner and the client to discuss the client's lifestyle.

At this point, the practitioner has had an opportunity to study the client's response to the lifestyle interview. In searching for lifestyle "threads" or overriding goals the helper relies on his awareness of modest probabilities of relationship between lifestyle variables (nomothetic laws). At the same time, he is trying to make deductions and identify logical patterns that will identify individual (idiographic) laws. While looking for tentative identification of the individual's network of goals, or cognitive map, the practitioner is, in a sense, attempting to put pieces of a jigsaw puzzle together. He is wondering as he reviews the lifestyle material: "if this person has drawn these conclusions about himself, others, and life, then what kind of overriding (future-oriented) goals would he have chosen to guide him in his striving to be a coping, significant person?" In addition to seeking to identify broad, overriding goals, the counselor keeps an eye out for specific convictions that relate to the client's present problem, such as adjustment to disability.

The focus is on the person's thinking patterns, notions, and goals and only secondarily on his methods of behaving that are in the service of lifestyle goals. Most Adlerians believe that the lifestyle reveals only limited probabilities about behavior patterns, which are often more changeable than basic goals. Information on behavior used to implement lifestyle goals is primarily obtained by other modalities, e.g., discussion with the client, counselor observations, others' observations. Material on lifestyle analysis can be found in the readings listed in the Appendix.

Once the practitioner has tentatively identified the client's lifestyle notions and goals, he shares his interpretations in a spirit of respect and exploration. He would use phrases such as "Could it be that . . . ," "A guess that I have is. . . ." Oftentimes, a client will respond with a "recognition reflex," a nonverbal indication that the practitioner has indeed hit a bullseye. Other times, semantic barriers are in operation and must be worked through. Occasionally, the helper misses the mark, regardless of semantic or communication barriers, and must simply return to the drawing board.

The practitioner must particularly keep in mind how the client's lifestyle operates when the client hears about his own lifestyle, e.g., those striving to please may be too agreeable, those striving for intellectual superiority may create a sparring match, etc. However, if the relationship is one of trust, if both parties are willing to cooperate and work toward understanding, agreement can usually be reached regarding major aspects of the client's lifestyle.

There are a number of frameworks for presenting lifestyle interpretations. The perspective of "I am . . . ," "Others are . . . ," "Life is . . ." is one approach. Another is to emphasize the "shoulds," e.g., "I am a person who should . . . ," "Others are people who ought to . . . ," "Life is a place that must . . . ." Often it is helpful to present the material in a goal-directed framework, which denotes a future orientation, e.g., "To . . . ." Mosak (1979) focuses on "Basic Mistakes," e.g., overgeneralizations, false or impossible goals of "security," misperceptions of life and of life's demands, minimization or denial of one's worth, faulty values. In addition, Mosak (1954) has divided lifestyle convictions into four groups: the self concept, the self ideal, the picture of the world, and ethical convictions. Another framework (Rule, 1982a) utilizes the perspective of the individual's private logic within a social context; the technique involves reframing the practitioner's interpretations in a positive and socially acceptable manner and with the imaginary context of the client's ideal self as viewed by important others. Lifestyle interpretations can also be incorporated into modalities of communication developed from other perspectives, e.g., parables and fables (Pancer, 1978), metaphors (Gordon, 1978; Rule, 1983), trance formations (Grinder & Bandler, 1981; Bandler & Grinder, 1975; Grinder, Delozier & Bandler, 1977), and Ericksonian teaching tales (Rosen, 1982).

In facilitating the interpretation process, the helper should encourage the client to take responsibility for identifying relationships between lifestyle and daily living. Sometimes clients are curious about how the practitioner arrived at the lifestyle interpretations. In response the helper may want to render brief explanations, all the while giving the client the opportunity to make the associations between past and present goals and behavior. The efforts by the counselor during the interpretation stage go a long way in enhancing client self-acceptance and feelings of OKness. The ripening of a positive attitude toward one's lifestyle is a key variable in the next and final phase, which focuses on the client and his difficulties.

REORIENTATION

Reorientation Goals

In the reorientation phase, the accent is on change. Upon achieving a measure of insight into the client's lifestyle, both the practitioner and the client are able to use this framework as a springboard for discussing change.

The primary goal in the reorientation phase is, of course, to help the client resolve his present difficulties. In attempting to accomplish this foremost goal, the practitioner often has in the back of his mind a number of related goals. Examples are:

1. To identify those self-serving decisions of the lifestyle that are contributing to the present difficulty by working to the client's disadvantage, and, in addition, to pinpoint those lifestyle advantages that can be used as assets in the reorientation process.
2. To assist the client in setting specific and realistic personal goals that are related to diminishing the self-defeating dimensions of the present difficulty, e.g., adjustment to disability.
3. To explore the interrelatedness of thinking, feeling, and doing. From an operational perspective, to explore the thinking processes related to the lifestyle in relationship to the associated feelings and behaviors. Although the past was utilized in order to understand the present better, the adjustment emphasis is on present responsibility for self.
4. To devise homework strategies, related to lifestyle assets wherever possible, that are a means to attaining the specified goals for change.
5. To encourage the client to believe in a significance of self that is not a function of comparisons with others or self-rankings.
6. To foster an increased other-directedness in the client. This is important because increased self-esteem seems paradoxically related to increased acceptance, empathy, and social interest in others (O'Connell, 1976).

Reorientation Strategies

Strategies for implementing many of these goals for change will be discussed below. The strategies are divided into three areas: (1) broad considerations the practitioner may keep in mind during the overall reorientation process, (2) specific goal-oriented interventions, and (3) supplemental techniques from other approaches.

Broad Considerations

The practitioner continually strives to be aware of the goal-directed nature of the client's behavior and expression of emotions. This focus characterizes the client's lifestyle goals as related to his current difficulties, his interaction with the practitioner, his decision-making procedures, and so on. As appropriate, the helper either provides the opportunity for the client to get in touch with his own goals that underly certain behavior and feelings or he takes a more direct role by gently pointing out how the client creatively implements goals and their usefulness to his lifestyle. This awareness is conveyed to the client, not in an accusatory manner, but rather in a framework that respects the individual's creativity in devising and implementing such a goal.

The responsibility is therefore placed on the client for creating his own approach to a given situation. Moreover, the focus is kept on the (future-oriented) goals of a behavior or feeling because this reduces the likelihood that the client will feel burdened by—or use to his "advantage"—the "whys" or "causes" of behavior. The "whys" or "causes" reflect past, unchangeable reasons; "goals" indicate future-oriented, changeable targets. Since the helper creates an opportunity for the client to have an increased awareness of his goals, the client is less likely to pursue those goals that ultimately work to his disadvantage. (Adler is said to have expressed this point in an unforgettable metaphor: once the therapist has spit into the client's soup, the client can continue to eat the soup, but it won't taste as good.)

Sometimes it is helpful to view this change process as one of "reframing." Bandler and Grinder (1979), speaking from the neuro-linguistic programming perspective, stated that "The heart of reframing is to make the distinction between *intention* . . . and the *behavior*. . . . Then you can find new, more acceptable behaviors to satisfy the same intention" (p. 138).

An awareness of the client's lifestyle enables the practitioner to consider other broad variations. The helper now has additional guidelines, as noted before, for varying his responses at critical periods. For instance, an authoritative, how-to-do-it approach may annoy a client who is heavily invested in intellectual superiority or in self-control, whereas an understanding, respectful approach would be apt to enlist cooperation more quickly. An increased lifestyle awareness may also help the practitioner recognize how different clients, with different lifestyles, may feel either encouraged or discouraged by the same behavior on the part of the helper.

The practitioner may use the lifestyle awareness to suggest change in aspects of the client's environment. These suggestions, designed to be in keeping with sensitivities inherent in the client's lifestyle, might be made to family members, medical personnel in an institution, supervisors in a work setting, and so on.

Sometimes an increased understanding of the purpose for artificial aids, such as alcohol or drugs, can result from lifestyle awareness. An individual may believe within his private logic that the artificial aid either increases the flow of his style or permits him to engage in options that are not within the flow of his lifestyle. For example, the charmer may feel more charming under the influence of drink or drugs; the self-controlled person may feel able to give up some control in his altered state.

The practitioner continually looks for opportunities to encourage the client to believe in a significance of self that is not a function of vertical rankings or comparisons with others. This awareness can be helpful to a client in learning to do a mental checkup when he experiences an unwanted negative emotion and then trying to discover how the lifestyle is dictating the message of inadequacy. This daily awareness of individual functioning can also be instrumental in avoiding future pitfalls.

In addition to encouraging the client to monitor and challenge himself on OK-ness in his daily functioning, the practitioner uses various broad strategies to accomplish the same purpose within the counseling setting. For instance, the helper may employ many uses of humor in the form of parables, fables, biography, quotations, cartoons, anecdotes. Or, the practitioner and the client may devise homework assignments designed to help the client accept himself while laughing at the exaggerated lifestyle demands he is making on himself. The use of Polaroid photographs (Rule, 1979) and nightly audio-tape recordings (Rule, 1977b) has been effective.

Adler believed in the potency of humor, as Rychlak (1973) has summarized below:

> . . . Adler believed in the advisability of using a series of fairly dramatic illustrations in making his point. If the therapist is too sober all he succeeds in doing is worrying the client needlessly, overvaluing the severity of the case, and establishing an authoritarian relationship. He must not make light of the client, of course, but the proper mood Adler sought was that of spontaneous cooperation in a joint effort which could assure success if they did not as therapist and client take themselves altogether too seriously. A hopeful person is not without a sense of happiness or lightheartedness, even in the face of some rather agonizing challenges. (p. 129)

Broad strategies are often necessary in facilitating change in a client who creatively uses a mental, emotional, or physical disability. These strategies are part of the intervention process for facilitation of adjustment to disability and will be later discussed in detail.

Encouragement should be a major part of the practitioner's overall attitude undergirding whatever broad strategies he selects. This important Adlerian procedure has far-reaching implications for process and outcome. As Dinkmeyer (1972) noted:

> Encouragement on the part of the counselor is comprised of both verbal and nonverbal procedures that enable a counselee to experience and become aware of his own worth. The counselor expresses faith in and total acceptance of the counselee as he is, not as he could or should be. Encouragement as defined here does not imply that the counselor rewards, bribes, or praises; it means rather that he places value on the counselee's uniqueness and humanness and indicates to him that because he is human he is of worth and value. Counselor encouragement

helps to correct the counselee's mistaken assumption that he is inferior to or not as able as others. The counselor demonstrates encouragement with a strong, empathic attitude that emphasizes health rather than illness, strength rather than weakness, ability rather than inability. He completely accepts the counselee as a person of real value. (p. 177)

Specific Goal-Directed Considerations

Upon having achieved awareness of a particular lifestyle goal (or belief), the client is in a position to make a decision regarding change, continuation, and related behavior. The next step after awareness might be to identify the parameters of desired change, after which point the individual is in a position to consider various alternatives for action or nonaction. The following is a variation of a framework developed by Rule (1980) that details various goal-change orientations and suggests possible solutions:

1. The client *likes* and wants to continue this goal (and the resulting feelings). In addition, he does not wish to change a related goal dimension (situational specificity, frequency of occurrence, or felt intensity). Nor does he wish to change the behavior used to implement this goal. Moreover, for having this goal, (1) he accepts himself or (2) he rejects himself.
   Possible solutions: For (1) no solution appears to be needed. For (2) consider: (a) monitoring and/or rating thoughts, feelings, and/or sensations; (b) a rational-emotive approach (Ellis, 1974); (c) self-directed humor for self/other acceptance; (d) practitioner encouragement and humanistic sharing.

2. The client *likes* and wants to continue this goal (and the resulting feelings). In addition, he does not wish to change a related goal dimension (situational specificity, frequency of occurrence, or felt intensity). However, he does want to behave differently in order to implement the goal more effectively and not to rate self-worth in the process.
   Possible solutions: (a) a rational-emotive approach; (b) self-directed humor for self-other acceptance; (c) specific cognitive self-management strategies; (d) overt behavioral strategies; (e) specific homework assignments, including utilizing community resources; (f) practitioner encouragement and humanistic sharing.

3. The client *somewhat likes* this goal (and resulting feelings). In general or in specific situations, he wishes to value the goal less or more often and/or more strongly. In addition, he wants to behave in keeping with the changed goal dimension and not rate his self-worth in the process.
   Possible solutions: (a) monitor and/or rate thoughts, feelings, and/or sensations; (b) explore and establish change goals; (c) a rational-emotive

approach; (d) self-directed humor for self/other acceptance; (e) cognitive self-management skills; (f) overt behavioral strategies; (g) specific homework assignments, including utilizing community resources; (h) practitioner encouragement and humanistic sharing.

4. The client *dislikes* this goal (and the resulting feelings), yet he does not wish to change the goal or a related dimension of the goal. Nor does he wish to change the behavior used to implement the goal. But, for having this contradiction he either (1) accepts himself or (2) rejects himself.

   Possible solutions: For (1) explore no-change secondary gains and maintaining conditions in the spirit of practitioner encouragement and humanistic sharing. For (2): (a) additional self-awareness experiences; (b) monitor and/or rate thoughts, feelings, and/or sensations; (c) explore no-change secondary gains and maintaining conditions; (d) increase decision-making skills; (e) explore and establish change goals; (f) a rational-emotive approach; (g) self-directed humor for self/other acceptance; (h) practitioner encouragement and humanistic sharing.

5. The client *dislikes* this goal (and the resulting feelings). In general or in specific situations, he wishes to value this goal much less often and/or less strongly. Yet, he does not wish to change any of the behavior that is related to the goal or rate his self-worth.

   Possible consideration: it is often more rewarding to change behavior as well (see 6 below).

6. The client *dislikes* this goal (and the resulting feelings). In general or in specific situations, he wishes to value this goal much less often and/or less strongly. Also he wants to behave in keeping with the changed goal dimension and not rate his self-worth in the process.

   Possible solutions: (a) monitor and/or rate thoughts, feelings, and/or sensations; (b) explore and establish change goals; (c) a rational-emotive approach; (d) self/other acceptance; (e) cognitive self-management skills; (f) overt behavioral strategies; (g) other specific homework assignments, including utilizing community resources; (h) practitioner encouragement and humanistic sharing.

Supplemental Techniques from Other Approaches

As we have seen, the lifestyle can provide the context within which the client's problem "deficit" is viewed. Expressed another way, lifestyle awareness can illuminate how the client's deficit (what he is wanting that he is unable to do for himself) fits into his broader life goals. Many techniques exist in addition to the Adlerian action-oriented ones. For instance, other counseling approaches, although sometimes theoretically incompatible with the overall lifestyle perspective, nevertheless offer many supplemental techniques that fit into various phases, particularly the reorientation phase. Some of these are discussed below.

Rational-Emotive Therapy (RET). The rational-emotive approach, developed by Ellis (1962, 1974), focuses on identifying and overcoming irrational thinking. It fits well into the reorientation phase of the lifestyle approach in that it helps clients reduce the intensity or frequency of identified lifestyle notions or goals that are working to one's disadvantage. In this educational approach, the counselor teaches the client how to dispute the importance that he is attributing to a real or imagined occurrence. The emphasis is on the should's, must's, ought to's, and other self-mandates that the person, often dimly consciously, upsets himself with. Both RET and the Adlerian lifestyle approach emphasize that it is desirable for self-acceptance not to be a function of achievement, comparison with others, or any form of self-rating. Moreover, both approaches assert that we mostly create our emotions rather than are possessed by them—an important counseling perspective. Additional reading in Walen, DiGiuseppe, and Wessler (1980) is suggested.

Behavioral Counseling. Behavioral counseling emphasizes learning new ways to think, feel, or act in designated situations. This essentially educational approach is especially useful in the final lifestyle reorientation phase when the client has identified a very specific problem he wants to work on. Broadly speaking, the sequence of behavioral counseling proceeds as follows: identification of problem, formulation of counseling goals, monitoring of client behavior, implementation of counseling intervention, and evaluation of goal attainment. Some useful techniques include assertive training; progressive muscle relaxation; modeling, including self-as-a-model; self- and contingency management programs; behavioral contracting. Further information may be found in Hosford and de Visser (1974).

Gestalt Counseling. The Gestalt perspective, pioneered by Perls (e.g., Perls, Hefferline, and Goodman, 1951; Perls, 1969), focuses on awareness of what a person is sensing, feeling, and, to a lesser degree, thinking, in the present moment. The assumption is that by being challenged to draw from one's own resources, coupled with the spontaneity of the now, problems and issues that need to be dealt with will emerge into awareness. The techniques can be useful in the early phases as well as in the reorientation phase, especially in teaching clients the direct relationship between many facets of awareness and thinking processes as well as in teaching clients self-responsibility for feelings. These interventions include nonverbal awareness, fantasy, use of language, feelings (past and future as related to present centeredness), and so on. Additional discussion of the uses of Gestalt techniques within a counseling framework may be found in Passons (1975).

Miscellaneous Approaches. Sheldon and Ackerman (1974) and Lazarus and Fay (1975) offer a wide variety of techniques for the very important dimension of client homework. Transactional analysis (Berne, 1961) may provide the client with descriptive concepts of understanding interpersonal dynamics; reality therapy (Glasser, 1965) presents a systematic perspective on assuming responsibility; stress management offers helpful ideas, either from a somewhat cognitive perspective (e.g., Woolfolk and Richardson, 1978) or a more physiological vantage point (e.g., Selye, 1974) on to a broad-based eclectic orientation (e.g., Schafer, 1978). Neuro-linguistic programming (Bandler and Grinder, 1979; Dilts, Grinder, Bandler, Bandler, and Delozier, 1980) offers many techniques for structuring subjective experience and is discussed within a lifestyle framework in Chapter 11.

Before concluding this section, it is worth noting that the importance of relationship factors cannot be minimized. The relationship factors, especially respect for another's rights and responsiveness to another's internal frame of reference, get the whole process moving and keep it moving. An appropriate metaphor might be that the complex interaction of relationship factors (feeling-oriented) is the key that opens the door to the dark room; the lifestyle self-understanding (thinking-oriented) creates light in the room; and the reorientation methods (action-oriented) rearrange the room and polish the furniture according to the wishes of the individual.

ADAPTION TO GROUP SETTINGS

Lifestyle counseling, based on a holistic approach, emphasizes the interrelatedness of man to himself and to others. As such, the lifestyle approach views man as a social being who is not—although he may at times behave differently—an island unto himself. Correspondingly, the lifestyle perspective regards personal problems as basically social problems, a concept that ideally lends itself to the social setting of group counseling. The overall group process would be generally consistent with the four phases of individual counseling.

Sweeney's (1975) observations about group participation and contribution are noteworthy. In groups, participants are:

1. inherently equal and may expect to behave as such, i.e., have a place that no one can rightfully challenge.
2. considered to be capable of assuming responsibility for their behavior.
3. individually understood best in a holistic, unified way as creative, purposive beings.
4. considered as social beings meeting the same life tasks as others.
5. capable of changing their attitudes and/or behaviors.
6. able to help as well as be helped in the process of giving meaning to life.

Discussion during the initial meetings should explore expectations of the group members and misconceptions about group counseling. Ground rules such as confidentiality, the fact that the group is not simply "a confessional," and that members will not be forced to do anything should be covered. Moreover, at this time, logistical matters should be dealt with, such as meeting times, length (approximately two hours is recommended), duration of group, replacement of members, etc.

Relationship techniques are useful not only in the initial phase of group counseling but also as a means of maintaining the cohesiveness, meaning, and productivity of the group. Dinkmeyer, Pew, and Dinkmeyer (1979) recommend techniques such as encouragement and focusing on assets and positive feedback. In addition, facilitating participation by utilizing nonverbal cues (e.g., seating place, seating posture, facial expression, voice, hand gestures, etc.) is often beneficial. Here and throughout the whole process consideration can be given to facilitative confrontation of discrepancies in what members think, feel, and do (e.g., what was said vs. what is being said; what one is saying vs. what one appears to be feeling; what one is saying vs. what one is doing, etc.). Furthermore, much can be gained by encouraging as much here-and-now interaction as possible (except for learning about the past from lifestyle exploration) as opposed to "there and then" orientations.

In facilitating the beginning stages of lifestyle group counseling, as well as in maintaining productive relationships throughout the complete group process, leader interventions are often necessary. These interventions not only enable the group process to continue productively but also provide effective modeling for other members to emulate. Dyer and Vriend (1975) suggest that intervention may be necessary when:

1. A group member speaks for everyone.
2. An individual speaks for another individual within the group.
3. A group member overfocuses on persons, conditions, or events outside the group.
4. Someone seeks the approval of the counselor or a group member before and after speaking.
5. Someone says, "I don't want to hurt his feelings, so I won't say it."
6. A group member suggests that his or her problems are due to someone else.
7. An individual suggests that "I've always been that way."
8. An individual suggests "I'll wait, and it will change."
9. Discrepant behavior appears.
10. A member bores the group by rambling.

Insofar as group lifestyle investigation and interpretation are concerned, each group member would have—needless to say—different expectations of himself and others and would have learned different behaviors for implementing the dimly conscious goals of the lifestyle. Thus, each person's self-understanding and other group members' understanding of a given individual's private logic would be enhanced by the lifestyle approach.

The lifestyle information can be gathered by the group, a partner, or the leader and then distributed to all of the members. Then the members and the leader offer their interpretations of the group members' lifestyles in a spirit of tentative sharing and exploration. They use phrases such as "Could it be that . . . ," "A guess that I have is . . . ," etc. If the interpretations are in the ballpark, if the group relationship is one of trust, and if the group member and others are willing to work toward understanding, major agreement can be reached regarding major aspects of the group member's lifestyle. This procedure is continued for each member and the leader. Throughout the process, the leader and other members refer to examples from the group experience (e.g., first impressions, group exercises, etc.) that supported the lifestyle interpretation.

Because the group is a social microcosm, the lifestyle is apt to express itself in the group as well as on the outside. Thus, the group member would get feedback on how he creatively and subtly has used and is using his lifestyle in relating to others in his attempt to strive for a place of self-determined social significance. Sometimes replaying a video tape of a member's interactions with others increases this self-understanding and serves to highlight certain lifestyle behaviors that otherwise would be hard to accept. Another approach is the absurd exaggeration of lifestyle characteristics by using masquerades (Rule, 1979); the group input into determination of each individual costume as well as the group masquerade itself can result in increased self-awareness, self-acceptance, and group cohesiveness.

Lifestyle introspection, group observations and encouragement, videotaping, and the lifestyle masquerade all serve to facilitate the process of a group member saying to himself, "Hey, this is me!"

The final phase is lifestyle reorientation. Upon achieving a measure of self-awareness, the members of the lifestyle group counseling process focus on positive change that will be helpful presently and in the future. The continued emphasis is, as O'Connell (1975) noted, on personal thinking patterns or goals, not on the common stereotype of a "drive-release" group that aims simply for the expression of emotions as a curative factor. In broadening one's insight or understanding of self in relationship to others, the group members move toward achieving "outsight" or "the learned ability to see, hear, and feel along with others" (O'Connell, 1976, p. 157). Expressed in another way, the attempt is to "free them from the intoxication of a private interpretation of the world" (Ansbacher & Ansbacher, 1956, p. 348) and encourage a spirit of cooperation or "common sense versus private sense" (Ansbacher & Ansbacher, 1956, p. 253).

H.S. Sullivan (1940), whose ideas have considerable overlap with Adler's, saw the powerful relationship between the interpersonal and intrapersonal realms and concluded that one achieves mental health to the extent that one becomes aware of one's interpersonal relationships. So, during this fourth and final phase, the group member develops his goals for change and refines methods he will continue to use for change and for broadening his sense of self in relation to others.

CONSIDERATIONS REGARDING THE DISABLED

As we have seen, the lifestyle approach contends that people are social beings by nature and are inclined to establish individual self-identity by relating with and comparing self with others. The comparison process for the disabled, especially on an ongoing basis, can have severe repercussions. Usually, the resulting inferiority feeling, based on comparisons with others, is coupled with a feeling of social isolation or not belonging. As Mosak (1977) notes, a goal for the practitioner, then, should be to decrease inferiority feelings and to increase feelings of belonging. An additional dilemma resulting from comparisons involves the concept of near-normalcy. Paradoxically, clients with mild disabilities can sometimes actually have, according to Eisenberg (1977), a more difficult adjustment because they are almost normal. Consequently, these individuals may try to deny or hide the disability beause it is marginal. The topics of family reaction and involvement are also self-in-relation-to-others issues, which will be later discussed in detail.

The practitioner should not overlook the implications of possibly one of the most obvious conditions imposed upon many disabled individuals—the loss of liberty. Perhaps the existence of the physical restriction is less serious than its consequences (Eisenberg, 1977). Relationships, architectural barriers, sexual adjustment, community reaction, loss of autonomy, dependency are all factors that may be sensitive problem areas. A reverse situation can also occur in which the client relates many other problems—old and new, personal and interpersonal—to the disability. In making the disability responsible for a host of difficulties, psychosocial adjustment to the disability is correspondingly delayed.

After reviewing a variety of investigations, which found that, on the average, disabled persons report lower self-esteem than nondisabled persons, Roessler and Bolton (1978) concluded that many disabled individuals' views of themselves "may militate against successful rehabilitation, unless modified through adjustment training" (p. 40).

Kir-Stimon (1977) noted a common fallacy on the part of both the client and the helper:

That he (the client) must be either nobody or somebody worthwhile. In this either/or situation in which the severely disabled person frequently finds himself, he fails to realize that he is important simply because he exists, despite societal standards of productivity—creation, invention, even procreation. For the severely handicapped person who is labeled totally and permanently disabled and considered unable to earn his own livelihood, this becomes a distinction between being and not being. Personal unproductivity in our society is literally "un-becoming." Whereas, as a matter of fact, personal creativity need not involve a product or an object but might relate more to the very craft of living. (p. 367)

This perspective, although not written in direct support of the lifestyle counseling approach, is consistent with the encouragement of self-acceptance and the discouragement of vertical rankings, both of which are efforts that are heavily emphasized in lifestyle counseling.

Resistance

During any phase of the helping process, the practitioner may encounter resistance. Dreikurs (1967) asserts that "resistance" essentially is a discrepancy between the goals of the practitioner and those of the client. Therefore, a keen awareness of the practitioner's expectations and the client's lifestyle goals increases the likelihood of working through the resistance in a spirit of cooperation. At times, however, facilitative confrontation may be in order; Shulman (1972, 1977) has suggested helpful techniques for this purpose. The controversial concept of resistance will be discussed more fully in Chapter 7. Perhaps here, a wise psychological attitude in rehabilitation, as stated by Mosak (1977), is "acceptance of the patient as he is" (p. 54), which is the basis in general for all lifestyle counseling techniques.

One way to respect the client "as is," yet respond in a facilitative, useful manner to what can be broadly termed "negativism," is to use responses that combine respect for the client's present internal frame of reference with the flow of a major lifestyle goal (Rule, 1977a). Typically, in working with clients, practitioners are often stunned or baffled at expressions of client negativism. Negativism can be broadly defined as verbal and/or nonverbal expressions that convey the message that self, others, or life are at fault because one's expectations are not met. This may be expressed in the form of hostility, resentment, aggression, etc., and could be directed at the practitioner. Again, in viewing emotions as goal directed, the helper is in a better position to understand the negativism. By having an awareness of the client's lifestyle, the practitioner has insight into the goals and, consequently, how the expression of negativism is useful to the individual. The helper can act facilitatively by responding in terms of the relationship between what the person is now wanting that he is not getting, his unmet lifestyle goals, and his feelings about the deficit.

Along a similar vein, sometimes clients feel threatened because of perceived "dangers." These perceptions can greatly interfere with client cooperation. The likelihood of occurrence of each of the perceived dangers is related to the degree of correspondence to the overall individual lifestyle. The following dangers perceived by clients were noted by Shulman (1973): being defective, incurring disapproval or enmity, being ridiculed, being taken advantage of, not getting necessary help, submitting to order, having to face responsibility, and having to face unpleasant consequences. In addition, Shulman cites possible defensive patterns or forms of behavior that may be used to ward off the dangers. These devices may be at either a conscious or dimly conscious level; they may be used either almost continuously or only occasionally at a time of stress:

A. Externalization ("The fault lies outside of me")
   1. Cynicism ("Life is at fault")
   2. Inadequacy ("I'm just an innocent victim")
      a. sickness
      b. a bad background
      c. victimized by cravings and impulses
      d. possessed by demons or supernatural force
   3. Rebellion ("I can't afford to submit to life")
   4. Projecton ("It's all their fault")
B. Blind Spots ("If I don't look at it, it will go away")
C. Excessive Self-Control ("I will not let anything upset me")
D. Arbitrary Rightness ("My mind is made up; don't confuse me with the facts")
E. Elusiveness and Confusion ("Don't pin me down")
F. Retreat ("Nothing ventured, nothing lost")
G. Contrition and Self-Disparagement ("Mea Culpa") and Good Intentions ("I didn't mean it")
H. Suffering ("I feel bad")
   1. Suffering as manipulation ("If you don't do what I want, I'll die and then you'll be sorry")
   2. Suffering as justification ("I have a right to my own way. Look how much I suffer when I don't get it")
   3. Suffering as self-glorification ("The amount of my suffering proves my nobility")
I. Sideshows ("I can't take care of anything else until I have slain my dragon")
J. Rationalization ("I really didn't fail")

Some Reminders

The practitioner must keep clearly in mind as he works with clients the purpose of emotions. As we know, the Adlerian viewpoint is that emotions are goal directed. That is to say, feelings are largely the byproducts of our goals, which are reflected in the way we perceive, evaluate, and regard various situations. As Dreikurs (1967) noted, we need our emotions because they provide the steam and fuel for our actions. Thus, our feelings are in the service of our thoughts. This functional relationship puts responsibility on the individual for his emotions; he cannot accurately say that he lost control of them, was a prisoner of them, or the like.

Another barrier to effective understanding is the imagined distinction between "intellectual" and "emotional" insight. As Mosak (1979) asserted, this dualism can be an avoidance maneuver created by the client. Such antagonistic forces (e.g., "I know it in my head, but can't accept it emotionally") can be creations by the client in order to acceptably delay action. Thus, at a dimly conscious level, he is victimized—in his private logic—by conflicting forces that absolve him of present responsibility for taking a position on the issue at hand. Mosak (1979) suggests an exercise, referred to as the "push button" technique, for teaching a client self-responsibility for his emotions. By closing his eyes and imagining a pleasant incident, then an unpleasant incident, and then repeating the first pleasant incident, the client realizes that he can create whatever feeling he chooses simply by deciding what he will think.

In regard to the broad area of symptoms, the Adlerian approach takes the position that the main significance of the symptom lies in its service to the individual. Just as symptoms serve purposes for the person biologically, they can also serve purposes for him psychologically. According to Shulman (1973), symptoms can serve as safeguards for self-esteem or as excuses. These symptoms are viewed as being in accord with the individual's lifestyle. The use of various methods for struggling with the symptoms in order to maintain face is an example of individual lifestyle creativity. Specific examples will be discussed further in subsequent chapters.

In addition to the creative use of symptoms, individuals can employ lifestyle creativity in gamesmanship maneuvers with the counselor. Adler (1964) would usually use a countertactic, such as a paradoxical bind, a maneuver to avoid the intended power struggle, or a shrewd cultivation of the client's sense of social interest.

Lifestyle information can sometimes broaden the counselor's understanding of how a client might either react to or use a mental, emotional, or physical disability (Ansbacher & Ansbacher, 1956). An example is a client whose lifestyle is such that feelings of being significant as a person exist only when recognition is gained for being number one. Perhaps this person may be especially determined not to let a newly acquired disability stand in the way. Or, on the nonproductive side, the individual may even try to make a special mark by being the number one unmanageable client. The counselor may want to consider how a client may be using a disability. For example, a client who has a congenital handicap and who was the only boy among seven sisters may well have developed many secondary gains from his handicap and hopes to continue using it in this manner. Sometimes, clients pursue what may be termed "elusive" goals. Gray-area goals such as this may be ones that are too broad, too lofty, too unclear, or incompatible with another important goal or ephemeral by nature. These elusive goals have been distilled into the three U's: *U*nfocused, *U*nrealistic, and *U*ncoordinated (Rule, 1982b). Sometimes, as Woolfolk and Richardson (1978) observed, when an individual is pursuing incompatible (seemingly uncoordinated) goals, especially if one of the goals is distinctly selfish or socially unacceptable, the person may experience "troublesome" emotions at a dimly conscious level. The purpose of these "troublesome" interfering emotions may be to enable the person to view himself as having altogether good intentions that were interfered with by the unwanted emotions, rather than to admit that these emotions are in the service of selfish or less-than-noble goals.

Finally, from a broader perspective, we might add that respect should be given to the client's short-term and long-term dreams. However, as Kir-Stimon suggested (1977), let the practitioner not confuse dream and illusions with hallucination. Dreams are useful, perhaps at times necessary, as a means for achieving satisfaction, and, after all, as Trieschmann (1974) succinctly concluded, "The key to coping with one's disability is to receive enough satisfactions and rewards to make life worthwhile" (p. 558).

SUMMARY

The overall counseling process for adjustment to disability was discussed within a framework of four phases: Relationship, Lifestyle Investigation, Lifestyle Interpretation, and Reorientation. This process is based on a facilitative, cooperative relationship and emphasizes client self-awareness and self-responsibility. Contributions of selected other counseling approaches and a group approach were overviewed. In addition, attention was given to specific considerations for working with the disabled.

REFERENCES

Adler, A. *Problems of neurosis: A book of case histories*. New York: Harper & Row, 1964.

Ansbacher, H.L., & Ansbacher, R.R. (Eds.), *The individual psychology of Alfred Adler*. New York: Basic Books, 1956.

Bandler, R., & Grinder, J. *Patterns of the hypnotic techniques of Milton H. Erickson, M.D.* (Vol. 1). Cupertino, Calif.: Meta Publications, 1975.

Bandler, R., & Grinder, J. *Frogs into princes*. Mohab, Utah: Real People Press, 1979.

Berne, E. *Transactional analysis*. New York: Grove Press, 1961.

Carkhuff, R. *The art of helping IV*. Amherst, Mass.: Human Resource Development Press, 1980.

Dilts, R., Grinder, J., Bandler, R., Bandler, L., & Delozier, J. *Neuro-linguistic programming: The study of the structure of the subjective experience* (Vol. 1). Cupertino, Calif.: Meta Publications, 1980.

Dinkmeyer, D. Use of the encouragement process in Adlerian counseling. *Personnel and Guidance Journal*, 1972, *51*(3), 177–181.

Dinkmeyer, D., Pew, W., & Dinkmeyer, D., Jr. *Adlerian counseling and psychotherapy*. Monterey, Calif.: Brooks/Cole, 1979.

Dreikurs, R. *Fundamentals of Adlerian psychology*. Chicago: Alfred Adler Institute, 1953.

Dreikurs, R. *Psychodynamics, psychotherapy, and counseling*. Chicago: Alfred Adler Institute, 1967.

Dyer, W.W., & Vriend, J. *Counseling techniques that work*. Washington, D.C.: American Personnel and Guidance Association, 1975.

Eisenberg, M. *Psychological aspects of physical disability: A guide for the health care worker*. New York: National League of Nursing, 1977.

Ellis, A. *Reason and emotion in psychotherapy*. New York: Lyle Stuart, 1962.

Ellis, A. *Humanistic psychotherapy*. New York: McGraw-Hill, 1973.

Glasser, W. *Reality therapy*. New York: Harper & Row, 1965.

Gordon, D. *Therapeutic metaphors*. Cupertino, Calif.: Meta Publications, 1978.

Grinder, J., & Bandler, R. *Trance formations*. Mohab, Utah: Real People Press, 1981.

Grinder, J., Delozier, J., & Bandler, R. *Patterns of the hypnotic techniques of Milton H. Erickson, M.D.* (Vol. 2). Cupertino, Calif.: Meta Publications, 1977.

Hosford, R.E., & de Visser, L. *Behavioral approaches to counseling: An introduction*. Washington, D.C.: APGA Press, 1974.

Kir-Stimon, W. Counseling with the severely handicapped: Encounter and commitment. In R. Marinelli & A. Dell Orto (Eds.), *The psychological and social impact of physical disability*. New York: Springer, 1977.

Lazarus, A., & Fay, A. *I can if I want to*. New York: Morrow, 1975.

Mosak, H.H. The psychological attitude in rehabilitation. *American Archives of Rehabilitation Therapy*, 1954, *2*, 9-10.

Mosak, H.H. *On purpose*. Chicago: Alfred Adler Institute, 1977.

Mosak, H.H. Adlerian psychotherapy. In R. Corsini (Ed.), *Current psychotherapies* (2nd ed.). Itasca, Ill.: Peacock, 1979.

O'Connell, W. Adlerian aphorisms. *The Individual Psychologist*, 1976, *13*, 18–28.

Pancer, K. The use of parables and fables in Adlerian psychotherapy. *The Individual Psychologist*, 1978, *15*, 19–29.

Passons, W. *Gestalt approaches in counseling*. New York: Holt, Rinehart & Winston, 1975.

Perls, F. *Gestalt therapy verbatim*. Lafayette, Calif.: Real People Press, 1969.

Perls, F., Hefferline, R., & Goodman, P. *Gestalt therapy*. New York: Julian Press, 1951.

Roessler, R., & Bolton, B. *Psychosocial adjustment to disability*. Baltimore: University Park Press, 1978.

Rosen, S. (Ed.). *My voice will go with you: The teaching tales of Milton H. Erickson*. New York: Norton, 1982.

Rule, W. Corrective reactions to client negativism using a combined facilitative and Adlerian–based approach. *Corrective and Social Psychiatry and Journal of Behavior Technology Methods and Therapy*, 1977, *23*, 7-10. (a)

Rule, W. Increasing self–modeled humor. *Rational Living*, 1977, *12*, 7–9. (b)

Rule, W. Increased internal–control using humor with lifestyle awareness. *The Individual Psychologist*, 1979, *16*, 16–26.

Rule, W. What next after self–awareness?: A rational apothecary. *Rational Living*, 1980, *15*, 24–25.

Rule, W. Life–style interpretation using imagination of the ideal social self. *Individual Psychology: The Journal of Adlerian Theory, Research and Practice*, 1982, *38*(4), 339–342. (a)

Rule, W. Pursuing the horizon: Striving for elusive goals. *Personnel and Guidance Journal*, 1982, *61*(4), 195–197. (b)

Rule, W. Family therapy and the pie metaphor. *Journal of Marital and Family Therapy*, 1983, *9*(1), 101–103.

Rychlak, J.F. *Introduction to personality: A theory–construction approach.* Boston: Houghton Mifflin, 1973.

Schafer, W. *Stress, distress and growth.* Davis, Calif.: International Dialogue Press, 1978.

Selye, H. *Stress without distress.* New York: Signet, 1974.

Shelton, J.L., & Ackerman, J.M. *Homework in counseling and psychotherapy.* Springfield, Ill.: Charles C Thomas, 1974.

Shontz, F.C. *The psychological aspects of physical illness and disability.* New York: Macmillan, 1975.

Shulman, B.H. Confrontation techniques. *Journal of Individual Psychology*, 1972, *28*, 177–183.

Shulman, B.H. *Contributions to individual psychology.* Chicago: Alfred Adler Institute, 1973.

Shulman, B.H. Encouraging the pessimist: A confronting technique. *The Individual Psychologist*, 1977, *14*, 7–9.

Sullivan, H.S. *Conceptions of modern psychiatry.* New York: Norton, 1940.

Sweeney, T.H. *Adlerian counseling.* Boston: Houghton Mifflin, 1975.

Trieschmann, R. Coping and disability: A sliding scale of goals. *Archives of Physical Medicine and Rehabilitation*, 1974, *55*, 556–560.

Walen, S.R., DiGiuseppe, R., & Wessler, R.L. *A practitioner's guide to rational–emotive therapy.* New York: Oxford University Press, 1980.

Woolfolk, R., & Richardson, F. *Stress, sanity and survival.* New York: Sovereign, 1978.

Part II

Family and Lifespan Considerations

Chapter 4

Lifestyle and the Family of the Disabled

Martha Stover Barlow

Lifestyle has been described as "that unity in each individual, in his thinking, feeling, acting, in his so-called conscious and unconscious, in every expression of his personality" (Ansbacher & Ansbacher, 1956, p. 175). This concept can be very useful in understanding how families work. If I may take some liberties with this cornerstone of Adlerian theory, I would like to extend it to describe that force that operates within families at an under-the-surface level, directing the family toward unarticulated family goals and sometimes limiting the autonomy of individual family members. I will use as examples families of psychosomatic children as well as families that adjust inadequately to a family member's disability. The focus will be on how this family force or "systemic" lifestyle can exacerbate physical symptoms that already exist, or in some cases, actually contribute to the onset of physical symptoms.

THE SYSTEMIC LIFESTYLE

The "systemic lifestyle," as the term will be used in this chapter, can be understood as the goal-directed philosophy of the family system. This philosophy manifests itself in the pattern of interactions that a family evolves over time in its efforts to solve problems. It is a product of its parts (i.e., the individual lifestyles from which it was created), although it is actually more than a sum of these parts. Just as problems may arise for the individual when his subjective interpretation of life distorts reality, so also do symptoms appear for families when the idiosyncratic pattern they have evolved prevents necessary change and growth.

Some systemic lifestyles are healthy creations in which the strengths of the individuals are enhanced by the union. Other couples connect in such a way that the resulting "familial stamp" is even more constricting for themselves and for their children than the adults' lifestyles have been for themselves individually.

Consider, for example, the systemic lifestyle created by the following couple: the husband's lifestyle is characterized by a need to be perfect, as well as an intolerance for the imperfections of others; consequently, he tends to distance himself emotionally when he or others do not live up to his expectations. His wife's overriding goal is to take care of, to nurture, and, as a supplemental goal, to take charge. Understandably, the husband frequently feels discontented with the flawed quality of his life. His wife, in response, tries harder to get close and tries to nurture him out of his discontent; he feels smothered and withdraws through alcohol. She feels guilty that she's not doing enough. ("It's my fault that he drinks.") She tries harder; he drinks more—the classic alcohol-focused couple is born.

The interlock of these individual lifestyles, neither of which is inherently "bad," has thus produced a destructive systemic lifestyle, which progressively develops a life of its own. In destructive interlocks such as the example just cited, the individual family members caught in this new creation are unable to see other options; they believe that the specific method they employ to resolve crises is the best or the only way, even if it no longer works. Ford and Herrick (1974) suggest that family lifestyles tend to perpetuate themselves. They take on qualities and powers that were not originally intended and that do not currently serve any constructive purpose.

Fogarty (1980) speaks of this systemic lifestyle when he writes: "Families have organizational elements that sort of sprout up and grow . . . over the years." He conceptualizes these organizational elements as "a philosophy, a purpose . . . a theory underlying the sphere of family thinking, feeling, and activity . . . beliefs, concepts, and attitudes" (p. 92).

Although Fogarty sees this theory as evolving in a "planned way," I see it as operating at a dimly conscious level, as is the case with Adler's individual lifestyle. Fogarty believes that family difficulties arise from the lack of a coherent family philosophy. However, for the families to be discussed here, the symptoms did not erupt because of the lack of such a philosophy; rather they occurred because the family philosphy or collective lifestyle was "faulty" or excessively rigid.

In 1945, H.B. Richardson suggested that rigid families are more vulnerable to disease, and emphasized that the duration or chronicity of the disease is especially related to family relationship factors (in Lewis, Beavers, Gossett, & Phillips, 1976). Since that time, there has been increasing support for the idea that family factors, to a greater degree than was ever suspected, impose themselves upon the functioning of the individual—mentally, emotionally, and physiologically.

Kerr (1980) has proposed a "unidisease" concept, in which diseases are seen as manifestations of a more basic process related to family interactional patterns. This emotional "background process," which is transmitted from one generation to the next in a family, influences the onset of an individual's disease as well as the evolution of that disease over multiple generations in a family. It may be reflected by one illness or disease repeating itself over generations, giving the appearance that one disease "runs" in a particular family, or it might be reflected by a number of apparently unrelated illnesses in a family. Thus, even if it appears that the current generation has created a lifestyle opposite to that of their parents, one would find that the multigenerational family's emotional background process (systemic lifestyle) contains common themes. For example, the systemic lifestyle may lead to obesity and body aches and pains in the grandparent generation, a health food and exercise focus in the parent generation, and finally pyschosomatic symptoms in the current generation.

Bowen (1980) suggests that symptoms, such as childhood psychosomatic symptoms, are most likely to be found within families whose adult members are not highly differentiated. In other words, these adults are relatively less able to maintain a consistent and responsible "self" within an intense relationship, because of a continuing lack of resolution within their families of origin. These individuals feel the need for current family to "fill the gaps." Psychosomatic symptoms can result then from the anxiety that is generated when unmet "togetherness" needs are focused upon one family member. This anxious focus can render that person (usually the weakest link in the family system and often a child) vulnerable to symptoms.

THE ROLE OF THE SYSTEMIC LIFESTYLE IN ADJUSTMENT TO DISABILITY

The next four sections of this chapter will discuss the role the systemic lifestyle can play in adjustment to disability. The focus will be upon four specific family problem areas: (1) a family's adjustment to a child's physical disability; (2) the role of the systemic lifestyle in the exacerbation of physical symptoms in a child; (3) the role of the systemic lifestyle in the onset and maintenance of physical symptoms in a child; and (4) the role of the systemic lifestyle in an adult's adjustment to disability.

Family Adjustment to a Child's Physical Disability

Some diseases or conditions seem to occur at random within a family, and the family interactional pattern does not seem to be implicated in the onset or the maintenance of the physical symptoms. Epilepsy is such a condition. The seizures are often unpredictable, and sometimes not completely controllable with medication (Zeigler, 1982). Although sometimes the etiology can be determined, quite often it remains unknown, and parents anguish over the time "he fell off the counter" or the time "we (or "you" or "I") didn't realize his fever was so high." Although many families have a family lifestyle that is sufficiently flexible to incorporate the impairment without centralizing it or disabling the child further, other families find it difficult to adjust to such handicapping conditions. For example, parents who are sensitive to issues of "control," "protectiveness," or "blame/guilt" find that an epilepsy imposition can shift what seemed to be functional individual lifestyles and well-working interactional patterns (systemic lifestyles) into discouraging, stifling, anxious styles of relating to the world and to each other. The adaptive process that the family evolves is crucial because it then provides the context within which the child shapes his own lifestyle. The following case example illustrates how the systemic lifestyle can affect the evolving individual lifestyle of an epileptic child.

Jerry C., an 11-year-old only child, experienced his first epileptic seizure when he was eight years old, approximately six months after his parents' separation preceding divorce. Jerry had suffered several life-threatening illnesses as an infant and had fallen into an empty swimming pool when he was two years old; however, the actual etiology of the seizure disorder is unknown. Although Mrs. C. admitted having always "spoiled" Jerry, she and her mother, who lived next door, increased this pampering and overindulgence after the divorce and the onset of seizures. For the past two years, Jerry has been throwing temper tantrums whenever he is frustrated, and his mother, terrorized and tyrannized by these "fits" of anger, relates them to the "fits" of epilepsy and vacillates in her response to them. Initially she placated him until he calmed down; more recently, though, she has tried to discipline him by removing his privileges and/or his toys. This has not worked very well, as Jerry runs, in tears, to the grandmother. The grandmother takes Jerry's side because she worries that getting Jerry "all worked up" will bring on a seizure. She criticizes her daughter for making Jerry cry, and Mrs. C., as a result, feels guilty and gives back whatever toys or privileges she has taken away. The mother then expends even greater efforts to protect Jerry from potentially distressful situations.

Mrs. C. regards Jerry as damaged, not only by the epilepsy, but also by the trauma she had allowed him to suffer during their years with the husband/father. Mr. C. had been emotionally distant from Jerry and had abused his wife in Jerry's presence.

From an Adlerian standpoint, Jerry is a discouraged child; discouraged by years of pampering and the current indulgent, overprotective, anxious attitudes of his mother and grandmother. The lifestyle he is creating probably also incorporates a position of incompetence related to his past inability to protect his mother, as well as his own failure to get his dad to love him. His unpredictable seizures, his temper tantrums, and his mother's anxiety prevent Jerry from being more autonomous, e.g., riding a bike, walking to school, playing ball. Negotiations that are developmentally appropriate for an eleven-year-old are delayed for Jerry, and he is likely to have difficulty moving into new developmental arenas. Fewer opportunities are afforded him to interact with peers, and his position of incompetence is increasingly confirmed. Intervention strategies for Jerry's family will be discussed later in the chapter.

The Exacerbation of Physical Symptoms in a Child

Unlike an epileptic seizure, which probably cannot be precipitated or averted by external circumstances, relapses of chronic asthma are often closely related to the affected child's patterns of interaction with his family. Chronic intractable asthma is defined by the structural family theorists as "a psychosomatic disorder in which the primary allergic disorder has been profoundly complicated by emotional factors, especially chronic unresolved conflicts in the family" (Liebman, Minuchin, & Baker, 1974, p. 536). It is also worth noting that about 10 to 12 percent of children with asthma experience recurring severe attacks, which often respond poorly to medical management (Liebman et al., 1974). The following case example illustrates the powerful role that the systemic lifetstyle can play in the exacerbation of severe asthmatic symptoms in a child.

Timmy B., an eight-year-old, is the third of four children from a middle-income family. Timmy has an older brother, Tom, age 16, a sister, Lisa, age 15, and a younger brother, Jason, age 6. Timmy's asthmatic attacks have increased in frequency and severity over the past three years, and his family is now so involved in preparing for and handling the necessary emergency procedures that they have "put on hold" many other individual and family activities. The older two children, now well into their teens, have been discouraged from inviting friends in because the house must be kept thoroughly clean and free of dust. None of the children have pets, nor do family members visit in homes where pets reside since Timmy is highly allergic to animals.

Since Timmy's attacks usually occur late at night or in the early morning hours, tension in the family begins to rise at bedtime, and family members have made several modifications in their routines as a result. For example, the family has an implicit rule that Tom and Lisa leave their bedroom doors open, as their rooms are closest to Timmy's. As the acute attacks have become more frequent, Mr. and Mrs. B. also leave their door open, which restricts the spontaneity of their sexual relationship. In addition, Mr. and Mrs. B. rarely go out without the children. On one recent occasion, Mr. B. did convince his wife to leave Timmy and Jason with Tom and Lisa so that they could attend a social function associated with his work. While they were gone, Timmy suffered a severe attack, and Lisa panicked and was unable to find the number where the parents could be reached. Tom was nowhere to be found. Lisa ran to the home of a neighbor who transported Timmy to the emergency room. The parents were convinced that they could never absent themselves again.

Seldom does one family member get into an open argument with another. Whenever a serious argument looms, Timmy (the family barometer) begins to wheeze, so that attention shifts from the argument back to Timmy. In addition, Timmy's three siblings are aware that Timmy "gets away with murder." There is an unwritten rule, though, that nobody says anything about it since Timmy starts to wheeze if he gets upset. Whenever Mr. B. speaks harshly to Timmy, he suffers an attack; Mrs. B., Lisa, and Jason come running to help, and Mr. B. feels humiliated and intimidated by Timmy and his wife's nonverbal reprimand.

A better understanding of this couple's systemic lifestyle may be gained by a discussion of their families of origin. Mrs. B. was the oldest of five children in her original family. Her father was a marginally functional alcoholic, and the systemic lifestyle that evolved around his drinking alternated between states of severe conflict and stringently adhered-to denial. For lengthy periods of time, she and her mother colluded (implicitly and not at a fully conscious level) to cover for the husband/father and to take charge when he was not available. Periodically, though, after months of festering hurt on both sides, Mrs. B.'s mother and father would go at each other with a rageful vengeance. Mrs. B., as a child, was frightened by these periodic eruptions. In fact, one of the themes reflected in her early recollections was: "people lose control when they argue," and "any emotionally charged talk hurts and is not worth it."

Mrs. B.'s two younger brothers rebelled at adolescence, and she keenly remembers her mother's inability to ever get them under control. One is now severely alcoholic. Mrs. B. is determined not to make the same mistakes in her family. Her lifestyle, containing threads of "need to control self and others," suggests that she would be hesitant to discuss highly charged issues; moreover, the likelihood exists that she will be especially sensitive to her children's arrival at adolescence.

Mr. B. was the youngest of three children of a stoically religious midwestern couple. His family subscribed to the traditional, paternal authoritarian family structure. He seldom saw his parents argue, and, in fact, was taught that overt disagreement within the family was unnecessary and indeed wrong.

Although Mr. and Mrs. B. have come from two very different family situations, both have created individual lifestyles that tolerate high levels of nonresolution. It is not surprising then that the systemic lifestyle that was created by their union placed a high premium on "peace at any price." From the early days of their marriage, Mr. and Mrs. B. had difficulty acknowledging disagreement, resentment, and anger at the other. Mrs. B. had never worked outside the home, and their early married life was fairly stress free, although they both felt tension due to unresolved differences.

The family might have been able to continue with this style of relating had normal life events and developmental phases not converged to render this interactional style maladaptive. Though Timmy had always been a sickly child, and Mrs. B. was especially close to him, his asthmatic symptoms did not become severe until he was five years old. Just prior to the onset of these severe symptoms, Mrs. B. was offered a teaching position in the local high school in her field of home economics—a position that is rarely available in her community. When the opportunity came up for Mrs. B. to work full time at a job she had always wanted, she and her husband both felt ambivalent, worried, and uncertain about the changes it would require, but neither was able to discuss these worries with the other for fear he or she would disagree or take offense. Tom, at age 13, was becoming more adolescent in his behavior, and both Mr. and Mrs. B. were uncomfortable with his uncharacteristically rebellious attitude. Lisa, at 12, also was beginning to move into adolescence. When Timmy developed these acute, frightening symptoms, Mrs. B. gave up her plan to work (eliminating the need for her to deal both with her own ambivalence and Mr. B.'s possible disapproval). The couple continued to defer dealing with the mounting marital tension by shifting the stress and focusing intensely upon Timmy and his symptoms. In addition, the two teens were covertly recruited back into the home to help care for Timmy.

Although neither Mr. nor Mrs. B. were aware of it, Timmy's attacks were being reinforced; of course, neither realized the constraints they were putting on themselves and their children. Just as individual lifestyles are not entirely conscious, this newly created systemic lifestyle was also unarticulated, implicit, and not consciously available to family members. In treating this family, the major goal will be to see that they have experiences they have seldom had before; they must express anger and conflict directly, and not allow Timmy to be the defuser, distracter, and diluter. It is important, of course, that this painful experience be a safe one.

The Onset and Maintenance of Physical Symptoms in a Child

Anorexia nervosa, unlike the disabilities previously discussed, is a purely psychosomatic disorder. A physiologically disabling condition does not ordinarily predate the anorexia, and the anorectic condition itself can be in service to the systemic lifestyle.

Five interactional patterns have been postulated that characterize the anorectic child's family system: (1) enmeshment, (2) overprotectiveness, (3) rigidity, (4) lack of conflict resolution, and (5) the child's involvement in parental conflict (Minuchin, Rosman, & Baker, 1978). Meissner (1980) sees the psychosomatic family as mutually dependent, with much intrusion on personal boundaries, poor differentiation between self and others, much concern for others' welfare, and protective caregiving. He emphasizes the heavy commitment family members have to maintain the "status quo," which is highly resistant to change. Meissner depicts the sick child as "a conduit by which conflict is avoided or diverted into concern for the sick one" (p. 41).

The anorectic child (more often female than male) often grows up in a family that operates on the principle of "closeness." Although the boundary between the family and the rest of the world is often almost impermeable, the personal, sexual, and generational boundaries within the family are often fuzzy and easily crossed. Family members seem, in fact, to be so close that no one has an exclusive relationship with any other family member. Moveover, one family member would not be likely to have very close relationships outside the family that would exclude parents or siblings. A parent might say proudly, "There are no secrets among us." Because this "control" is seen by the family members as concern, protection, and love, any overt questioning or asserting oneself against the status quo is seen and felt as betrayal (Minuchin et al., 1978). Because the family is often "child focused," the youngster experiences the family as watching her and evaluating her behavior. Many times she is perfectionistic—usually not out of her own internal motivation, but instead to please her parents. Conflict does not surface except in a sort of circular form of bickering; certainly differences in opinion are not resolved.

The individual lifestyles that culminate in anorexia often seem to be characterized by blacks and whites, "Either you're for me, or you're against me"; "if you disagree with me, you don't love me." These individual lifestyles interlock to form a systemic lifestyle that has little tolerance for directly and clearly expressed conflict.

The developmental crises in family lifestyles can also be paralleled to those in an individual's lifestyle. An individual lifestyle might not be very constricting, and may in fact be comfortable, until the individual embarks upon a new developmental stage, which by its very nature requires growth or change. The requirements of the new stage may be incompatible with the individual's particular lifestyle, and behavior that worked well at an earlier stage may become dysfunctional. For example, a man whose overriding goal is "to please" is successful as an employee, but wreaks havoc when he becomes a boss. Similarly, a new developmental phase may precipitate a crisis in the systematic lifestyle. For example, the anoretic systemic lifestyle of excessive nurturing, protecting, and controlling may work well when the children are toddlers and need a high level of parental involvement. However, it may well be destructive and dangerous in families of adolescents when the developmental tasks required by adolescence run a collision course with the interactional style the family has come to depend on. Conflicts around the emerging need for individuation are not allowed to surface and the family system suffers from chronic subthreshold stress (Meissner, 1980).

An Adult's Adjustment to Disability

Children are not the only family members whose adjustment to disability is affected by the systemic lifestyle. Adults are also powerfully influenced by their family relationships. Many times these relationships strengthen the individual and help him adjust to a disabling condition, as evidenced by many reports of individuals overcoming tremendous odds because of the unwavering encouragement and support provided by family members. Other times, an individual's adjustment to a disability is handicapped by the family's patterns of interacting. A practitioner would be wise to keep in mind the power of the family—either in the push for health and growth or in the maintenance of an individual's dependency and discouragement. Obviously, the families and couples that support the strengths of their members do not usually require outside intervention.

Some couples begin their relationship at a time when one of them is disabled, and the durability of the relationship seems dependent on that one remaining disabled. An example is the J. couple, who met while Mr. J. was in the hospital recuperating from a spinal cord injury, where Mrs. J. was one of his nurses. They built their relationship upon their original roles, hers as nurturer and caretaker and his as recipient and "grateful one." If these parameters of the relationship remain important to their evolving systemic lifestyle, Mr. J. will have difficulty in ever achieving independence.

The individual lifestyles of the affected adults are also a crucial variable here. Does her lifestyle center around the need "to be needed" or "to help?" Does his lifestyle have elements of "being helped" or "being taken care of?" Sometimes seemingly obscure supplemental goals of an individual's lifestyle might increase in intensity or frequency during times of stress or may interlock with a mate who has a suitably complementary lifestyle. A possible example would be the hypothetical couple discussed earlier in the chapter whose systemic lifestyle came to be centered around alcohol. They began their relationship with relatively benign individual lifestyles, the interlock of which formed the building blocks of a mutually destructive systemic lifestyle.

Another variation on the same theme occurs when the nature of a couple's relationship serves to contribute to or to escalate the physiological distress in one or both of them. Jaffee (1978) calls these couples "lethal dyads." An example is a couple whose systemic lifestyle solidified around the dominance of the husband and the wife's submission and utter dependence upon him. He worked hard to provide for them, often late into the night and on weekends. At middle age, he developed severe coronary problems. His physician ordered him to slow down, and he consequently shifted some of his responsibility to his wife. She immediately developed physiological problems of her own, and, in effect, put the ball back into his court. He obligingly took back his old role and suffered another heart attack (Jaffee, 1978). Obviously, this couple's marital lifestyle was not sufficiently flexible to allow for expanding roles as they aged and their needs changed.

Earlier in the chapter, we noted the difficulties families can have in moving on to an appropriate developmental phase. Similarly, a couple or an adult's inability to move on developmentally can point to the deficits in a couple's systemic lifestyle. Sometimes those deficits are minor; for example, a couple's difficulty in adjusting to one member's new disabling condition might have to do with the couple's inability to share their grief about the physiological loss (Derdeyn & Waters,

1981). After they are able to mourn that loss, they move on in a flexible way, making the necessary adjustments to the changes in their family situation.

Individuals who have been disabled since childhood often have difficulty in ever being seen as an adult. The handicap (deafness, blindness, congenital deformities) sometimes comes to define the person as disabled. His label, in effect, disables him further, often to the extent that maturity and growth are impeded. Webb-Woodard and Woodard (1982) tell of a family in which a 33-year-old blind sister of the wife is the identified patient. She had recently moved to their home, and the family was resentful of her incapacity and the attention and care she was demanding of them. Although they criticized her for her childish behavior, they were not seeing her as a capable adult in any sense. She, of course, reciprocated by behaving childishly. The counseling focused upon the blind woman as an adult, experiencing adult emotions, capable of adult tasks. A key therapeutic maneuver was to highlight the strengths of the identified patient by having her teach the family various skills she had learned as a result of her blindness. This led to the family changing their perception of this woman from "blind and incompetent" to "adult and potentially capable." Daily living conflicts were then negotiated not on a pseudo-child/parental level but instead as a negotiation between peers.

The following section on intervention will focus primarily upon families who have a symptomatic child. However, the works of Madanes (1981) and Bowen (1978), among others, are possible resources for those who are particularly interested in the effects of family patterns upon adult functioning.

APPROACHING INTERVENTION

A counselor beginning treatment with a family that has adjusted poorly to a disability, or one that includes a psychosomatic child, can generally make the following assumptions, keeping in mind that as with all generalizations there are many exceptions:

1. The disability (or the psychosomatic symptom) serves a function within the family system. If the symptom were removed, family members would be confronted with the fallacies of their private logic and would face the frightening prospect of having to act against the dictates of their systemic lifestyle.
2. The centralized disability or psychosomatic symptom is often preventing the family's transition through successive developmental phases if the requirements of the developmental phase run counter to the systemic lifestyle.
3. A psychosomatic symptom in a child usually serves as a way to avoid and/or defuse conflict; this is most often manifested across generational lines.

4. A family with a psychosomatic child is usually a "nice" family that appears to be healthy except for the physical symptomatology in the child. This kind of problem often appears easy to treat. A counselor can be seduced into accepting their view of themselves as a big, happy, conflict-free family, thereby missing the subtleties of the dysfunctional pattern (i.e., enmeshment, lack of conflict resolution, cross-boundary alliances, etc.). Again, it is worth remembering that "a patient brings his lifestyle to therapy" (Mosak, 1973, p. 54).

As noted previously, two types of families can become imprisoned in the systemic lifestyle: families that mobilize around a symptomatic family member or families that, by way of their daily pattern or interactions, actually contribute to the onset or maintenance of symptoms in one of their members. Of course, some systems are not this influential in the lives of the family members. Sometimes the system exerts too little influence on its members, which results in problems of another sort. Other times, the system is a major source of the individual's strengths and creativity!

INTERVENTION STRATEGIES

Many different psychotherapeutic and medical approaches have been tried with children with psychosomatic symptoms. For example, it has been found that some asthmatic children, who were hospitalized for long periods and periodically exposed to the allergens from their own homes, continued to improve, only to relapse when they were discharged to their homes (Liebman, Minuchin, Baker, & Rosman, 1976). This phenomenon led some observers to suggest that the child would fare better without his family, and to advocate, therefore, for permanent removal of the child from his family. Those who take this stance fail to recognize the systemic nature of the symptoms, the complementarity of interactions within the family, and the child's vital, purposeful role in his family's systemic lifestyle. Furthermore, removal increases feelings of guilt, resentment, and helplessness in those family members who have been deemed "noxious," while similar feelings, plus a powerful sense of loss, are created in the "victimized" child (Liebman et al., 1976).

Historically, individual psychotherapy has not been very successful with these children. A practitioner's attempt to individually treat the child presents the child with more evidence to justify his feelings of low self-worth. "Individual intervention tends to sanction the stigmatization of the individual in distress, make the symptom chronic, and crystallize the system of family relationships around it" (Andolfi, 1979, p. 3). For these reasons, this chapter has focused heavily upon the systemic lifestyle and has given less attention to the workings of the individual family members' overriding goals and private logic. Individual lifestyles certainly contribute to the problems that have been discussed, and they need to be considered seriously as the counselor formulates intervention strategies. However, the first order of business for the counselor is to conceptualize the family as the patient, and to challenge the family's blind faith in the systemic lifestyle, providing them with a fresh way of seeing themselves and their family. Finally, the counselor must help the family members behave differently.

The Structural Approach

There are numerous family therapy methods one could employ to help a family make these essential changes in their systemic lifestyle. Some have been referred to earlier in the chapter; others will be addressed later. The therapeutic model that I will utilize most closely in the case examples below is the Structural Family Therapy model. This model is an active therapy utilizing the "here and now" behavior of the family members. This framework has been used extensively with psychosomatic families, among others, and has been found to be effective in treatment (Minuchin et al., 1978). Because I will be referring to some structural terms and techniques as I describe the intervention strategies, brief definitions are in order.

"Structure" itself refers to the system of the family and to the functional or organizational demands placed upon family members. Who has the "power," who is aligned with whom, who is distant or disengaged from whom, are all functions of the family structure. "Boundaries," also an important concept in this therapeutic model, serve to protect the separateness of the family members. The personal, generational, and sexual boundaries within a family need to be clear and explicit, but not rigid or impermeable.

Because "joining" is perhaps the most underrated part of this therapeutic process, I will describe it in more depth. Treatment with any family, regardless of their presenting complaint, must begin with an encouraging, validating, rapport between family and counselor. Adler's concept of encouragement, i.e., the act of instilling courage, can be compared to the act of "joining." Some miss the beauty of joining as a therapeutic experience and view it as a superficial "cocktail party" repartee occurring before the "real" therapeutic work begins. Instead, joining is inseparable from any other segment of therapy.

Joining is the constant use of self by the counselor to instill hope and confidence in the therapeutic process. Sometimes it might include a discussion about "last night's ball game"; at other times it might involve a touch to an adolescent's knee or a well-timed supportive eye contact with an overwhelmed mother. Sometimes, though, it is the necessary verbal confrontation with the family's unspeakable truths, the family's implicit private logic. The counselor joins most effectively when he communicates to the family his courage and willingness to caringly remove the family's blinders.

Joining from the counselor's perspective requires him to find something in the family to care about. If the counselor has difficulty liking any of the family members and cannot empathize with their pain and fear, then joining has not been accomplished, and the family's willingness to take important risks will be affected.

"Unbalancing" is defined as "challenging the family's power allocation" (Minuchin & Fishman, 1981). The counselor might side with a family member who has very little power or might ignore or side against other powerful family members. This throws the system out of balance and allows family members new freedom in their interactions.

"Reframing" is a frequently used technique that involves altering the family's view of the problem, making available to them a whole different set of responses. "Restructuring" involves any therapeutic operation that forces a change in the family's systemic lifestyle. This technique assists the family to interact with each other in new ways, so that symptoms are no longer needed as vehicles for family communication. The counselor helps the family formulate new rules for behavior that are explicit and congruent. "Stabilizing" is simply a solidifying of the new family structure.

The structural theorists have specialized in work with psychosomatic families. Minuchin, Rosman, and Baker's book, *Psychosomatic Families* (1978), describes the family dynamics and the structural family treatment approach to anorexia. Palazzoli, a psychiatrist from Milan, who with her Milanese colleagues made famous their paradoxical prescription model of family treatment, published *Self Starvation* in 1978. There are also other recent publications on anorexia, among them *The Golden Cage* (1978), written from a psychoanalytic perspective by Bruch. Because of the wealth of available literature, treatment specifically for anorectic families will not be included here. The following case examples will be used to illustrate methods one could use in helping a family that has adjusted poorly to a child's disability and one whose systemic lifestyle has exacerbated a child's physical symptoms, altering their dysfunctional lifestyles. Both families were introduced earlier in the chapter.

The C. Family

As discussed previously, Jerry's family system (including mother, grand-mother, and Jerry) had adjusted poorly to Jerry's epilepsy. Obviously, Jerry was as disabled by the interactions surrounding the disability as he was by the disability itself. This pattern of interactions led to Jerry's tantrums, his poor performance at school, and his immaturity among peers. These behavioral symptoms served an obvious purpose for Jerry and for his family; the major goal for Jerry, at a barely conscious level, was simply to avoid the tasks that lay before him—at school, at home and among peers. By keeping Jerry incapacitated, Mrs. C. could forestall his impending adolescence; by continuing to protect him, she could prevent or postpone his "leaving home."

The counselor began by joining with the family, then she unbalanced the system of interactions, providing the family new options and different methods of interacting, and finally, she helped the family to stabilize around a more complex field of interactional possibilities.

To unbalance the system of interactions, the counselor "reframed" the family's view of Jerry as "weak and vulnerable" to "the one who calls the shots." The counselor clarified for the mother and the grandmother the difference between a seizure and a tantrum, emphasizing that, unlike a seizure, a tantrum is an act of will, and that Jerry was being defiant: "Why do you let him jerk you around?" There were two purposes for this reframing. The first was to challenge the way the family saw themselves and each other, allowing a shift in existing alliances (i.e., that between the grandmother and Jerry). The second was to begin to erode Jerry's and others' perceptions of him as "incompetent."

The next step required Mrs. C. and her mother to face their disagreements without involving Jerry, since much of the undermining covert competition between mother and grandmother involved issues totally unrelated to him. Because the mother and daughter were unable to solve their differences directly, disagreements were played out through their mutual relationship with Jerry.

Another phase of restructuring occurred when the mother elicited the grandmother's support for her attempts to "help Jerry grow up." The counselor reinforced the grandmother's competency and good intentions ("You've raised your four children, you know how it's done, can you help Peggy get Jerry under control?"). The grandmother's genuine concern about Jerry then made it unlikely that she would continue to undermine the mother's disciplining efforts. During this stage, the mother's role as the primary parent was emphasized, while the grandmother was moved to a more advisory, consultative position. ("It's obvious that Jerry is defeating you two by dividing you; Jerry needs you, Grandmother, to support his mom's rules.")

The third step with Jerry's family involved stabilizing and further solidifying the emerging family configuration. During this phase, an appointment was made for Jerry and his mom with Jerry's pediatrician, who had been informed of Jerry's involvement in counseling. The session with the physician focused on educating the mother, grandmother, and Jerry about his seizure disorder and clearly informing them that a seizure is not likely to be brought on by anger or distress. The physician also talked to Jerry man-to-man about realistic precautionary measures. For the most part, he simply gave Jerry medical permission and, indeed, a "prescription" to get on with his life: to make friends, to play ball, and to help his mother around the house. Thus, the new view of Jerry as "adjusting well to a disability'' was reinforced. This also underscored for the family Jerry's general good health and prevented their return to their old patterns when Jerry again had tantrums or the family experienced stress.

Although Jerry initially made it very difficult for his mother as she tried to be more consistent and firm in her disciplining, eventually her persistence was rewarded. We then entered the final stage of counseling, as Jerry's behavior improved, and he became more interested in school and more involved with friends.

Mrs. C. was relieved and happy about Jerry's changes, but was puzzled by her own feelings of depression and emptiness. The counselor began seeing her alone to explore the void she was feeling in her life. With some encouragement, she joined a bowling league at her workplace and also became more involved with her peers at church. She also addressed in treatment the long-standing resentments and ambiguities in her relationship with her mother. In addition, Mrs. C.'s concerns about relationships with men, her problems in being assertive, and her feelings of low self-worth began to emerge.

In this family, the systemic lifestyle was characterized by the conviction that males were difficult, often unreasonable and abusive, but that a female should adapt and make allowances for them. Both males and females subscribed to this underlying belief. The therapeutic process challenged Mrs. C.'s adherence to this conviction. When this systemic lifestyle was diluted and discredited, Mrs. C.'s individual lifestyle (which included this same theme) became obvious to her, and she requested individual counseling to explore this further.

The B. Family

Although much has been written about psychological components of severe asthmatic conditions and reference has been made to the powerful role the family seems to play in these situations, until recently few interventions were aimed at the family system itself. Liebman et al. (1974) outlined the family characteristics that often accompany severe asthmatic symptoms in a child, noting mutually intrusive, overinvolved, overprotective family members. They found these families to have a low threshold for overt conflict, and intense parental concentration on the child's symptoms, allowing a detour of marital conflicts. Often, there are also resentful siblings whose own concerns and problems have been neglected.

These characteristics describe the B. family very well. This family also went through the therapeutic stages of joining, then unbalancing, restructuring, and finally, stabilizing at a new, more complex level of functioning. The following sequence traces, in a necessarily brief and skeletal way, the B.'s therapy using the model developed by Liebman et al. (1976) for treating the asthmatic child and his family.

As is the case with so many families presenting with a psychosomatic member, this family was articulate, witty, and truly a joy to be with. Tom, at 16, had an especially keen sense of humor, although his jabs often had a tinge of hostility. Social chatter did not suffice as a means of joining, because in a family like the B.'s, their social graces and likableness are their defenses against intruders. So, to join with the B.'s, the counselor needed not only to enjoy them but also to be willing to confront the niceness, to show the family that the counselor was aware of, but not afraid of, their discomfort.

It was obvious from the beginning that Mrs. B. was overinvolved with and overprotective of Timmy. Mr. B., in contrast, was distant, intimidated, and resentful. The counselor's task was to prescribe new ways of relating that would decrease the emotional involvement between mother and son, facilitate a better relationship between father and son, and make room for different supportive interactions between the parents.

During counseling, the father was directed to take charge of Timmy and his emergencies; the mother was instructed to help the father if he asked for help, but not to interfere or undermine. ("Your son is at the age when he needs his dad's help.") The father and Timmy were taught deep breathing exercises, which the father was to practice daily with Timmy to avert an asthmatic attack. In the event that Timmy did suffer a severe attack, the father was requested to take charge of the emergency procedures. The message was repeatedly given to the parents that they could only help Timmy master his symptoms if they worked together supportively. Though hesitant and self-conscious at first, Mr. B. educated himself about the medical aspects of asthma and eventually took great pride in his new-found ability to help Timmy decrease the frequency of his attacks.

The next stage of counseling began when Timmy's asthmatic attacks subsided. The family then came to treatment complaining about Tom, who had been suspended from school for continued disobedience. The next four sessions focused upon the neglected problems of the other three children. Tom was the major concern, as he was angry and resentful at his mother about many issues, but felt unable to talk to her about his feelings. Several sessions were spent helping Tom say what he wanted to say and helping his mother hear him. This segment of counseling, though difficult for the family, was crucial because the family members learned that disagreements can be resolved without adversely affecting the family's mutual caring. The children then expressed their resentment at Timmy's preferential treatment at home. Timmy acknowledged sheepishly that he could "get away with most anything," and certainly didn't get punished as much as Jason did. The parents renegotiated with the children their expectations of them all, including Timmy.

Thus, this phase emphasized Timmy's place among his siblings. Just as he had problems in growing up, so did they. And, just as they had responsibilities in the running of the household, so did he. The parent/child boundary was drawn clearly during this segment of the counseling process.

As Timmy became more and more involved with his siblings and more adept with peers, we entered the final stage of counseling. Mr. and Mrs. B. came without their children to explore the now apparent marital tension. Many unresolved issues from the past surfaced, such as their current emotional distance and their poor sexual relationship. Leaving out the children during this final stage further strengthened the parental/marital subsystem and emphasized Timmy's role as "one of the kids."

The Paradoxical Approach

The two families whose treatment is described above responded to the basically direct structural treatment approach. There are some families, however, that would respond more positively to a less direct approach. One example of a less direct technique that is useful with families whose rules are long-standing and engrained is called the "paradoxical method." This approach is often used when repeated attempts to intervene in a direct way are met with family resistance.

Just as an individual brings his lifestyle to therapy and asks, in effect, that the counselor ease his pain but leave his lifestyle intact, families presenting with a symptomatic child often expect the child to get relief from his symptoms with no interference with the family's ways of interacting. In such situations, the counseling sessions often become nonproductive power struggles. The paradoxical method involves defining and prescribing the family system accurately and unacceptably. This tactic makes explicit that which has been implicit, forcing a change in the family's pattern (Papp, 1981), while removing the counselor from the power struggle. This interventive tool is only effective when used thoughtfully and skillfully after the counselor has a thorough understanding of the purpose of the symptom within the family system. For example, if Jerry's mother and grandmother had strongly resisted the use of consistent discipline in response to Jerry's tantrums, the counselor might have said, "You know, I think you all need Jerry's tantrums; you, Mom and Grandmother, wouldn't have a relationship if you didn't have Jerry to fight about. Jerry is not only helping you two maintain contact by having tantrums, but he is also adding a little spice to your lives. Jerry, it's real important, then, that you try to have at least one good tantrum a day, and, Mom, you and Grandmother must have a good argument about Jerry at least once a day."

To the family, this is obviously an accurate and an unacceptable description of the symptom's role in their interactional pattern. The directive is not given facetiously or sarcastically. It is introduced to the family by the counselor as a phase of the family's treatment with the expectation that the family will take it seriously. If the family complies with the directive, the symptom's usefulness to the family has been made explicit, and the symptom is now under the counselor's control. As a result, it loses its effectiveness for the family and for the symptom bearer. If the family refuses to comply, the result of the noncompliance is a reduction of the symptom. Palazzoli, Cecchin, Prata, and Boscolo (1978), Hoffman (1981), Madanes (1980, 1981), Haley (1976), and Papp (1981), among others, have specialized in this complex therapeutic method.

The Family Systems Approach

Another approach to family-related problems is the nondirective, cognitive approach advocated by the Bowen (1978) family systems group. This group advocates directly treating only the adults (or the individual or individuals most capable of change) in the family. Practitioners utilizing this approach believe that a positive change in one important family member will result in reciprocal changes in other family members.

The counselor helps the individual adults differentiate themselves from their original families by encouraging them to learn a great deal about their parents and other members of their original families. This allows the individual to discover the themes in his own family of origin that might have culminated in the current family problems. The themes might be as simple and explicit as, for example, "The first-born male takes over the family business." Many family themes are less obvious, and genealogical research might be required to uncover them, for example: "Emotional stress seems to result in physiological symptoms for the males in this family, whereas females seem to react to stress with psychological symptoms." Once the individual has acquainted himself with his original family (parents, grandparents, great-grandparents, aunts, and uncles), he becomes keenly aware of his own "programming" and is thus less likely to unknowingly continue destructive family interaction patterns.

Many times, very little time and effort is expended on the presenting problem *per se*. If the problem is discussed, the counselor assists the parents to decrease their anxiety about the current problem, as well as to examine and change their own habitual responses to it (Bowen, 1978). For example, the counselor would have assisted Timmy's parents to examine each of their families' multigenerational themes. In so doing, Mrs. B. would have realized the she and Mr. B. tended to focus on Timmy when they were anxious or angry with each other, in much the same way that her parents focused on one of her younger brothers under similar circumstances. By becoming more highly informed about the lives of her ancestors, she also would have seen numerous incidences of physiological symptoms occurring simultaneously with emotionally stressful events (as is apparent in her current family). Mr. B. would also be encouraged to note patterns and themes in his original family. The counselor would help the couple discontinue those patterns that were maladaptive in their nuclear family, allowing them to be more objective with each other and with their children.

SUMMARY

This chapter has extended Adler's concept of "lifestyle" to increase our understanding of families whose interaction patterns inhibit the growth of individual family members. The systemic lifestyle themes most common among families of psychosomatic children include those of "control," "overcloseness," "lack of privacy," "avoidance of conflict," and "difficulty in resolving serious disagreements." In families that are having difficulty adjusting to a disability in a family member, the symptom is purposeful within the family system and often prevents developmental changes that would be appropriate for the individual, the couple, and/or the family. An understanding of the developmental task that is being avoided gives the counselor clues about the systemic lifestyle deficits.

This chapter does not conceptualize the symptomatic child as a victim; instead he and his symptom are seen as participants in the systemic lifestyle his family has developed to adapt to family stresses. Similarly, the success of an adult's adjustment to disability is also heavily influenced by his spouse's and/or his family's reaction to his disability. Consequently, a counselor is most effective if his primary goal is to help the family alter its dysfunctional lifestyle, rather than to simply eliminate the presenting problem.

REFERENCES

Andolfi, M. *Family therapy, an interactional approach.* New York: Plenum Press, 1979.

Ansbacher, H.L., & Ansbacher, R.R. (Eds.). *The individual psychology of Alfred Alder.* New York: Harper & Row, 1956.

Bowen, M. *Family therapy in clinical practice.* New York: Jason Aronson, 1978.

Bruch, H. *The golden cage.* Cambridge: Harvard University Press, 1978.

Derdeyn, A., & Waters, D. Unshared loss and marital conflict. *Journal of Marital and Family Therapy,* 1981, *7*(4), 481–487.

Fogarty, T.F. The family organization. *The Family,* 1980, *7*(2), 92–98.

Ford, F.R., & Herrick, J. Family rules: Family lifestyles. *American Journal of Orthopsychiatry,* 1974, *44*(1) 61–69.

Haley, J. *Problem solving therapy.* San Francisco: Jossey-Bass, 1976.

Hoffman, L. *Foundations of family therapy.* New York: Basic Books, 1981.

Jaffe, D.T. The role of family therapy in treating physical illness. *Hospital and Community Psychiatry,* 1978, *29*(3), 169–174.

Kerr, M.E. Emotional factors in physical illness. *The Family,* 1980, *7*(2), 59–66.

Lewis, J.M., Beavers, W.R., Gosset, J.T., & Phillips, V.A. *No single thread.* New York: Brunner/Mazel, 1976.

Liebman, R., Minuchin, S., & Baker, L. The use of structural family therapy in the treatment of intractable asthma. *American Journal of Psychiatry,* 1974, *131*(5), 535–540.

Liebman, R., Minuchin, S., Baker, L., & Rosman, B. The role of the family in the treatment of chronic asthma. In P. Guerin (Ed.), *Family Therapy.* New York: Gardner Press, 1976.

Madanes, C. Protection, paradox, and pretending. *Family Process*, 1980, *19*(1), 73–85.

Madanes, C. *Strategic family therapy*. New York: Jossey-Bass, 1981.

Meissner, W. The family and psychosomatic medicine. *Psychiatric Annals*, 1980, *10*(2), 36–49.

Minuchin, S., & Fishman, C. *Family therapy techniques*. Cambridge: Harvard University Press, 1981.

Minuchin, S. Rosman, B., & Baker, L. *Psychosomatic families: Anorexia nervosa in context*. Cambridge: Harvard University Press, 1978.

Mosak, H.H. Adlerian psychotherapy. In R. Corsini (Ed.), *Current Psychotherapies*. Itasca, Ill.: Peacock, 1973.

Palazzoli, M. *Self-starvation*. New York: Jason Aronson, 1978.

Palazzoli, M., Cecchin, G., Prata, G., & Boscolo, L. *Paradox and counterparadox*. New York: Jason Aronson, 1978.

Papp, P. Paradox. In S. Minuchin & C. Fishman (Eds.), *Family therapy techniques*. Cambridge: Harvard University Press, 1981.

Webb-Woodard, L.W., & Woodard, B. A case of the blind leading the "blind": Reframing a physical handicap as competence. *Family Process*, 1982, *21*, 291–294.

Ziegler, R. Epilepsy: Individual illness, human predicament, and family dilemma. *Family Relations*, 1982, *31*, 435–444.

Chapter 5

Using Selected Lifestyle Information in Understanding Multigenerational Patterns

Michael D. Traver

The family counselor's initial objective in the first session is to conceptualize the presented details in a manner that elucidates and organizes the data into some understandable familial patterns of interaction. First, before discussing objectives, consideration should be given to theoretical assumptions.

BACKGROUND

The systems counselors have been instrumental in pinpointing interactional systems within the nuclear family (Andolfi, 1979; Haley, 1967, 1971; Minuchin, 1974). In recent years theorists (e.g., Bowen, 1978; Guerin and Pandagast, 1976) have begun focusing on multigenerational patterns and the impact on the nuclear family. The concept "nuclear family" is defined, for the purpose of this chapter, as the first sociopsychological environment of the individual and/or the individual's immediate family. These theoretical ideas have been generally accepted by systems counselors and, as such, systems counselors generally focus on delineating nuclear or generation triangles. A triangle is a type of family structure that defines the membership, boundaries, and emotional process within a system (Minuchin, 1974). The objective is to detriangulate the dysfunctional triangles in an effort to establish more functional interpersonal relationships.

From a somewhat different perspective, Alfred Adler's (Adler, 1954; Ansbacher & Ansbacher, 1956, 1970) major focus was that of the child's first social environment and the interactional process that occurred. Adler concluded that it was not the specific situation in which the child was born that impacted on personality, but rather the perception derived from the interactions within the

---

To Roy F. Traver: I was confused while the patterns were being shaped—now I am beginning to understand.

family unit. A basic premise maintained by Adlerians is that all behavior is purposeful and goal directed. In addition, the most important motivator is considered to be a result of "felt" inferiority feelings. Hence, the child's ensuing struggle has the purpose of moving the individual from a perceived "felt" minus position to a "felt" plus position. The child is most likely to learn what works best for him through both observing his family (first social environment) and modeling their behavior.

Adler believed that by understanding the apperceptive schema of the individual, the counselor and client would be more likely to effect the desired change (Ansbacher & Ansbacher, 1956). Today, Adlerians frequently utilize lifestyle analysis to delineate the unconscious or dimly conscious goals of the individual and the purposes behind his behavior. The lifestyle inventory taps basically two forms of information: family constellation and early memories (see Chapter 2). The family constellation portion will be emphasized in this chapter.

THE FAMILY CONSTELLATION

The term "family constellation" is used to describe a family's sociopsychological configuration during the individual's formative years. Dreikers (1952) noted that:

> This investigation reveals his field of early experiences, the circumstances under which he developed his personal perspectives and biases, his concepts, and convictions about himself and others, his fundamental attitudes, and his own approaches to life, which are the basis for his character, his personality. (p. 109)

One would suspect that the Adlerian family constellation analysis might be highly instrumental in assessing the family in multigenerational systems. While much clinical information has been published on the use of this procedure in assessing nuclear familial interactional patterns (Mosak & Mosak, 1975), there is a dearth of information on the use of the lifestyle format in assessing multigenerational interactional patterns.

The purpose of this chapter is to offer the reader a new perspective in understanding personality dynamics and their retention by introducing one means of understanding established familial patterns from an Adlerian perspective. As noted previously, the lifestyle is viewed as a goal-directed set of behaviors that are purposeful in nature. Correspondingly, the interactional relationship in a marital dyad is determined directly by the qualities, skills, and possessions of each individual. Each individual brings to the relationship needs and resources that are thought to complement one another's style of life and to help maintain an equilibrium that was established in their first social environment, namely the nuclear family. Beckman-Brindly and Tavormino (1978) noted that a power-dependency exchange takes place as each individual needs something the other has to offer. The assumption is that the desired quality is difficult to obtain elsewhere. As such, there is an attraction that somehow relates to the other's lifestyle, which was generated in the first familial environment and which is likely to have originated in the interactional patterns of the parents with each other and the siblings.

The family constellation assessment procedure involves gathering information on the personality characteristics and emotional distance of each person; ordinal position and the relationship that existed among siblings, between siblings and the parents, and between parents (e.g., sibling allies and rivalries along with parent-child interactions); parental models; family atmosphere; and family values (Shulman, 1973). Assumptions in the helping professions include the influence of adult models on children (e.g., child abusers are likely to have been abused themselves as children) and the influence of family values (college-educated parents are most likely to have children who also obtain college degrees). Far less emphasized are generational patterns that may be sustained because of established triadic relationships within the family.

Adlerians have included within some versions of the family constellation questionnaire (e.g., Dreikurs, 1967) simple inquiries that have some far-reaching multigenerational applications. Although the individual is best understood through the analysis of the family constellation in its totality, one aspect of the family constellation will be discussed at this time. In the parental information section the client is requested to respond to the following inquiries as if he were five or six years of age. (Information is gathered on both parents.)

1. Parents' name, age, occupation.
2. What kind of person was the father/mother? Give as many descriptions as possible.
3. If the father/mother could have molded you to suit his/her notion of an ideal child, how would he/she have wanted to change you?
4. What could you do to make your father/mother the happiest with you? What could you do to make him/her the angriest with you?
5. Which sibling was father's/mother's favorite? Why?
6. What were father's/mother's ambitions for the children?
7. What was father's/mother's relationship to the children?
8. Which sibling was most like father/mother? In what ways?

A key question in this series is the identification of the favorite sibling. Shulman and Nikelly (1976) have noted that there are definite advantages and disadvantages in being bestowed with the position of "favorite" by a parent within the family unit. They suggest that the favored sibling may have an undisputed position in the family and, consequently, may struggle less and may find his place among others more quickly. He may also conform more easily and expect to be accepted by others. As a result of this special status, the favored sibling may never learn to fight for a cause and may find it difficult to accept situations where not viewed as the favorite. Conversely, the "nonfavorite" may never feel sure of his status, i.e., of being accepted. This may, in turn, promote the possibility of the unfavored sibling learning at an early stage of life to accept "second best." More probable also are the possibilities of learning to depend on himself and his own efforts without taking a sensitive position on the unfriendliness of others.

Frequently, parents who generally view the perspective of having a favorite as a negative parental characteristic are surprised to learn that it is a normal phenomenon. Occasionally, an individual is unwilling or unable to identify a favorite sibling. The counselor may circumvent this dilemma by highlighting the normality of favoritism within families and by emphasizing the age at which the proposed favoritism took place, i.e., five to six years of age. By obtaining the answer to who are the parental favorites, the systems counselor may find himself on the edge of discovering deeper generational patterns that may offer explanations to the presenting problem. The following is an example.

Case History

When George and Mary became engaged and were married, she was in her late teens and he in his early twenties. Within a year and a half Joan was born, followed by George, Jr., two years later. These births drastically changed the dynamics in the family from the original complementary relationship George and Mary shared immediately following their marriage. George must now work harder and progress upwardly in order to provide for his growing family, while Mary has the added burden of caring for two children.

Because of this process, the marital dyad changes and original expectations are more difficult to obtain. George becomes more distant and Mary experiences an isolation within her life. At the same time, the children are competing for their parents' attention, each hoping to obtain more than or at least an equal share. The parents gravitate toward a sibling, in this case George toward Joan and Mary toward George, Jr. Again, complementary relationships are established with the child being more flexible than the adult, molding himself or herself to the parent.

In the above situation, Joan learns to fulfill many of her father's expectations in reciprocation for his attention (as does Junior to Mom). To fulfill her father's needs, Joan must draw on either environmental models or trial and error for solutions. Shulman (1973) notes that the more narrow or distorted the parental models, the fewer the alternatives available to the youth. As such, if Mary is a submissive, indulgent mother and father is dictatorial and tyrannical, then Joan might be expected to assume the posture of her mother in an effort to complement the father (as did the mother at marriage).

As Joan begins to mature, she may assume many of her mother's characteristics without realization. This is essentially due to having replaced the mother in the complementary relationship with the father. For example, Joan may develop similar defense techniques as her mother in addition to similar fight techniques. Joan is apt to select those that have been demonstrated as most effective in confrontation between the parents. If this develops, then Joan and Mary will utilize similar arsenals and may complain about and dislike similar characteristics in one another. Outside the home each may also hold in disdain others who have similar characteristics, all along not fully realizing that they, too, possess similar qualities. This reflects the adage "Those things you dislike most in others are most likely possessed by yourself." It may be added that individuals are most likely to use weapons (for example, emotional distance, crying, yelling, hitting) that they most fear themselves. Another way of stating it might be "Your most powerful weapon is your most feared retaliation."

Later, as the differentiation process is stepped up and Joan begins to demand her independence, the father may experience intense reactions, similar to those he has experienced with his wife, which may force him to use emotional distance to obtain control, sporadically align with his wife, or sporadically align with the daughter. This is a particularly confusing period. The focus on the child will ultimately allow the spousal subsystem to express rage and/or anxiety through a disguised manner, around the topic of the child's behavior. Minuchin (1974) describes a family structure with chronic problems around generational boundaries where it is the "norm" to utilize a child in spousal conflicts as a rigid triad.

Joan, in reaction to her nuclear familial uproar, may attach herself romantically to a male peer whose characteristics are similar to her father's personality. Since Joan's personality development was, in part, due to the consistent attention of the father (coupled with learning through modeling her mother's interaction within the family constellation), she may now attempt to duplicate this relationship within her present social schema; after all, it is what she is both comfortable with and adequate at manipulating. A male who is most likely to be successful in complementing Joan's expectations might be one who has had his mother's attention and whose father has some personality characteristics similar to those of Joan's father. If Joan makes such a choice, then, unintentionally, or at a dimly conscious level, she will have established a new complementary relationship, which most fulfills her perceptions, as developed in childhood, of the world in general and which will likely closely resemble her nuclear family.

Joan's relationship between her and her parents may continue to be disruptive until Joan establishes herself as independent of the family unit, which may be most successfully delineated through marriage. Following marriage, Joan and her father may resume their previous relationship at some level, but not necessarily Joan and her mother. While marriage, which is an experience to which both mother and Joan can relate, may link the two women together briefly, there may not be a sustaining force. Rather, it may not be until the birth of children that Joan and her mother can establish an empathic relationship.

The generational patterning increases the possibility that Joan and her mother can relate to one another because of the similarities of their marital and familial relationships. As Joan experiences satisfaction or dissatisfaction similar to her mother's experiences, the possibility of an empathic and understanding relationship between the two increases. For example, when Joan and her husband begin having children, and if the pattern of favoritism continues, as in the parents' previous family, the similar dissatisfactions with the relationship and difficulties with the children may be expected to arise. The two women, Joan and her mother (or the husband and his father), will have experienced similar dissatisfactions and at this time Joan will be able to better empathize with her mother's previous position. As a result, Joan may turn to her mother for comfort (misery loves company?).

IN-DEPTH CASE HISTORY

What follows is a multigenerational case study that will expand on the above example. The study gleans evaluative techniques utilized by various systems theorists (e.g., Andolfi, 1979; Guerin & Pendagast, 1976; Haley, 1971, 1976; Haley & Hoffman, 1967) and lifestyle data developed by Adlerians (Ansbacher & Ansbacher, 1956, 1970; Dreikurs & Soltz, 1964; Shulman, 1973). The focus will be on favoritism, how favoritism extends across generations, and the impact that such a phenomenon has on familial interactional systems.

A genogram, as described by Guerin and Pendagast (1976), is a three-generational structural diagram of the relationship system. It is a tool utilizing symbols that aid the counselor to illustrate graphically the relationships and positions of various family members. (See Figure 5-1 for an explanation of the symbols.)

Jack and June have been married for 17 years. They entered therapy because of the psychiatric hospitalization of their firstborn daughter, Mary. This was the second hospitalization, with the previous hospitalization being in another facility. Jack and June have identical birth dates and are 45 and 37 years of age, respectively. Their marriage has produced three offspring: Mary, 15; Shirley, 12; and Moe, 8, with all three being full-term noncomplicated births. In addition, there have been two miscarriages, one (sex unknown) prior to Mary's birth and one (a female) following Moe's birth. Both parents deny any trauma as a result of the miscarriages. The following is a description of the nuclear family, as recalled by the children, at the age of five years.

Figure 5-1 Symbols Used in Family Diagram

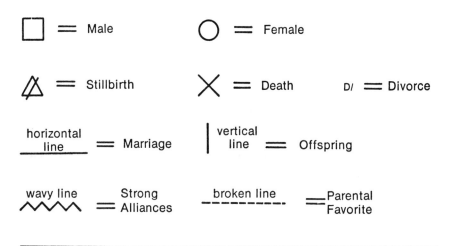

Mary

Description of:

Father: big, strong, bossy, took me bowling, happy, nice, with family much of the time.

Mother: busy much of the time, interested in us, disciplinarian, spent time at house, did things for the family, had lots of friends, got along with neighbors, associated with female neighbors, liked to be outdoors, liked flowers.

How I would have been molded by:

Father: He would not have changed anything. I did everything he liked.

Mother: Calm me down.

How I could have made my parents the happiest and angriest:

Father: Happiest by doing things with him and making him feel needed (listen to him read a story). Angriest by causing Mom to become upset (not responding to Mom's directives, not keeping my room clean).

Mother: Happiest by cleaning my room. Angriest by not listening to her and by running away.

Parental favorite and why:

Father: Me. I was more patient, did things with Dad.

Mother: Initially Shirley because they had the same interests like cooking and watching TV. Later it was Moe because he was a boy; they could afford this sibling and he was spoiled.

Parental expectations:
Father: To be happy, to do what we wanted.
Mother: To be accomplished and get high-paying jobs.
Which sibling was most like your parents?
Father: Me. Did things together, went to movies, went bowling, both patient, liked math.
Mother: Shirley. Did things together, dressed like Mom, was Mom's girl.
Describe yourself and your siblings:
Mary: Rambunctious, took care of Moe, outgoing.
Shirley: Shy and quiet, cautious, would hide things, throw things, sleep-walked a lot, never put things away, liked to be with female friends, liked to be outside and liked flowers.
Moe: Just gurgled.

Shirley

Description of:
Father: Nice, fun to be around, taller than me, happy.
Mother: Nice, busy doing stuff for everyone, happy, strong.
How I would have been molded by:
Father: I don't know (IDK).
Mother: IDK, like I was.
How I could have made my parents the happiest and angriest:
Father: Happiest by doing what I was told and helping in the house. Angriest by disrupting things, tearing up the recreation room and by fighting with siblings.
Mother: Happiest by helping her in the house and listening to her. Angriest by tearing stuff up and being disruptive.
Parental favorite and why:
Father: Mary. IDK, she was just closer to Dad than Mom.
Mother: Moe. He's the youngest and only boy.
Parental expectations:
Father: To be happy with what we did, to get a good job and have a family.
Mother: Same as father.
Which sibling was most like your parents?
Father: Mary. Liked the same things, did things together.
Mother: Me. Tried to do things as she did. Domestic—she'd show me how. Didn't always work out. Still have hard time keeping up with Mom.
Describe yourself and your siblings:
Mary: Not quiet and shy like me; outgoing, but not too outgoing; shy in some ways.
Shirley: Shy, quiet, followed big sister.
Moe: Lay around and was cute, tried to imitate people.

Moe

Description of:
Father: Kind of chubby, nice, gray hair, intelligent.
Mother: Kind of chubby, nice, black hair, understanding, lost temper some-
   times.
How I would have been molded by:
Father: Good.
Mother: Good.
How I could have made my parents the happiest and angriest:
Father: Happiest by being nice to others around me. Angry by breaking up
   things of my father's.
Mother: Happiest by being perfect and not stuffing my face. Angry by breaking
   something—maybe good glass.
Parental favorite and why:
Father: Mary. Because she watched me.
Mother: Me. IDK.
Parental expectations:
Father: Rich.
Mother: Rich.
Which sibling was most like your parents?
Father: Mary. Mean sometimes and sometimes considerate.
Mother: Mary. Yelled at me, understanding, lost temper easily.
Describe yourself and your siblings:
Mary: Nice, mean, understanding, serious, smart.
Shirley: Always joking, lost temper easily, smart.
Moe: IDK.

Parents:

Jack, their father, is the product of a single-child family. However, it is
important to note that two miscarriages occurred following Jack's birth, after
which his mother was informed by the family physician that another birth would be
detrimental to her health. Jack's father died of lung cancer at age 63 and his mother
is presently living and domiciles within a few miles of the nuclear family. Jack's
father was an alcoholic and Jack remembers him as frequently being intoxicated,
as being obnoxious and unconscious. His mother, who was apparently symbiot-
ically attached to Jack (for example, she continues to call each morning to wake
him), is presently retired.

June was adopted by her stepfather following her mother's remarriage when
June was two years old. In the interview, June's mother opted not to discuss this bit
of history as it was too painful. Later, June noted her natural father left the family

while in the service. June's parents have been married for 34 years and out of that relationship was born a son. This son was recently killed in an accident. Mary, during the discussion of this incident, became visibly upset (as did the maternal grandmother) and "cried," albeit no tears were evident. The maternal grandfather appeared to rescue his wife by entering and leading the discussion for this first time.

Further discussion revealed that June's family was influential, in contrast to Jack's family. The family's success was credited, to a large degree, to the maternal grandmother's persistence. Presently, Jack works in the family business for the maternal grandfather and is dependent on them for his family's subsistence. In discussing Jack and June's familial difficulties, the maternal grandmother noted that Mary's past behavior closely paralleled what Mary's grandmother and grandfather had experienced with June.

The following is a description of their families as Jack and June recall at the age of five years:

June

Description of:

Stepfather: Loved me, strict, always there, old-fashioned, wanted me to be perfect, big-hearted, family important, didn't like being lied to. (Natural father left family and June does not remember him.)

Mother: Pretty, loving, strict, stable (took care of all money), strong-minded (Dad feels she's fragile), moralistic.

How I would have been molded by:

Father: Nothing, I fit his notion of a perfect child.

Mother: To do as she said.

How I could have made my parents the happiest and angriest:

Father: Happiest by giving him a kiss and telling him I love him. Angriest by lying or disobeying him.

Mother: Happiest to be good, to love her. Angriest by talking back to her, acting out.

Parental favorite and why:

Father: Me. I was adopted by him and he loved me. My brother was very young then.

Mother: Jim. He was the baby.

Parental expectations:

Father: To be the best at whatever we did.

Mother: To have a good life, to be good.

Which sibling was most like your parents?

Father: Me. Belligerent and headstrong, lenient. Jim was sensitive, intelligent.

Mother: Me. Think things should be done a certain way (follow protocol), observe rules, be a good person in public.
Describe yourself and your siblings:
June: Pigtails, long ringlets, grandmother braided hair, brought in stray people, felt sorry for less fortunate, friendly, helpful.
Jim: Cute, just there.

Jack

Description of:
Father: Never disciplined me, alcoholic, close-mouthed, distant, not home.
Mother: Was not opinionated, she worked, disciplinarian, ran the household, was a strong woman.
How I would have been molded by:
Father: IDK, he was close-mouthed and never praised me and never indicated what he wanted.
Mother: I met her expectations by obeying her.
How I could have made my parents the happiest and angriest:
Father: Happiest—IDK. Angriest by getting in his way.
Mother: Happiest by being good, listening to her and by doing things for her. Angriest—I'm not really sure.
Parental favorite and why:
Father: No one (only child).
Mother: Me. I was there and I was special to her.
Parental expectations:
Father: IDK
Mother: Only that I do well and make a decent life.
Which sibling was most like your parents?
Father: N/A
Mother: Me. Excessively sentimental, family oriented.

DISCUSSION

The family history as discussed above is a description of a nuclear family consisting of two parents and three siblings whose interactional relationships have specific patterns. In addition, information is provided on the maternal grandparents and interactions that existed in those families. Figure 5-2 gives a graphic illustration of the family.

This chart indicates the establishment of a complementary pattern where favoritism is determined through the association and interaction between sexes. One would expect Jack and June to have been attracted into their present relationship,

Figure 5-2 Illustration of the Family

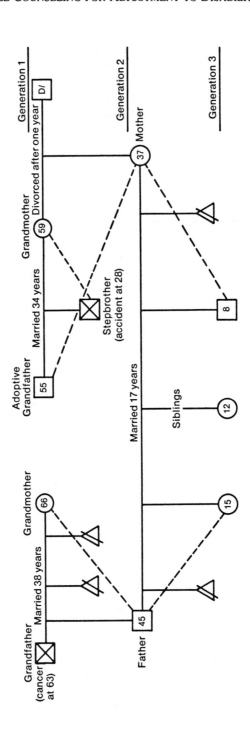

in part, as a result of their favored position within their own families. By becoming coupled with one another, they could effectively transfer their familial ties (and the unverbalized expectations) into the new relationship. It might also be noted that June was able to bring to the new relationship the strength that Jack's mother possessed in Jack's nuclear family. Jack, in turn, provided the sensitivity and awareness of rules that June appreciated in the maternal grandfather. The resulting union effectively transferred the relationships Jack and June experienced in their separate families to the new nuclear family, e.g., Jack portrays some qualities attributed to June's father (nice, big, happy, family oriented, bossy, intelligent), and June some of those of Jack's mother (busy, disciplinarian, children/family oriented, loses temper at times, strong).

Adler (Ansbacher & Ansbacher, 1956) noted that a dead sibling or miscarriage heightens parents' anxiety and this may be "caught" (Shulman, 1973) by the living children. This situation was experienced in both Jack's nuclear family and his present family. Both he and Mary were directly affected by these family losses (one might hypothesize that, upon learning of his wife's inability to have additional children, Jack's father withdrew further from the family). Mary's birth, following a miscarriage, may have, in part, compounded the intensity to which Jack transferred his attention to her. Evidently, Jack's efforts to fulfill his needs were, for some reason, foremost. His only alternative was to respond to this "new female" as he had responded to females throughout his life. As a result, a transference of the symbiotic relationship from his mother to his daughter appears to have ensued.

Given the limited environmental stimuli and models available, Mary was quick to learn what techniques were most effective in obtaining the desired goodies from her father by observing her mother. Those behaviors that were not effective became extinguished; those that were successfully orchestrated became strengthened. Hence, Mary developed fight techniques, e.g., seductiveness, bargaining from a position of strength, etc., and attitudes that closely resembled those of her mother. However, as will be discussed later, neither she nor her mother may ever be fully aware of this development.

Jack's desire to satisfy his needs through his daughter rather than his wife may have been heavily influenced by the nature of Jack and June's relationship. Multiple purposes for transferring his attention from June to Mary could exist. One might be a desire to dilute his wife's power as she may have asserted herself in a manner different from what he had previously experienced in his environment. An indication of this possibility may be detected in Mary's response to the lifestyle questionnaire. Here, Mary stated that father would not have changed her, whereas mom would have attempted to calm her down. However, Mary indicates that father became angry when mom was pushed to the point of becoming upset herself. This description may suggest that father, possibly at a dimly conscious level, could have encouraged the "rambunctious" behavior. Mother may have been the brunt of this behavior, which would have served to keep mother busy, thereby diluting her assertiveness with the father. In the process, Mary would have become aware of the power of pairing with her father. However, the disadvantage of such an alliance with father might be his abandonment when Mary exceeded the limits.

A second possible purpose for Jack's transferring his attention might be to increase the subjective feeling of being needed as his mother needed him (and as a newborn child needs an adult). Another possibility might include an effort to distance from the responsibility of being a husband (as did his father) and remain the baby or only child. Evidence to support this last hypothesis is found in Mary's remembrance of being closest to her father simply by listening to him as though to make him feel important.

Whatever the purpose of Jack's overinvolvement with his firstborn daughter, Mary swiftly responded and attempted to fulfill his needs in an effort to fulfill her own. The complementary interaction that ensued highly influenced her developing personality and the manner in which she would interact with her family and others in the future. As Beckman-Brindley and Tavormina (1978) might assert, a power-dependency exchange occurred as each, Jack and Mary, needed something that the other individual had to offer.

Now June was faced with a dilemma. She no longer possessed the individual attention from her husband that she had nonverbally contracted for (Sperry, 1978) in the marriage agreement. Hence, when Shirley was born, June spent much time encouraging this new sibling to be more domestic and sensitive by successfully allocating the type of attention that would facilitate a more passive development. Shirley responded to this challenge but, as she noted in her lifestyle questionnaire, she was never quite able to match her mother's capabilities. If she had, the relationship would have been more conflictual than complementary, as June needed to maintain the dominant role.

Following her son's birth, June turned her attention from Shirley to Moe with such intensity that Shirley, in the interview, described herself as being left out and as having no place. As intensely as Shirley experienced the dethronement, Moe experienced the specialness of his position. His personality, as described by his sisters, exemplifies that of a gurgling baby who imitated others. Indeed, as a young adolescent, Moe presents much like his father, i.e., placid, less effectual than the females, dependent, resistant to others' opinions, and passive-aggressive. Here, Moe's personality appears to have evolved, as did Shirley's, to complement his mother's more dominant nature. In so doing, Moe's resultant personality closely resembles his father's.

When interviewing a client who occupied a favored position, the counselor may expediently determine characteristics that the client may be only dimly aware of and that may work to his disadvantage. The client may be unaware of his behaviors or attitudes, so much so that he may identify them in others as unattractive or undesirable without ever realizing that he, too, is guilty of presenting himself in the same manner. The counselor is apt to discover these characteristics by encouraging the client to describe in detail how the nonpreferential parent (or parent figure) was perceived when the client was five to eight years of age. It will be these characteristics that the client will likely abhor but retain as his own.

In the above case, Jack perceived his father as distant, ineffectual, as not disciplining the children, and as being unclear. Jack contributed to the dysfunction within the present family through his desire to be liked by his children, which was played out through undermining his wife's disciplinarian action, by giving unclear messages to the children and his wife, and by maintaining a dependent relationship with his in-laws. On the surface, Jack's behavior may appear unlike his father, who remained aloof from his family through noninvolvement and dependency on alcohol. However, Jack's interaction with his family had the identical consequences, i.e., both he and his father were ineffectual. Moe appeared to approach life in a similar manner as his father in that he was dependent, ineffectual in obtaining and maintaining friendships, overly sensitive, passive-aggressive in his relationships with his siblings, and tended to put others in his service through having family members speak for him and fulfill his desires.

June's mother was characterized as being stable, strong-minded, the financial organizer, strict, and moralistic. Indeed, June maintained a similar stance within her home (which was supported and encouraged by her husband's lack of participation), which eventually contributed to the conflict between her and Mary. The conflict was compounded by Mary's having developed in a similar manner as her mother, i.e., strong-willed, powerful, and determined. Indeed, within the hospital milieu and away from the familial conflict, Mary presented herself as strict and moralistic when confronting her peers for their inappropriate behaviors. June was described by the maternal grandmother as presenting similar antagonistic behaviors within her home when June was an adolescent.

The conflict between June and her daughter and between June and her mother is not surprising; rather, the paradigm presented above would predict the resulting relationships. As indicated earlier, these females in their privileged positions with their fathers had to acquire power to assert their demands. The techniques, adopted prior to the age of five years, had to be modeled from their first social environment. The mother was the most available model who possessed experience with conversing or manipulating the father. Seemingly, as the sibling became older and began to differentiate from the family, thereby asserting certain demands, the mother and her child became conflictual. The volatility was compounded as a result of highly specialized weapons or techniques learned from one another. Since, in mortal combat, individuals tend to use the most destructive weapon they perceive themselves to possess, Mary, June, and the maternal grandmother fought one another with the most effective weapons they possessed, i.e., those they themselves most feared.

It is probable that Mary, June, and the maternal grandmother utilized the most effective defensive and offensive techniques they possessed. It is also probable that these maneuvers were ones they themselves perceived as most unpleasant, i.e., in mortal combat one does not attack the enemy with a weapon that in turn would not be destructive to oneself. In this situation, all three women used strength, alliances with important males, determination, and overt resistance. This behavior in comparison with the less overtly effective behavior of the males (passive resistance, bravadoism, and distancing) and Shirley's behaviors (compliance, shyness, and not being vocally assertive) has more overt effectiveness within this family and is therefore dominant. There is a high probability that this learned dominance results from the complementary power dependency relationship and compensation through modeling of behavior within the first social environment, i.e., the family.

PREDICTING FAMILY DEVELOPMENT

The paradigm of familial behavior we have examined is softly deterministic, as opposed to Freud's deterministic model (Ansbacher & Ansbacher, 1956). Adler believed that while future behavior may be predicated by past behavior, the individual has the creativity to change directions. The patterning of behavior through the third generation of this case study has been observed to be similar within the three generations. As a result, the counselor may guess that the siblings in the present generation will continue the sequence. Mary might be expected to marry at an early age if she is successful in locating a male peer who complements her dominant and demanding style. Her new husband will tend to be the favored male of a dominant mother (or some similar combination such as a second-born male with a much older sister who took favor with him and who was a parental figure). Upon the birth of their first child, depending on sex, one or the other will transfer their affection, thereby completing the cycle.

One might predict that Moe may also follow a similar route. However, Moe may experience difficulty in detaching from his mother, which may delay his involvement with another female. Much of the differentiation from the mother-child symbiotic relationship would depend on the parental diadic spousal relationship. The longer the child can depend on the mother for nurturance, the more retarded will be the transference of the dependency to a spouse.

Shirley's future is equally predicated by her development within this family system. Shirley experiences herself as inadequate and not quite living up to her own or others' standards. Her priorities may involve coupling with an assertive male who will assume a more traditional masculine role, or she may attempt to compensate through academic achievements and eventual occupational success. However, she may never fully shake her deep feelings of inadequacy or desire to gain heightened reassurance of her place.

The family is likely to continue to influence the lives of all the children and their families long after the children leave home. If Mary follows the established familial pattern, by 30 years of age she will have children and a husband who does not support her as she desires. As a result, Mary may come to empathize more with her mother's previous problems within the family. The shared experience between Mary and her mother may bind them into a tighter alliance than they had previously shared. Moe may very likely continue his close relationship with his mom, never quite being able to relinquish entirely. As for Shirley, she may always feel unable to live up to her mother's example. Her gnawing self-doubt and the mother's future criticism may have a paramount influence on Shirley and her future family. Finally, the family's dependency on the maternal grandparents' wealth has the potential to box in any of the siblings and/or their families.

The maternal grandparents' success in acquiring wealth has had an important and far-reaching impact on the family. Presently, not only the nuclear family's existence is dependent on the grandparents, but also any fringe benefits including social interaction and community recognition. The influence on the children is apparent through examining their perspective of their parents' future expectations, i.e., to be "rich" and to "get high-paying jobs." This expectation to achieve through the acquisition of wealth, if not achieve through occupational success or marriage, may lock the children into the family web, where they may remain dependent on another's actions. Certainly, such circumstances are pregnant with the potential for dissatisfactions, unhappiness, and covert hostility.

COUNSELING STRATEGIES

The counselor's objective is to reduce the stress within the family unit or alleviate the negative felt experience of the client. Following the reduction of stress, the counseling focus may then be oriented toward resolving the issue that originally necessitated and maintained the stress. The first intervention might be, particularly when the entire family is available, rearranging familial interactions so as to force new patterns of interaction designed to alleviate the immediate stress. As for the individual, the counselor may elect to encourage a new behavior so that the client may experience success. Following the successful implementation of these interventions, the focus may then be narrowed to a reeducation process (Ansbacher & Ansbacher, 1956) and/or reinforcement of the new patterns of behavior.

Adler (Ansbacher & Ansbacher, 1970) saw the individual's most important motivation as being subjectively felt inferiority feelings. In addition, Adler believed that it was not the situation in which the individual found himself but, rather, the individual's perception of the situation that ultimately influenced the nature of the striving. Therefore, behavior is viewed as purposeful and as designed subjectively by the individual to move him from a less favored position to a more favored position.

Dreikurs and Soltz (1964) described four types of maladaptive behaviors that are learned and employed in early childhood to gain advantage: undue attention getting, power, revenge, and a display of inadequacy. Once well rehearsed and adopted as a style of interacting, these types of behaviors are apt to become well ingrained. If so, then the individual will utilize the behavior to struggle against or with other individuals to gain some advantage. This behavior becomes particularly significant when viewed in light of the "pairing," i.e., closeness, between a favored child and the parent.

The pairing that develops between the preferential child and parent is a durable and complementary relationship. This relationship may be designed to jointly maintain the advantageous position within the triangle or avoid resolving difficulties between the two of them. The pairing ultimately deprives another individual (or part of a system) and/or protects at least one of the paired individuals from the third or one of the pair. Therefore, it is necessary to view exhibited behavior within the family or system as an interaction among individuals or factors, i.e., a triadic interaction or combination thereof.

The above discussion may be more clearly delineated by focusing on the pairing that might occur between the preferential child and parent when considering Dreikurs' typology in understanding children's behavior. Shulman (1973) noted that children always reflect some facet of the parents' attitudes and values. Further, "One can assume that a power-drunk child has at least one parent to whom force and forcefulness have a high positive or negative value" (Shulman, 1973, p. 48). Shulman's position might be applied to all of Dreikurs' four observed behaviors of children. For example, a favored child who utilizes revenge as a compensatory behavior may be paired with a parent who feels inadequate and repressed by the spouse or a parent who craves attention and feels neglected. By coupling, the duo may create a unified complementary relationship designed to forestall, get even with, or somehow change the behavior of the third party. Control, then, becomes the central issue and pairing is the technique utilized against a strong opponent to maintain this control.

It is quite evident that in the above case study, Mary (the identified patient) and her father would tend to support one another, either covertly or overtly, against perceived interfamilial threat. But just how extensive is this network and how does it generalize to other contacts within the family? Figure 5-3 may, in part, better explain the patterns that may emerge in such a system.

The broken lines indicate favoritism and wavy lines denote strong alliances. Note how these alliances with one exception (Shirley and her mother) are between males and females. In this particular family, power is of paramount importance. Here, Mary was able to struggle the power away from other females by aligning with males. For example, if Mary were able to align with her mother's father (i.e.,

Figure 5-3 Family Relationships

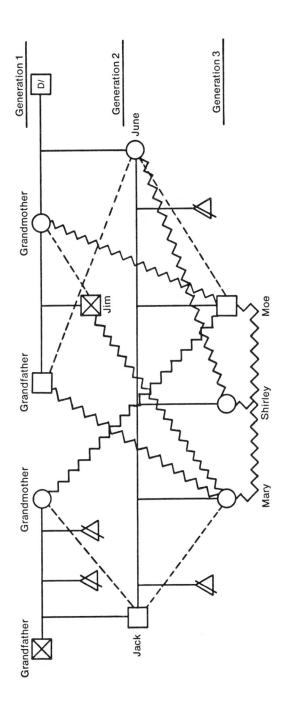

complement him) more effectively than her mother over some pertinent issue, then Mary would maintain the advantage.

This modus operandi, shared by all females in this family (with the exception of Shirley), strategically gave the advantage of power to the females. At the same time the males are able to manipulate and utilize this resource to their advantage. As noted earlier, Jack's alliance with Mary may have been an effort to dilute his wife's power, to increase the subjective feeling of being needed, or an effort to be taken care of or babied. Mary's relationship outside the family and eventual marriage is likely to assume a similar complementary flavor.

One might suspect that Shirley has the potential to reverse this process. By experiencing herself as more inadequate and less powerful than other females, she may attempt to attach herself to a perceived adequate and strong male figure. This may, in part, explain her lack of camaraderie with males in her family, i.e., they do not complement her needs. However, her mother does and a potential mate may be expected to exhibit similar characteristics.

The counselor's task, following his understanding of the triadic relationships, is to rearrange the interaction in an effort to align individuals in a more functional manner. There are several assumptions that need to be accepted. First, parents need to jointly have control over the offspring. Second, to most effectively accomplish this task, there must be a certain amount of shared responsibility and support for one another. Third, generational contamination, i.e., familial decisions influenced by grandparents, dilute the parents' effectiveness. Another assumption is that there must be some mutual sharing and caring between the spouses. Finally, clear parental expectations and consequences need to be established.

In the initial phases of counseling, primary efforts are made to resolve the presenting problem (Haley, 1971), which generally entails the disruptive child. Alignment of the parents to agree jointly on the expected behavior and consequences (Dreikurs, 1964) for noncompliance will effectively withdraw the child's favored position and implant the control into the more experienced hands of the parents. Predicting failure and the probable intensified efforts of the child to reinstate the status quo may be reassuring to the parents when difficulties do arise.

The counselor may begin to facilitate mending the deteriorated marital dyad and separate the dysfunctional parent-child relationship in the initial sessions. The process might best be performed without the family's conscious awareness. In the presence of the children, the counselor might encourage parents to discuss shared premarital activities. In so doing, old emotions and remembrances are rekindled, it provides the favored offspring and parents a glimpse of the potential unified force, and cues the counselor to possible reinforcers for parental success in assignments. The parents are encouraged during the session to agree upon a reward for themselves (to be obtained following the successful execution of some specified assignment or objective) that would extract them from the duties of parenting and provide an opportunity to recapture and/or practice displaying the previously suppressed caring emotions.

Cross-generational influences are of particular importance. As in Mary's case, she was especially adept at encouraging the grandparents to influence the parents, thereby effectively maintaining the control within the family herself. The counselor may need to jointly interview all three generations if the parents are unwilling or unable to set limits on the grandparents. Often, getting the family to discuss and agree on the roles of grandparents (e.g., to spoil grandchildren, to be a resource to parents when asked) and the roles of parents (to discipline the children, to provide consistent expectations) will accelerate this process.

The above tactics coupled with other interventions (for a more detailed explanation see Andolfi, 1979; Bowen, 1978; Haley, 1971; Haley and Hoffman, 1967; Palazzoli, Cecchin, Prata, Boscolo, 1978) allow the counselor to facilitate the separation of the favored dyad. With continued success in cooperativeness, the presenting problems may be virtually resolved. However, a relapse into old patterns of interacting might be expected if the marital dyad is neglected.

Sperry (1978) maintains that individuals during the attraction phase preceding their marriage develop a private pact that might be best described as an unspoken and likely unconscious alliance. These expectations are probably reflective of the mates' early social environment and may be an effort to maintain some predictability experienced in that environment. To assess the nature of these expectations, the counselor might inquire as to what attracted the mate to the spouse, what did this mate see in this person that was different from other perspective mates? (Sperry, 1978). Often physical attraction is mentioned. However, further probing may offer the counselor a glimpse of a characteristic reflective of the preferential parent.

Counseling may focus on an educational process in an effort to help the client understand how problems in his immediate family are reflected in that of his original nuclear family. By recognizing patterns in their interaction and how they are both complemented and contrasted within the family interactional system, the couple may be better equipped to remediate their marital conflicts. The mates, following the revelation of their inner expectations, may then be able to assess if these expectations are rational; if they are attainable, and, if so, how; and, finally, how the couple can more adequately communicate a need for fulfillment. Counseling may then focus on building a better relationship.

SUMMARY

The preceding pages have attempted to weave an Adlerian assessment technique designed to better understand the individual with more global patterns of behavior observed across generations. Essentially, the focus has been on the parental favored child and the complementary interfamilial and intrafamilial relationships that emerge. The favored child and respective parent are viewed as complementary pairs designed to maintain control over a third party who may present some perceived threat or to avoid resolving some conflict between themselves.

Marriage is viewed as a complementary relationship where each individual brings to the relationship something of value to the other. As children are added to the family unit, new relationships develop and old ones are redefined. When a spouse selects a sibling as a favorite, the child develops in a manner that would complement the personality of that parent. The child draws from individuals within his first social environment, i.e., the nuclear family, as interactional models. The most effective model the child would likely mirror would be one that complements the parent, e.g., the spouse or possibly a live-in grandparent.

Further attention was given to the ramifications of the pairing process and its "contagious" effect across generations. The learned responses of the sibling are thought of as ingrained and as predicating future responses to others. As such, the sibling will likely mate with a spouse whose personality complements that of the sibling and resembles the favored parent. By establishing such a relationship, the cycle is completed and the stage set for its continuance.

REFERENCES

Adler, A. *Understanding human behavior*. Greenwich, Conn.: Fawcett, 1954.

Andolfi, M. *Family therapy: An interactional approach*. New York: Plenum Press, 1979.

Ansbacher, H.L., & Ansbacher, R.R. (Eds.). *The individual psychology of Alfred Adler*. New York: Basic Books, 1956.

Ansbacher, H.L., & Ansbacher, R.R. (Eds.). *Superiority and social interest: Alfred Adler* (2nd ed.). Evanston, Ill.: Northwestern University, 1970.

Beckman-Brindley, S., & Tavormina, J.B. Power relationships in families: A social-exchange perspective, *Family Process*, 1978, *17*, 423–435.

Bowen, M. *Family therapy in clinical practice*. New York: Jason Aronson, 1978.

Dreikurs, R. The psychological interview in medicine, *American Journal of Individual Psychology*, 1952, *10*, 99–122.

Dreikurs, R. *Psychodynamics, psychotherapy, and counseling*. Chicago: Alfred Adler Institute, 1967.

Dreikurs, R., & Soltz, V. *Children: The challenge*. New York: Hawthorn, 1964.

Guerin, P.J., & Pendagast, E.G. Evaluation of family system and geneogram. In P.E. Guerin (Ed.), *Family therapy*. New York: Gardner Press, 1976.

Haley, J. *Changing families*. New York: Grune & Stratton, 1971.

Haley, J. *Problem solving therapy*. San Francisco: Jossey-Bass, 1976.

Haley, J., & Hoffman, L. *Techniques of family therapy*. New York: Basic Books, 1967.

Minuchin, S. *Families and family therapy*. Cambridge: Harvard University Press, 1974.

Mosak, H.H., & Mosak, B.A. *A bibliography for Adlerian psychology*. Washington, D.C.: Hemisphere, 1975.

Palazzoli, M., Cecchin, G., Prata, G., & Boscolo, L. *Paradox and counterparadox*. New York: Jason Aronson, 1978.

Shulman, B.H. *Contributions to individual psychology*. Chicago: Alfred Adler Institute, 1973.

Shulman, B.H., & Nikelly, A.G. Family Constellation. In A.G. Nikelly (Ed.), *Technique for behavioral change*. Springfield, Ill.: Charles C Thomas, 1976.

Sperry, L. *The together experience*. San Diego: Beta Books, 1978.

Chapter 6

Developmental Considerations in Counseling for Lifestyle Adjustment

Beverly Marie Momsen

The explosion in the area of adult development and life stages has caused counselors and helping professionals to become increasingly aware of the importance of these concepts in working effectively with clients. As developmental issues are universally experienced, they are no less important to counselors working with disabled clients. An understanding of adult development processes and family stage dynamics, together with knowledge of one's lifestyle orientation, can increase considerably the rehabilitation practitioner's effectiveness in helping disabled clients.

ADULT DEVELOPMENT

Until very recently, adult development, particularly in the middle and late years of life, was largely neglected by researchers and theorists in the behavioral sciences. One reason for this void may be the prevailing view that saw adulthood as a period of stability during which very little growth or development occurs. Once a person survived an oftentimes turbulent adolescence, he or she was thought to "settle down" into adulthood. However, research findings in the last decade suggest that psychological growth and change occur continuously throughout the life cycle (Gould, 1972; Levinson, Darrow, Klein, Levinson, & McKee, 1977; Lowenthal, Thurner, & Chiriboga and Associates, 1975; Neugarten, 1976). Adults, like children and adolescents, progress through life in rather predictable and most often sequential stages. Adults, as well as family units, seem to experience conflicts, urges, frustrations, and difficulties that are shared by others at similar points during the life cycle. The way individuals or families respond to

---

Special appreciation goes to Janice M. McMillan, Ph.D., for her contributions to this article through a workshop and seminar presentation.

developmental tasks and transitions is dependent upon the complex mixture of personality variables, lifestyle orientation, past experiences, and extraneous events or circumstances.

Basic Assumptions

The developmental perspective emphasizes that growth and change occur continuously over time. The life cycle is seen as divided into stages that typify or describe general experiences and issues that are commonly shared by people within a particular stage. Below are the assumptions basic to a framework embracing adult and family development (Aldous, 1978; Brim, 1976; Erikson, 1963):

1. Growth and development can be characterized by sequential stages and is continuous throughout the life cycle.
2. In each stage of development, critical issues and development tasks become the central focus for individuals in that stage.
3. Developmental tasks require mastery and resolution before the individual or family can successfully move on to the next stage. If the issues are not resolved successfully, they typically result in further difficulties at a later time.
4. Transitions to subsequent stages require some major shifts that produce disequilibrium.
5. Individuals are part of a family system, an interacting network in which every member influences and is influenced by the system. A change in one part will lead to change in all parts.

These assumptions establish a conceptual base for understanding individual and family growth. The developmental processes of individuals and families are very much interrelated. If a composite systems and lifestyle perspective for human behavior is accepted, then a practitioner cannot completely understand a client without assessing the individual's stage of development, unique lifestyle orientation, and where the family is in its life cycle.

Stages of Development

Several theorists have delineated stages of adulthood and stages of family growth and development. A synthesis of developmental patterns and stage characteristics basic to most individuals and families is presented below, drawing from Aldous (1978), Duvall (1971), Erikson (1963), Havighurst (1972), Hill and Rodgers (1964), Levinson et al. (1977), Neugarten (1976), Lowenthal et al. (1975), and Sales (1978). It is important to point out that these stages reflect a life cycle for what has been considered representative or typical for adults in the past several decades. Several circumstances and changing trends will no doubt produce variances in the individual and families issues that come into focus. These include but are not limited to (1) postponed marriage and a delay in having a family, (2) alternative family arrangements (single-parent, blended families, dual-career, multigenerational), and (3) for the disabled individual, the nature of the disability. And to mention again, the lifestyle of the individual and the collective personality of the family will also account for variations within each stage. The following framework does typify trends and patterns for most adults with children.

Individual Autonomy: Pulling Up Roots

Preceding the first stage of adulthood, adolescents are confronted with the task of establishing identity (Erikson, 1963). When young adults feel comfort and satisfaction in their struggle for identity as separate individuals, they are better prepared to face future developmental tasks. As an adult, the individual begins to make decisions with minimal outside help. These decisions are based on the young adult's values, needs, goals, and aspirations, and influence the remainder of that individual's life.

Events that typify this first phase of adulthood may include leaving one's family of origin, attending college or vocational training, and choosing or embarking on a career. Some of the developmental tasks that young adults face are (1) separating emotionally and physically from the home; (2) becoming independent and financially responsible; (3) appraising one's self-concept, values, and abilities and making decisions based on this appraisal; (4) making a commitment to and caring for friends; and (5) learning to relate as an adult to others of varying ages.

The first stage of adulthood requires new levels of intimacy and interpersonal functioning for both men and women. Intrapersonal conflicts may occur as this new level conflicts with previous values and methods of behavior. Moreland (1979) points out, for example, that during adolescence boys are typically excused for lacking emotional sensitivity and responsiveness. Up until this time, acceptable means of status acquisition for boys have been through athletic competition and sexual prowess. When adolescent boys then move into adulthood, a redefinition of this concept of masculinity is required as these behaviors are no longer appropriate.

Stress during this stage may emanate from different sources for men and women. Campbell (1975) reports higher stress and lower life satisfaction levels for young men during this stage. The pressures result from the required selection of a permanent occupation choice, which will strongly influence all other lifestyle components: economic, marital, and social. While women at this age may be less burdened by this demand (Sales, 1978), they may experience conflict as professional or vocational goals collide with societal expectations for marriage and family. Both young men and young women may experience frustration stemming from the mixed messages concerning sex role expectations that they are faced with today.

The additional stress of adjustment to disability makes the first stage of adulthood a complex one. Reframing one's identity in terms of altered self-image, potential, needs, ability, and motivation will impact on separation issues, including independence as well as the intimacy concerns that young adults face. Furthermore, the disability may interfere with the developmental tasks and cause them to progress more slowly.

Intimacy: The Couple Stage

The two major events that characterize the next stage of adulthood are launching a career and getting married. It is during this stage that young adults begin to set goals and make plans for marriage and career. Many changes occur as the newly married couple begins the task of developing patterns for their life together. These patterns include tasks concerning (1) role differentiation, (2) determination of work patterns, (3) development of mutual friends and recreational activities, (4) determination of authority lines and decision-making processes, and (5) decisions about the role of the extended family in the couple relationship.

Each spouse comes from a different family of origin with unique expectations and styles of interacting. Thus, completing the above tasks involves negotiation and compromise. The successful mastery of these tasks requires that both partners have developed some secure sense of their own identity and independence.

Achieving intimacy also implies some fusing of one's identity with that of another. If one has not developed a sense of comfortable identity, relinquishing part of one's independence may be very frightening. The subsequent reduction in personal freedom may be too much for the immature individual (Cox, 1974). Women who have not developed some sense of their own identity, and who merely shift their dependence from their parents to their husbands, may experience difficulty with successful self-satisfaction at this stage, as well as with subsequent stages. Unrealistic expectations and perceptions about one's spouse must also be resolved during this stage. The couple must learn interdependence and develop a satisfactory system of mutual support (Rhodes, 1977). The inability to resolve these issues can create problems later in the family life cycle and may contribute to the high rate of divorce for couples in this stage (Duvall, 1971).

Launching careers may be an area of stress for both the individual and the couple. The new rules, demands, and energy required to work in the adult world may temporarily create self-doubt and disillusionment. In particular, women may experience role conflict if their career aspirations run counter to their husbands'.

Adults adjusting to disability in this phase may experience a change in terms of independence, financial needs, work roles and expectations, and role differentiation. They need to strive to be sensitive to the importance of equal input into decision-making/authority issues and relationship building.

Early Parenthood: A Turning Point

The critical tasks of early parenthood most often concern work and intimacy: (1) reevaluating one's career choice and (2) the maintenance of a viable marital relationship. The introduction of children adds a new dimension to the couple relationship, as roles are expanded and are juggled to mesh with existing roles of spouse and worker. Since establishment in a satisfactory career is a major individual developmental task that often conflicts with the tasks of parenting, a satisfactory balance between work and family roles is often difficult to achieve. The concept of "role overload" has often been applied to the young wife/mother who is also trying to maintain a career (Sales, 1978). Today's college-educated man may experience the same double expectations: those of being a successful provider as well as sharing in household tasks and childrearing (Veroff & Feld, 1970).

Economic issues can strain family relationships. At a time when additional finances are required for the raising of children, typically the second income provided by the wife has stopped. Economic frustration, career demands on the husband, and the wife's loss of self-esteem after leaving work can generate stress and tension for the couple. If the couple has not previously developed satisfactory intimacy and support systems, distancing may occur. If there is no method in the family system for each of the couple to "re-fuel" themselves, then each will slowly be consumed with ideas of self-interest that run counter to family interests (Rhodes, 1977).

Married couples report the highest stress when children are preschoolers (Campbell, 1975), and subsequently, there is a marked decline in marital satisfaction (Aldous, 1978). During this stressful time, many adults become critical of the life structure and patterns developed in the preceding stages. The husband and wife question earlier decisions concerning career and marriage choices, as well as their own interests and activities. Both may be experiencing their own individual stagnation versus generativity crises (Erikson, 1963). The husband may find that his career is no longer rewarding and may attempt to resolve this dilemma by either deepening his commitment or by changing careers. Typically, the wife's "stagnation crisis" results from a relatively thankless period of high demand (house, husband, and dependent small children) and low self-esteem (Kimmel, 1974). Bernard (1973) and Lopata (1971) point out that being a housewife is not personally rewarding for most women. They may try to thwart stagnation through involvement in home or outside activities. In early marriage, women often deemphasize their own personal needs for marital closeness and emotional involvement to avoid interference with the husband's career establishment

(Sheehy, 1976). However, during this early parenthood stage, the wife may be more likely to express her needs, which places even more demands on the husband.

Middle Parenting: Settling Down

Many of the same tasks present in early parenthood that concern both individuals and families continue into the next stage. Marriage may continue to be strained, work concerns grow deeper, and care of children may be replacing care of the spouse (Gould, 1978). Spousal distancing increases and marital satisfaction is reported to be at its lowest point (Aldous, 1978). Individually, the husband and wife may be experiencing different developmental pulls. The husband (1) is making a deep commitment to his career in anticipation of his BOOM period (Becoming One's Own Man), (2) is considering a break with his mentor, and (3) is preparing for crucial career promotions (Levinson et al., 1977). His preoccupation with shaping his own visions into long-term goals may be at the expense of time shared with his wife and family. The wife's daily parental responsibilities usually decrease, and she may be considering her own reentry into the job market. The low self-esteem and stagnation of the housewife period typically evolves into a new search for identity and independence for the woman in her thirties (Bernard, 1973). Her role exploration at this time may resemble the role exploration of the younger man during his earlier identity crisis, and she may begin a shift from passivity and dependence to activity, self-assertion, and independence (Sales, 1978).

For both parents, there are increased role responsibilities as children enter school. It now becomes essential to develop a role with the community and become involved with parents, teachers, and other adults involved in school and community activities. Important tasks for all family members at this time include reorganization to provide for the growth of individual members and maintaining a viable marital relationship at a period when continued strain makes it difficult.

As children become teenagers, stages of individual development may conflict with family stage development and cause considerable tension. As younger individuals begin to develop their independence and identity, it is important that the family system recognize this growing separation and begin to shift family relationships and patterns. Parental authority lines need to change from the arbitrary rule of younger childhood to more negotiation. Parents, however, are approaching a point of their own development where it is important for them to maintain some continuity in their lives. This makes it a difficult time to face the fact that one's children are growing up—parents have their own developmental stake in minimizing family change (Bengstrom, 1971). However, the disengagement of children that begins at this time must not be impeded by parental fears of isolation. A developmental task for this period is for parents, as couples and individuals, to develop new relationships and friendships as the parent-child relationship is redefined.

Late Parenting

The reorganization of parent-child relationships continues as children begin the transition into the adult world and leave home. The departure of children from the home is a natural and necessary part of life. If the family does not reorganize, the child may either be held back in the system or expelled prematurely because of conflict over independence (Rhodes, 1977). The husband and wife may be facing some very salient issues in their own lives, which can make this period a difficult one.

A widespread misconception formerly held that women experienced a negative "empty nest" period when grown children left home. However, current evidence suggests that this may be a very positive time for women, as opposed to a time during which women experience depression and feelings of uselessness (Neugarten, 1976; Lowenthal, 1975; Deutscher, 1964). Women tend to become more assertive and turn outward from the home, viewing life as "getting better" (Glen, 1975). The need for personal achievement is at its highest point for women at this stage of life (Baruch, 1966), and women in the work force may begin to break into their own period of Becoming One's Own Person (Sales, 1978). However, as Perrucci and Targ (1974) point out, women who define themselves primarily as mothers may face some difficulties at this time. As this period continues through middle age, women tend to develop a more positive sense of identity, may play a more dominant role in marital decision making, and generally adjust better to aging than the husband.

This period may be slightly more difficult for the husband. Having reached a plateau in his career, he may begin to question his own life accomplishments (Targ, 1979). The gap between aspirations and accomplishments may become very apparent (Brim, 1976). At this time, men turn inward toward home and family for support and reassurance. The concern for one's own mortality along with the threat of changes in the family seems to underscore the husband's sense of decreasing influence (Brim, 1976). With family support and readjustment, men can begin to accept and enjoy their lifestyles. Goals can be modified to fit with reality in preparation for retirement and the onset of other roles—grandparenting and contributing to the next generation.

If the marriage has maintained its viability through the previous more difficult stages, marital happiness may rise considerably at this point (Feldman, 1964; Glen, 1975) for both men and women. Marital support at this time helps each spouse deal with a major issue concerning aging, which may intensify by the aging or death of their own parents or the addition of grandchildren.

Aging

The last phase of adulthood is most often characterized by retirement, loss of energy and health, and experiencing the death of close friends or one's spouse. Older adults must learn to (1) cope with physiological aging, (2) adjust to loss of income and potential financial hardship, (3) adjust psychologically to role loss through retirement, and (4) develop new activities and friendships to combat loneliness.

The need for aging adults to maintain an independent identity is as important as maintaining a sense of continuity (Lowenthal et al., 1975). These tasks may be particularly difficult if the threat of health or financial difficulties forces a dependence on extended family members. A family system of exchange, in which everyone benefits, fosters a feeling of self-worth for older adults and is essential to maintaining identity and continuity.

Most aging persons face changes that may be stressful (Kimmel, 1974). Older adults have an increased awareness of death. As they experience the gradual loss of their peer group, they face a significant decrease in their own meaningful relationships. In addition, aging adults may also experience a decrease in their physical life space as they move to smaller living areas (apartment, retirement homes, in with children, etc.). Thus, adjustments to new surroundings and the establishment of new relationships are important tasks. Struggling to remain productive, being able to accept one's past life, and valuing the choices made during that earlier life are critical to adjustment at this time (Erikson, 1963).

Aging adults also must contend with the process of disengagement in which the individual and the social system mutually release and separate from one another (Cummings, Dean, & Newell, 1960). Role disengagement should be a gradual process or else feelings of uselessness and loss of self-esteem may develop. The maintenance of bonds with the family and friends and renegotiation of family roles are necessary for successful adjustment at this stage.

Family attitudes toward aging and elderly relatives will impact on all family members. One's attitudes and experiences will influence how one views aging adults (the extent they are valuable, useful, etc.), as well as how successfully one can master the tasks of this later stage.

Stage Transitions

Practitioners helping clients adjust to disability must also consider factors impacting on stage transitions. The stress or difficulty within each stage or between stages may be minimized or intensified by the person's lifestyle orientation: the distinctive way one strives for significance and approaches the problems of life. The conclusions a person draws about self, the world, and consequent goals for belonging and superiority will indeed influence the perception and resolution of tasks inherent in each phase of life.

Problems surrounding developmental issues and transitions may be intensified for any of the following reasons. One may be the client's fear of an impending stage, such as apprehension about committing to marriage, fears about parenthood, fear of aging or senility. Another problem may be the client's reluctance to leave a gratifying stage. An example might be a couple or family that doesn't want its children to grow up and leave the home. Unresolved earlier issues also create problems in stage transitions, as when an individual moves on before psychological readiness. Examples might include marrying before one has the capacity for intimacy or leaving home before one can assume self-responsibility.

Another factor that can create difficulty for clients is a cumulative erosion of energies. Clients may be worn down from facing too many issues at once—a disabled client making physical and psychological adjustments as well as marital, career, and financial adjustments. Experiencing off-time events such as the unexpected death of a spouse, forced early retirement, or delayed grandparenting roles may also impede task resolution.

IMPLICATIONS FOR COUNSELING

In helping clients adjust to disability, counselors must be aware of where their clients and families are in their own developmental cycles. In addition to diagnosing the rehabilitative process and tasks to be addressed, practitioners must be sensitive to developmental issues clients may be facing.

Dynamic presenting symptoms may often mask a developmental issue. For instance, an individual may act out a family stage difficulty with dynamic symptoms (Haley, 1973). An example of this may be a delinquent or truant teenager who misbehaves because the marital relationship in the family has disintegrated. Counselors should be able to use developmental knowledge in conjunction with lifestyle assessment to sift through symptoms and pinpoint the real issues.

When counselors help clients view their problems from a developmental perspective as those issues that are natural and predictable, much of the clients' anxiety can be "defused." Understanding the universality of the difficulty and its transitional status can help clients take a more positive "growth experience" approach.

Developmental concepts emphasize change and we must keep in mind that adults and family units are constantly in the process of evolving and growing. Growth and development are not easy; they often involve struggle and trial-and-error behavior. Vines (1979) suggests that some adult behavior that may have been previously viewed as pathological should be seen as an "adult-unfolding." The behaviors may be more positively viewed as trial-and-error struggles to adapt to life change. This concept of growth should impress upon us the potential and the resources available in our clients and their family systems and may require us to reevaluate our strategies for intervention.

DEVELOPMENTAL GOALS AND STRATEGIES

In a broad sense the goal of a developmentalist is to enhance the self-potentiating capabilities of the client. A developmental stance would focus on the client's awareness of his or her resources, alternatives, competence, and lifestyle orientation and would emphasize growth and assets instead of deficits. The following guidelines are offered to practitioners as they assist clients in resolution of developmental issues.

1. Help clients explore and understand the scope of their concerns and the relationship to other issues. Reassure clients that growth and change throughout the life cycle is normal and necessary.
2. Identify the client's psychological, physical, and social resources and competence.
3. Explore with clients ways in which their lifestyle orientation works to their advantage in task resolution and how it impedes or becomes a liability.
4. Help individuals view their problems in the context of their own developmental growth as well as their family system and help them understand the mutual impact and change that is produced.
5. Help clients plan strategies for helping themselves, developing decision-making/problem-solving skills where needed.
6. Encourage clients to view transitions as a positive opportunity for growth. Help them prepare for changes to come in a proactive light.

Specific interventions and activities may be employed at various stages according to the issue or task at hand. These may include values clarification, parenting skills, role negotiation, career exploration, structural family therapy, goal setting, etc.

SUMMARY

As growth and development continue throughout the life cycle, individuals are faced with new tasks to master, new issues to resolve, and new roles to try on. Clients adjusting to disability will experience points of stress during their lives in a predictable sequence that may or may not be related to their disability. An awareness of normal changes and growth patterns in concert with a lifestyle assessment will give practitioners a more comprehensive understanding of issues affecting their clients. Counselors, together with their clients, can pinpoint problems, alleviate anxiety, and develop intervention strategies that can produce meaningful growth in their clients' lives.

REFERENCES

Aldous, J. *Family careers: Developmental changes in family*. New York: Wiley, 1978.

Baruch, R. The interruption and resumption of women's careers. *Harvard Studies in Career Development*, 1966, p. 50.

Bengstrom, V.L. Interage perceptions and the generation gap. *Gerontologist*, 1971, *11*, 85–89.

Bernard, J. *Women, wives and mothers: Values and options*. Chicago: Aldine, 1973.

Brim, O.G. Theories of the male mid–life crises. *The Counseling Psychologist*, 1976, *6*, 2–9.

Campbell, A. The American way of mating: Marriage si, children only maybe. *Psychology Today*, 1975, pp. 31–47.

Cox, F.D. *Youth, marriage and the seductive society*. Dubuque, Ia.: Brown, 1974.

Cummings, E., Dean, L., Newell, D., & McCaffrey, I. Disengagement, a tentative theory of aging. *Sociometry*, 1960, *23*, 23–35.

Deutscher, I. The quality of postparental life: Definitions of the situation. *Journal of Marriage and the Family*, 1964, *26*, 52–59.

Duvall, E. *Family development*. Philadelphia: Lippincott, 1971.

Erikson, E. *Childhood & society*. New York: Norton, 1963.

Feldman, H. *Development of the husband–wife relationship: A research report*. Ithaca, N.Y.: Cornell University Press, 1964.

Glen, N.D. Psychological well–being in the post–parental stage: Some evidence from national surveys. *Journal of Marriage and the Family*, 1975, *37*, 105–110.

Gould, R. The phases of adult life: A study in developmental psychology. *American Journal of Psychiatry*, 1972, *129*, 521–531.

Gould, R. *Transformations: Growth and change in adult life*. New York: Simon & Schuster, 1978.

Haley, J. *Uncommon therapy: The psychiatric techniques of Milton H. Erikson, M.D.* New York: Norton, 1973.

Havighurst, R. *Developmental tasks and education* (3rd ed.). New York: McKay, 1972.

Hill, R., & Rodgers, R. The developmental approach. In H. Christianson (Ed.), *Handbook of marriage and the family*. Chicago: Rand McNally, 1964.

Kimmel, D.C. *Adulthood and aging*. New York: Wiley, 1974.

Levinson, D., Darrow, C., Klein, E., Levinson, J., & McKee, B. Periods in the adult development of men: Ages 18–45. In N. Schlossberg, & A. Entine (Eds.), *Counseling adults*. Monterey, Calif.: Brooks/Cole, 1977.

Lopata, H. *Occupation: Housewife*. New York: Oxford University Press, 1971.

Lowenthal, M.F., Thurner, M., & Chiriboga, D., and Associates. *Four stages of life: A comparative study of women and men facing transitions*. San Francisco: Jossey–Bass, 1975.

Moreland, John. Some implications of life–span development for counseling psychology. *Personnel and Guidance Journal*, 1979, *57*, 299–302.

Neugarten, B.L. Adaptation and the life cycle. *Counseling Psychologist*, 1976, *6*, 16–20.

Perrucci, C., & Targ, D. (Eds.). *Marriage and the family: A critical analysis of proposals for change.* New York: McKay, 1974.

Rhodes, S.L. A developmental approach to the life cycle of the family. *Social Casework*, 1977, *58*, 301–311.

Sales, E. Women's adult development. In I. Frieze, J. Parsons, P. Johnson, D. Ruble, & G. Zellman (Eds.), *Women and sex roles*. New York: Norton, 1978.

Sheehy, G. *Passages*. New York: Dutton, 1976.

Targ, D.C. Toward a reassessment of women's experience at middle age. *The Family Coordinator*, 1979, *28*, 377–388.

Veroff, J., & Feld, S. *Marriage and work in America: A study of motives and roles*. New York: Van Nostrand, Reinhold, 1970.

Vines, N.R. Adult unfolding and marital conflict. *Journal of Marital and Family Therapy*, 1979, *5*(2), 5–14.

Part III

Interventions for Disabilities in General

Chapter 7

Lifestyle Approaches and Resistance to Change

Gail Fitzpatrick Scott

Traditionally, resistance is thought to be a marshaling of forces in the unconscious to protect the individual from painful material repressed in the unconscious. According to this line of thinking, the very defenses the person created to keep painful, conflictual material from awareness will now work against the person as he struggles to make conscious these repressions. The difficulties encountered in the course of treatment, once an appropriate contract has been negotiated, are the work of these unconscious forces. In this framework, resistance is limited to those defenses that are manifest while the client is actively engaged in counseling. This definition would exclude as "resistant" clients who were unmotivated for treatment, who honestly felt they had achieved their treatment goals and wished to terminate, or who had a real basis for determining that the counseling was not productive (Weiner, 1975).

Examples of resistance can be seen in a client's attempts to manipulate appointment times or dates, use of constant focus on issues and situations outside the counseling session, continued lack of focus or agreement on treatment goals, missed appointments, too much or too little talk, focus on the counselor and his credentials or personal life, confusion, anger, tears, etc. These defenses affect the client by influencing the degree to which—if at all—he will allow himself to be a client.

Resistance is evident at every stage in counseling and reflects the client's use of self and interpersonal style. According to Weiner (1975), resistance always serves to impede communication and it was because of this that Freud first saw it as something to be overcome at all costs. Later the concept was expanded to include a need to understand and utilize these forces in the counseling process. As a here-and-now phenomenon, resistance is actually seen as enhancing the process.

I wish to gratefully acknowledge the assistance of Robert N. Glenn, Ph.D., in the editing of this chapter.

Traditionally speaking, however, the unconscious forces are still seen as inhibiting growth by blocking access to the unconscious, and, as such, ". . . it is one of the critical psychoanalytic tasks to uncover and overcome these resistances" (Loew, Grayson, & Loew, 1975, p. 28).

THEORY OF COHERENCE

Adler and, more recently, Dell (1982a) view resistance in a different light. Although the word "resistance" is found throughout Adlerian literature, the general underlying assumption is that there is no such thing as a truly "resistant" client, but rather a "discrepancy between the goals of the counselor and those of the patient" (Dreikurs, 1967, p. 65).

Dell also sees resistance as an immanent and integral part of the system (i.e., the person, family, or institution, etc.); an appropriate metaphor is the act of pushing against a brick building and failing to make it move—the "resistance" is due to the nature of the building and not the building "being resistant." This view involves a shift from the traditional definition of a part of the system as defender of the status quo (homeostasis), which resists all pulls to disrupt that stability, to one where the system is seen as holistic and homeostasis as the nature of it.

Dell (1982a) proposed to replace both the concept of homeostasis and the traditional views of resistance with a theory of coherence. Central to his theory is the concept of a "coherently organized system" that includes both apparent stability at times as well as the creative ability to change. That is, the system will continue to move toward a steady state (homeostasis) in accordance with its own coherence until something is introjected that is disruptive to its present organization. Every behavior of the person emanates from this coherence and in turn affects the coherence; hence, the system is constantly in a state of evolution. Homeostasis is, therefore, seen as a fluid state that either evolves in a fashion dictated by the coherence of the person or as a result of disruption. Once disrupted, the system will seek a new steady state (homeostasis). The system will change with disruption, but until then, it continues to behave in the fashion in which it is organized. The system can only behave in a manner dictated by its coherence. Put very simply, the result is a theory that proposes that the system is "what it is."

LIFESTYLE

This concept of a coherently organized system is the cornerstone of Dell's theory and of Adler's lifestyle concept. The lifestyle is essentially the compilation of the "what is" as understood and experienced by the child. As such it contains much that is distorted, biased, and idiosyncratic. As the child struggles to make sense out of chaos, he develops an idea of what life is all about and how best to meet its demands. Over a period of time all behavior becomes organized in a unified pattern (i.e., the lifestyle) around these early convictions about life.

The lifestyle is the blueprint of the overall movement of the person toward a subjectively determined goal (to be number one or on top, to be inadequate or protected, always to be right, never to make a mistake, etc.). According to Adler, the overall movement of the person is from a minus to a plus, that is, in the direction of feeling OK about oneself (Shulman, 1973). The subjectively determined goals are in the service of the overriding goal. An individual determines, for example, that the best way to feel good about himself is to always be number one, to be taken care of by others, to be disruptive or inadequate, etc. The lifestyle becomes progressively more selective as it is refined by the person. The coherence of the system determines how and what new experiences will be perceived. Of interest here is the contention that this internal coherence allows for a constancy from situation to situation, so that if the lifestyle is understood, behavior can often be predicted. Shulman (1973) notes that "what remains flexible is the ability to find new and better ways of striving toward the goal inherent in the existing lifestyle" (p. 7).

According to Shulman, "The lifestyle provides an overview of personality in several dimensions; the concept of the self, the view of the world, the basic motivations and the usual methods of operation" (p. 42). Components of the lifestyle are revealed through the convictions a person holds—life is, I am, people are. The convictions are the expression of reality, the "what is" as experienced by the person. The person responds to life "as if" the internal reality were, in fact, reality.

LIFESTYLE IMPLICATIONS

The goals established by a child clearly will not allow for a smooth transition at all developmental stages. The lifestyle by its nature limits the data the person perceives, serving to narrow options and stifle creativity. Obviously, in those areas where the lifestyle and reality coincide there is little or no dissonance. Conversely, when they do not reflect one another accurately or there is no complementarity, there is pain and disruption in the system. Since the person is coherently organized, disruption or complementarity (i.e., interaction that allows the system to continue "as is") must occur as a result of interaction with other systems (individuals, groups, institutions, etc.). However, it is the coherence (lifestyle) of the individual system that is the main determinant in the interactional process and not the coherence of the larger system. Therefore, the individual is always the key to change no matter how large or complex the system with which the counselor is faced.

The coherence of the system will indicate those disruptions that will begin the process toward the desired changes. This is a crucial concept. Translated to counseling it means that a client is not seen as resistant. Rather, the client is seen as being organized in a way that includes a coherent set of goals and concomitant behaviors. Counseling then becomes a matter of understanding and appreciating the underlying goals and behaviors and helping the client decide whether or not he wants to change them. To understand the lifestyle of the person is to understand the coherence that dictates his reality.

REALITY PRINCIPLE

The reality principle states that "things are what they are, not what we want or expect" (Dell, 1982a, p. 30). The system is governed by the reality principle because it can act only in accordance with its own coherence and never in a way in which it is not organized. It can only be what it is. The more adaptive the lifestyle the more in touch with reality. Adler states that lifestyles that are "more sound are in accordance with common sense" (reality), while those that are less sound are more founded in "private idiosyncratic logic" (Shulman, 1973, p. 201).

To maintain a reality base a system needs to rely upon its own internal organization and its connection with other systems. The more aware and accepting a person is of his own lifestyle (internal organization) and of other systems (external organization), the more easily he can maintain his own identity in interactions. By accepting that he is what he is and that they are what they are, he can avoid the pitfall of either refusing to accept things as they are or of feeling he must do something to change the way things are (Dell, 1982a). The ability of the system to productively connect and disconnect with other systems is closely related to its ability to accept its self as it is.

The higher the level of adaptability within the system, the more amenable it is to change. The opportunity for change is provided when responses to new demands are not available. The client is usually not aware of this potential for change. Creativity is a key concept in the process, allowing perception of new patterns in response to new data. It is here that counselor interventions can be the catalyst for change. Before moving to a discussion of the change process, it is important to look at some of the implications for the counselor of viewing resistance in this way.

IMPLICATIONS FOR THE COUNSELOR

As noted previously, resistance is seen as the nature of the particular organization (lifestyle) of the person and cannot be separated from the whole. It is simply the system being itself. This interpretation of resistance carries with it some clear indications for counseling.

The system appears resistant when its reality is denied. Understanding the lifestyle is the first task the counselor must undertake after a treatment contract has been agreed upon. Incidentally, without a contract there is no counseling. The process of establishing a contract will help weed out the unmotivated client who has applied for services only because of external pressure to do so. An example is a rehabilitation client who receives a monthly disability check because he is too nervous to hold a steady job. He will be referred to counseling as part of the rehabilitation process. However, the secondary gains of his disability (not having to work for a living) if coupled with certain lifestyles (e.g., I am weak and need someone to take care of me) are reinforcing and leave him unmotivated to change. Unmotivated clients employ such tactics as missing scheduled appointments, repeatedly arriving late, failing to establish an appropriate treatment contract, constant avoidance of ownership of problems, marked lack of anxiety or intensity while discussing problem situations, etc. Counseling will not work in these cases, unless something in the system changes.

Understanding the lifestyle will prevent attempting to effect change against the flow of the system thereby creating a "resistant client." This knowledge may be of particular importance to the rehabilitation client who, along with significant others, struggles to adjust to a debilitating disease or injury that demands major changes in his life. These clients often seem to "resist" what medical science and reality dictate. For example, a high-ranking civilian in the military became blinded by a freak accident while overseas. Following his recovery and return home, he became progressively less active in the family and made few attempts to do anything for himself. A lifestyle possibility is that he was a man who felt good about himself when he was in charge and had others in his service. Following his accident he continued in this mode but now as an invalid who controlled others by being totally dependent and depressed.

The temptation here for the counselor is to either become the "eyes" of the client and find out all about the resources available or to push him to take advantage of the resources offered. In reality, however, the more active the counselor becomes, the more passive or resistant the client will seem.

Indications to the counselor that treatment is not progressing are twofold: (1) signs of resistance on the part of the client and (2) counselor attempts to take responsibility for the client, i.e., to convince the client of necessary changes, to push him in a certain direction or toward a particular goal, or to problem solve with the client. When this happens, the client, his support system, and, particularly, the counselor become discouraged and frustrated. They may be tempted to give up and see the client as either unmotivated or unready for counseling. However, in the context presented here, what this indicates is that the lifestyle is not understood and that the counselor needs to back up and learn more about the coherence underlying the client's behavior. A rule of thumb is that if the counselor feels stuck or if he perceives the client as resistant he needs to go back and get more data.

Resistance in counseling indicates simply that the counselor has insufficient or inaccurate information about the coherence.

The focus of the counselor is therefore on understanding the overriding goals of the system and not on selected behaviors. This focus will remain throughout treatment as individual behaviors and patterns gain meaning in the course of being seen as attempts to meet the overriding goals. All behavior is purposeful. The payoff to the counselor is that he does not have to have an agenda. The client contains all the elements necessary for his own cure.

CHANGE PROCESS

The disruption that is essential to the change process occurs first prior to entry into the mental health system. It is this disruption that propels a person to seek counseling. Systems that are more amenable to change are those where the disruption is constant to the coherence (as with the loss of a limb). Disruption must be continual for the system to want to change. Consciously the person may not "know" that his coherence has been violated, but he will demonstrate it subjectively by an affective expression, i.e., anxiety or depression. If feelings remain intense and pervasive enough, the system will be disrupted and will seek a new homeostasis. People generally respond to a crisis by making an immediate effort to change. When typical problem-solving techniques do not produce the desired results and the pain continues, the individual is most open to change.

Change is an arduous process that requires a clear commitment toward a steady course of action, a commitment to constancy. Thus, if a client wishes to be a nonsmoker he must first make that decision and then constantly reinforce that goal by thoughts and actions. Over a period of time if he continues practicing being a nonsmoker, there will emerge a new coherence in his thinking, behavior, and biological functioning that is consistent with his nonsmoking (Dell, 1982a). This commitment to new behaviors practiced over a period of time will lead to a system change. This represents change. It is a slow process of which the person is often unaware. Keeney and Sprenkle (1982) maintain that "one can choose to be different or, 'see differently' only by a commitment to a different context in which one patiently practices and waits" (p. 13). It is the job of the counselor to help the client clarify for himself what he is willing to do to reach his stated goals. Change can even include not changing "problem" behaviors. The acceptance of oneself as is can be enough of a resolution to allow for a new homeostasis.

THE ROLE OF SYMPTOMS AND CONFLICT

Central to this is a view of symptoms as creative attempts by the person to reach his goals. In this vein, Morita Therapy suggests that "once you are friendly with your symptoms and accept them as a reality, you will find yourself cured—able to function—whether or not you still have them. . . . One of the main aims of the treatment is to persuade the patient not to eradicate his symptoms by force of will'' (Mozdzierez, Macchitelli, & Lisiecki, 1976, p. 169). Once the purpose of the symptom is understood by the client, the options for a more appropriate response can be considered and the decision to change be made.

A client can remain symptomatic after accepting his lifestyle and after understanding the purpose of his symptom. In these circumstances he does so because he feels unable to meet his established goals. The symptom or conflict keeps him from facing his goals and provides the benefit of secondary gains. For example, a client feels he must do a perfect job and yet is faced with certainty of a poor performance on the GED pre-exams that he needs to take for assessment purposes. The method he uses to avoid this is to be too nervous to study for the exam and/or too busy in his daily life to make time to study. As long as he does not study and does not take the exam, he does not need to face the failure he anticipates. If the counselor can help his client see and accept the protective qualities of his symptom or conflict, then he can give permission to the client (or have the client give himself permission) to continue doing what he is doing until he no longer needs the protection. The key is to tell the client that he will know when he can stop. This puts the client in charge of the symptom. By encouraging the client to do as he already was doing, i.e., not studying, the counselor avoids a resistant client who would have found a reason not to study. As it turned out in an actual case, sometime later the client announced that he had made arrangements to take the test. Prior to this decision, the exam had not been an issue in the counseling for quite some time.

A variation of this idea that is beneficial at times is symptom prescription. The symptom is encouraged by prescribing it and increasing its frequency—the client need not be aware of the purpose served by the behavior. For example, a client complained of not falling asleep for several hours after retiring and of then waking early. She was feeling very stressed about her relationship with her boyfriend and could not stop thinking about it especially at bedtime. She was told to spend two hours every night prior to bedtime at the kitchen table (no TV, radio, calls, etc.) in concentrated worry about this worrisome situation. She was further told that if she awoke during the night clearly she had not spent enough time thinking about this problem and should arise and spend one hour again at the kitchen table before going back to bed. The counselor respectfully accepted the client's assessment that this was an enormous problem that required an excessive amount of worry. She was instructed to save her worrying for these special times when she could really concentrate on them and not to bother with them during the day.

Initially, the client followed the instructions although she found them somewhat inconvenient. Within a few weeks she reported that she no longer had any sleep disturbance. She was told to repeat this procedure if the problem reoccurred. Whereas prior to the symptom prescription, she had spent a good deal of energy trying to avoid the worrisome thoughts she had, with the prescription she was told that her worry was justified and should be done more purposively and consciously. An added benefit in this case was that it helped the client verbalize her fears.

By going with the flow, symptom prescription will often result in the client decreasing the behavior he has been instructed to maintain or increase. As a result this technique has been erroneously labeled as paradoxical intention. A paradox is defined as a statement or a doctrine that is "seemingly absurd or contradictory but possibly or demonstrably true" (*Funk & Wagnalls New Standard Dictionary of the English Language*, 1963, p. 1790). Dell (1982b) challenges the existence of a paradox, maintaining that the phenomenon "exists only in the crack between human expectation on the one hand and the actuality of the world on the other hand" (p. 40). By debunking the myth of the paradoxical intention, one is left with the reality principle. Things are what they are and it is only our faulty understanding that causes them to appear paradoxical to us.

The acceptance or the accentuation of the situation as it is can disrupt the system enough to allow new solutions to emerge. Acceptance provides an opportunity for the therapist to "spit in the client's soup" (to borrow Adler's phrase) by reminding him of the choice he is making, thereby depriving him of the secondary gains of the symptom or conflict, i.e., not being in control of the symptom. These techniques make the process more conscious and less effective and, thus, pave the way for change.

Before moving to the discussion of the role of the creative process in counseling, it would be helpful to review the treatment process to this point. When resistance is seen as something to be overcome, the counselor is primed to do battle with the client no matter how subtly. This sets up a win/lose framework with defeat a certainty for either the counselor or the client. However, assuming that only the system can elect to change within the limits of its organization, then all seemingly "resistant" behaviors can be accepted as integral parts of the system rather than a response to counseling. The counselor cannot be defeated if he goes with "what is" and works to uncover the coherence.

The primary task of the counselor is to understand the lifestyle and the problem areas defined by the client. The resistance he meets is really an adherence to an internal organization (i.e., lifestyle/coherence) that allows the client to reject avenues of change that are not in accordance with that coherence. The client who enters counseling is experiencing a disruption in his coherence or in the avenues he has chosen to maintain that coherence. The individual needs to recognize this disparity and decide what he wants to do about it. Knowledge of the lifestyle will clarify both the coherence and the supporting behavior patterns. The major tool the counselor has in preparing the client for a decision and the creative process is educating the client as to the purposes of the maladaptive behavior. Interventions that move away from a control (other) focus and toward an internal (I) focus are effective in the education process.

THE CREATIVE PROCESS

Respect for the creative process is an important theme for Adlerians. They see the lifestyle as a creative response to the system's need for a holistic, coherent, unifying blueprint for behavior. Symptoms are viewed as a creative response by the system to the perceived or real inability of the system to meet its goals. Change is the creative process whereby new solutions or ideas are incorporated in the lifestyle.

Brain Functioning

Adlerians purport that the lifestyle operates at a "dimly conscious" level. With an increased awareness of the goals and attendant behavior patterns, the client is in a better position to decide how he wants things to be. However, because of the complexity of the system and the systems with which it interacts, "conscious knowing is limited to our awareness of a fragment of the whole system or context within which we are an interactant" (Keeney & Sprenkle, 1982, p. 15). The lifestyle will always remain to some degree unknowable and therefore unavailable to the client except at a dimly conscious or unconscious level (i.e., right brain). The creative process allows the client to tap into the vast material and processes of the right brain and utilize this wisdom in meeting his goals. Just as the coherence is only partly knowable, so too are the solutions or answers the client seeks. Keeney and Sprenkle (1982) argue that "any attempt to *know* the answer involves translating it into a left brain, manipulative side" (p. 15), thereby reducing it to a problem-solving activity. Keeping the client focused in left brain activities enhances refinement and building in problem-solving skills and is an appropriate adjunct to counseling. However, focus on left brain functions is only the first step in the creative process, i.e., preparation. Motamedi (1982) explained that

> much of the mental activity critical to the creative process emanates from the unconscious. However, it is likely that . . . the journey requires the flexibility to shift between and across different styles of thinking and working. The successful outcome seems to depend on the ability to integratively use the two hemispheres of the brain. Both the analytic left hemisphere, specializing, by and large, in language and reduction, and the holistic right, specializing in visual tasks, rhythm and composition, contribute to the creative outcome. The creative journey necessitates the concretization and abstraction of events, as well as mutual interaction of past and present experiences. (p. 82)

The implications here for the counselor are that once the lifestyle has been defined, the counselor may be most helpful by not pushing the client toward specific goals or outcomes. Believing and behaving as though one has no control over the choice the client will now make often results in the client moving toward a decision, thus avoiding resistance (Keeney & Sprenkle, 1982). This approach relies on the assumption that at a deeper level (i.e., right brain), the individual already "knows" how best to respond to maintain or change his coherence. This allows the counselor to let things remain vague and unhurried while the client struggles to make sense out of it all. Keeney and Sprenkle (1982) propose that the counselor's "participation in therapy has more to do with being alive than creating specific outcomes" (p. 16).

A CASE EXAMPLE

Essential to the treatment contract is trusting the system (i.e., individual, family, etc.) to fashion responses that can best meet its needs. A case involving a young single woman illustrates this premise. Her presenting problem was chronic depression. The approach used in this case was threefold: (1) to use the lifestyle as a tool to demonstrate her primary goals, which were "I want to be special and protected" (Daddy's little girl), "Life is full of demands, therefore, I have to avoid displeasing others;" (2) to provide ample opportunities for her to experience how the behavior patterns she had developed to meet these goals worked both for and against her; and (3) to utilize the anxiety she experienced as an aid in pushing her to dig deeper for her own answers.

The client's lifestyle was presenting difficulties for her in her relationship with her parents, her boyfriend, and on the job. She regularly chose to relate to people whom she felt were more knowledgeable than she and then felt angry and resentful when she felt she could not live up to their expectations. This became an issue early in our relationship as she tried to get me to be the expert and then berated me for judging her. The temptation here was to be the competent one and provide answers that would have ended up with her either dropping out of counseling (as she had in the past) or becoming resistant. Instead my interventions were geared to have her gain in competency as treatment progressed. For example, I would be confused or unsure and ask for more information, thereby putting her in the position of explaining to me.

The focus throughout was to have her explore and to understand increasingly from an internal (I) reference what the problems she had meant to her. She entered counseling because her usual patterns of pleasing others were not working in several areas of her life and this was causing her to feel suicidal. With her focus on pleasing others, she felt panicked when she could no longer pull that off. Even while gathering the lifestyle information, I pushed her to explore what that meant to her and what she wanted for herself. Her panic increased when I refused to give her answers. A basic premise that was reinforced often was that she was in control and would generate better solutions to her problems when the time came. Her panic was normalized and she was given permission to back out of counseling at those points if she so desired. Each time that happened she declined to drop out, reaffirming her intention to resolve her difficulties. One response, when faced with her panic at not knowing an answer, was that she could be curious instead of panicky. The first few times the panic was overwhelming and immobilizing. However, she did begin to explore the feelings, and the realization that she could tolerate them allowed her the freedom to continue to do so. After the initial breakthrough, most of this work was done outside the sessions.

Once she made the decision to take the risk to shift her focus (i.e., when it presented a problem) from pleasing others to pleasing herself, the educational phase was intensified. I instructed her to be aware of certain behaviors or patterns on a regular basis and to be curious rather than judgmental about the way she interacted. This allowed her to formulate for herself what kept her repeating painful, nonproductive interactions and to consider what behaviors or consequences she wanted to change. Again the emphasis was on having her interpret and define and tell me. Opportunities were provided in the session for her to explore the fears she identified through the interventions of role playing, guided fantasy, and the empty chair procedure (see below). These techniques allowed her to explore more fully the things she feared and to formulate possible responses. The purpose was to increase her flexibility in situations she previously avoided or felt stuck in and to encourage her sense of mastery as she refined her responses.

One way to neutralize fears presented is to have the client tell the counselor if he could survive such an ordeal and, if so, what would be the consequences. This forces him to go beyond the surface response of panic and most often he will grudgingly admit that he could survive. The counselor now has an opportunity to encourage him and to explore resources not previously known. Pat answers at this stage may provide immediate relief for the client but circumvent the creative process and hamper change by strengthening the notion that the counselor and/or others have the solution. Rather, suggestions or interventions offered by the counselor should encourage the use of internal resources to find answers.

Underlying this approach is the assumption that change is decided by the person and not by the counselor. As long as the counselor's interventions are in the direction of a healthier organization, he can relax knowing the client will respond to whatever makes sense to him. This reinforces the notion that the counselor is more effective when responding from his own internal reference than in following "cookbook cures."

The approach presented in this chapter can be used in the vast majority of counseling cases. To summarize: it requires (1) knowledge of the lifestyle, (2) exploration of the problem areas to determine the discrepancies between the established goals of the system and the client's current reality, (3) decision by the client to work to correct the discrepancies or to accept things the way they are, and

(4) commitment to practice regularly those behaviors that will bring about the desired changes in the system. Creativity is the silent partner in this process and is present any time change occurs. Sengel and Shurley (1978–79) found that with the increase of pertinent data there is a greater probability of a "significant new combination or synthesis" (p. 222). This means that even when the focus of treatment is on left brain input (e.g., problem solving, educational activities, guidance), the counselor is, in fact, preparing the client for the creative process and, therefore, change. Change is the inherent goal of counseling.

COUNSELING STRATEGIES

Once the decision to change has been made, there are numerous interventions available to help the client in this process. The techniques discussed here will have the common theme of encouraging the client through creative use of internal resources to fashion his own solutions or directions. Although people regularly and naturally fluctuate in and out of the right brain, they do so with limited awareness. The counselor's task is to make the transition more explicit, more available, and more focused when change is required.

The creative process requires integration of the functions of the left and right brain. Gowan's (1979) description of the creative process is the basis for this discussion. The left hemisphere prepares the person for the creative journey by accumulating adequate information about the problem. It completes the process by synthesizing concretizing, and applying the creative insights achieved during the middle phase. The middle stages are dominated by the right brain and require the ability to shut down the input and activity of the left brain and to attend to internal stimuli. Without the integration of the hemispheres, the middle phase would be nothing more than a pleasurable activity. Leaffer (1982) maintains that "hemispheric interaction contributes to a higher level of consciousness, to a heightened aesthetic appreciation and creativity and to integration of the mind" (p. 250). Therefore, techniques that combine the verbal abilities of the left hemisphere with the imagery of the right brain will be most effective in achieving this end. The intent of the counselor is to disrupt the normal flow—typical ways of thinking—of the client, creating an "unusual condition" that can often initiate the creative process (Sengel & Shurley, 1978–79). The techniques described here encourage the use of both hemispheres and provide opportunities for the client to experience the problem in a new way.

Humor

The use of humor in the Adlerian lifestyle approach is extensive. Elevating the lifestyle to its absurd conclusions and prompting the client to act "as if" it were a reality allows the client to face the consequences or discrepancies of the choices he has made in a less intense way. Humor should never be at the expense of the client but rather with full respect for the lifestyle he has fashioned. Biondi (1981) cited research that has shown that when information is followed by a humorous anecdote it is more often remembered; furthermore, ''when the joke or humorous anecdote was in some way relevant to the key learning point, the greatest degree of retention was registered'' (p. 75).

Rule conducted several quasi-experiments that indicate that the ability to laugh at the dysfunctional elements of one's lifestyle leads to decreased negative feelings (1977) and increased internal focus of control (1979). His research in this area is related to the notion that an unhostile sense of humor is a significant indication of the healthy individual. Ellis (1976) also utilizes humor to help crack the ''musturbatory,'' absolutizing way clients have chosen to think, act, and feel about life.

Imagery

With the technique of imagery the focus is on accessing the right brain directly, using guided fantasy, dreams/daydreams, relaxation, and meditation. The more aware of and comfortable with himself the counselor is the freer he will be to trust his internal processes and respond to the client from his right brain. This reinforces the earlier discussion regarding the counselor's main tool being his humanity and use of self.

Using guided fantasy the counselor suggests an experience for the client to participate in with focus on feelings and sensations. Wenger's (1981) variation of this technique has the client develop his own fantasy and then describe it out loud in minute detail as he is experiencing it. He feels this will expand and refine the client's ''conscious awareness of the response and behaviors of the right parietal lobe and what that lobe shows (the client) at every moment about all that matters'' (Wenger, 1981, p. 77). Verbalizing develops and embellishes the ''language'' of the right brain so that it is more accessible.

Relaxation and meditation serve to minimize the left brain input. This allows the person to focus inwardly and attend to internal feelings, fluctuations, and stimuli. Gowan (1979) contends that the right brain is always functioning, but that we must stop to hear it. The client should be encouraged to describe feelings and the ensuing images. These descriptions can provide metaphors that will facilitate a cooperative interaction between the left and right brain. Such cooperation expands the client's awareness of the complexity of the system that is intuitively understood at the right brain level. (This reaffirms the conviction that the client ''knows'' at some level what is best for him and that the role of the counselor is to prepare him to hear it.) Facilitating an inward focus is the most powerful tool we have as counselors in helping clients create a more satisfying life.

Mosak and LeFevre (1976) proposed a number of techniques that enhance the use of self in conflict resolution. These include the following four techniques:

1. The empty chair technique helps clarify the bipolar, circular structure of conflict (i.e., a "damned if I do and damned if I don't" situation) and enables the client to go beyond the intellectualization of it. The client defines the two sides of the conflict and speaks from a different chair when supporting each side. This can also be used when the conflict is an internal one, e.g., around the "good me" and the "bad me." As he develops the argument to support each side, the client is forced to go inward and will become aware of previously obscured thoughts and feelings. One chair will begin to feel more right than the other. The nonverbal right brain input of feeling and movement are the most valuable feedback from this exercise.

2. Another technique is to have the client imagine himself at some point in the future (6 months, 3 years, etc.). As the client is imagining this, the counselor asks him to visualize meeting him on the street and explaining where he would be vis-à-vis the conflict. This use of fantasy can help bring the person out of the currently stuck position by reviewing how things will be different in the future. It has the added value of establishing a time limit accepted by the client for enduring this conflict. An example would be a college freshman in conflict over a career choice. He may state that in six months he would still be confused but intends to declare his major at the end of his sophomore year. He has allowed himself a period of over a year to come to a resolution. The counselor can point this out and suggest that he stop pressuring himself to make a decision and use the energy and time more productively.

3. Techniques such as the one mentioned above foster emotional distance from the conflict. This allows the client to assess the situation more realistically. A variation on this theme is to have the client imagine himself as a little bird perched on his tombstone and reading the epitaph. Would the conflict be long forgotten or is it important enough to get final notice? This technique involves some ability on the part of the client to laugh at himself, which decreases the intensity of the emotions that maintain the conflict.

4. The counselor can have the client guess at the probability of his deciding the conflict one way or another. The counselor can insist that a 50-50 probability is, in reality, a vote for no change, a resolution that likewise involves a decision on the part of the client.

Role Playing and Psychodrama

Both role playing and psychodrama allow the client to act in an "as if" manner that can shed light on aspects of himself and/or others that may have remained obscured. Role playing allows a client to "try on" a new role or to experiment with an existing one in a safe environment. This may pave the way for a healthier adjustment to that role by helping the client identify problem areas he had not been aware of previously. Role playing also can provide a greater appreciation of the demands of the role of a significant other with whom the client is experiencing difficulties. Psychodrama offers a facilitative "extra" by encouraging the client to create a new ending to an old conflict. This can provide powerful reframing or closure experiences that one might not be able to duplicate in reality but that may satisfy needs at a deeper (right brain) level.

A clear omission to a list of techniques designed to involve the right parietal lobe in the counseling process is the use of hypnosis and trance. Hypnosis provides a direct path to the imagery of the right brain. However, a discussion of the level of sophistication and training required to utilize this technique is beyond the scope of this chapter.

What we have considered is a partial list of techniques, suggestions, and exercises that could be utilized by the counselor without specialized training. These interventions produce results in the more normal states of consciousness, i.e., "daydreaming, fantasy, meditation creative spells, relaxation, sensory deprivation and the like where the ego and full memorability are present" (Gowan, 1979, p. 42). The role of the counselor is to help the client tap into and develop or refine those creative spaces he normally fluctuates through. The client struggles during this stage will often be painful, frightening, and confusing. There will be a strong temptation for the counselor to "rescue" the client by providing him with the answers. He can best resist this urge by reminding himself and the client that the best answers will come from the client's internal creative process. This belief is central to the ideas presented in this chapter.

SUMMARY

A theme of unity and integrity is central to both Dell's theory of coherence and Adler's lifestyle concept. It is a marriage of ideas that allows for both the simplicity and clearness of theory as well as the complexity of the system that is inherent in both approaches. The lifestyle is viewed as the blueprint of the coherence of the system. The reality principle dictates that the system is what it is and not what the person or the counselor would like it to be or thinks it should be. Given this framework, resistance can be seen as the system's adherence to its internal organization. Therefore, when resistance is encountered in counseling, it suggests a misunderstanding based on insufficient or inadequate data. This can best be rectified by further exploration. Furthermore, this approach streamlines and focuses counselor interventions.

Once the lifestyle is understood and the problem areas defined, the client is ready to make the decision about what changes he wants to make. The targeted behaviors or patterns are then explored in a manner consciously geared to push the client inward toward his creative resources. The solutions and ideas generated are then carefully examined using left brain functions (i.e., verbalizing, describing, concretizing) to determine their validity and the best way to operationalize them.

It is hoped that the framework suggested here will stimulate exploration of the extensive literature available on creativity and change. The usefulness of any counseling approach is in its ability to facilitate change. It is in the creative phase that the real value of these theories lies, because they both allow for change as a natural, evolving process within the confines of the coherence as established by the system.

REFERENCES

Biondi, M. On the magic of your mind. *Journal of Creative Behavior,* 1981, *1*(2), 75.

Dell, P. Beyond homeostasis: Toward a concept of coherence. *Family Process,* 1982, *21*(1), 21–24. (a)

Dell, P. Family theory and the epistemology of Humberto Maturana. *Family Therapy Networker,* 1982, *6*(4), 26, 39–41. (b)

Dreikurs, R. *Psychodynamics, psychotherapy, and counseling.* Chicago: Alfred Adler Institute, 1967.

Ellis, A. Paper presented at the national convention of the American Psychological Association, Washington, D.C., September 1976.

Funk & Wagnalls New Standard Dictionary of the English Language. New York: Funk & Wagnalls, 1963.

Gowan, J.D. The production of creativity through right hemisphere imagery. *Journal of Creative Behavior,* 1979, *13*(1), 39–51.

Keeney, B.P., & Sprenkle, D.H. Ecosystemic epistemology: Critical implications for the aesthetics and pragmatics of family therapy. *Family Process,* 1982, *21*(1), 1–21.

Leaffer, T. Left brain–right brain: Domination or cooperation. *Journal of Creative Behavior,* 1982, *16*(2), 75–88.

Loew, C.A., Grayson, H., & Loew, G.H. (Eds.), *Three psychotherapies.* New York: Brunner/Mazel, 1975.

Montamedi, K. Extending the concept of creativity. *Journal of Creative Behavior,* 1982, *16*(2), 75–88.

Mosak, H.H., and LeFevre, C. The resolution of "intrapersonal conflict." *Journal of Individual Psychology,* 1976, *32*(1), 19–26.

Mozdzierz, G.J., Macchitelli, F.J., & Lisiecki, J. The paradox in psychotherapy: An Adlerian perspective. *Journal of Individual Psychology,* 1976, *32*(2), 169–184.

Rule, W. Increasing self-modeled humor. *Rational Living,* 1977, *12*(1), 1–4.

Rule, W. Increased internal-control using humor with lifestyle awareness. *The Individual Psychologist,* 1979, *16*(3), 16–20.

Sengel, R.A., & Shurley, J.T. Stability and creativity: Modeling a psychoneural mechanism. *Journal of Altered States of Consciousness,* 1978–79, 4(3), 217–225.

Shulman, B.H. *Contributions to individual psychology.* Chicago: Alfred Adler Institute, 1973.

Weiner, I.B. *Principles of psychotherapy.* New York: Wiley, 1975.

Wenger, W. Creative creativity: Some strategies for developing specific areas of the brain used for working both sides together. *Journal of Creative Behavior,* 1981, *15*(2), 77–89.

Chapter 8

Medical Information and Lifestyle Counseling for Adjustment to Disability

Patricia C. Franco

Darwin's "survival of the fittest" takes on new meaning in light of recent medical and technological advances. An increasing number of people are surviving traumatic events and life-threatening illness to an extent never before realized. The price for survival often is physical disability and psychological sequelae that vary considerably according to the cause, treatment, and outcome of the medical condition.

THE COUNSELOR'S ROLE

Regardless of theoretical orientation or practice setting, today's counselor, in becoming an integral member of the treatment team, is faced with a greater demand to be conversant with the medical aspects of disability. The movement toward a holistic approach to rehabilitation requires an understanding of inter-disciplinary roles and more meaningful communication. The counselor must be able effectively to incorporate incoming medical information into counseling goals and to provide other professionals with psychosocial information consistent with their treatment objectives.

The consumer movement in rehabilitation fosters a spirit of self-determination as the disabled assume greater responsibility for their care. More frequently individuals are being asked to participate in treatment decisions that ultimately influence the quality of their lives. To keep pace with these changes, the counselor must know the factors that precipitated the disabling condition and the unique problems it poses immediately and over the long run.

The counselor is the one professional whose primary vested interest is the patient's adaptation to these new circumstances. His charge is to explore recommended treatment options and the possible consequences of each. If, indeed, alternative solutions exist, or if there is confusion related to expected outcome, the patient must be referred back to appropriate professionals for clarification. In some instances the counselor may be asked to take a more active advocacy role, for example, helping the patient phrase questions designed to get specific information, or, if necessary, becoming the patient's spokesman.

Finally, the very essence of lifestyle counseling is to establish a linkage between the patient's subjective view of his situation and an objective impression gleaned from medical data. With a given disease process or disabling condition, despite variations relative to individual physiologic response, there are certain realities derived from available medical information. How a person processes this information and whether or not he uses it advantageously may be the primary focus of counseling intervention. The reverse also is true in that knowledge gained from an understanding of premorbid personality may be used to enhance the medical management of a specific case.

ASPECTS OF DISABILITY

There are significant differences in the etiology, diagnosis, and treatment of most disabling conditions. Accordingly, the course and outcome of each may vary considerably. Such factors bear heavily on psychosocial adjustment, making it a more fluid process to be considered across the continuum of a lifespan. Just as each normal developmental period superimposes different tasks, which, in turn, create different problems, many disabilities in fact change over time, either as a result of this development, or because of the nature of the condition itself.

Onset

Facts about the onset of disability may present issues for counseling. If the disability was trauma related, what role does the individual assume or assign to himself or others in bringing about this unfortunate event? What are the feelings related to this role—guilt or anger—and how does this response fit one's lifestyle?

Take, for example, the middle-aged homemaker who suffered mild facial scarring secondary to burns sustained in a kitchen fire and who refused to leave her home years after the incident. Despite the availability of special cosmetics with which she could achieve a reasonably good appearance, she consistently relied on family members to get groceries and so on. This minor inconvenience became a constant reminder of her suffering and kept others in her service long after it was necessary.

The onset of disability may also be insidious, as in a malignancy, unjustly causing feelings of guilt, self-blame, regret ("If only I had done this or that") or anger ("How did the physician overlook these symptoms?"). The time lapse between discovery of symptoms and that of seeking medical attention, especially if there is an unreasonably long delay, may be important issues to explore. Some diseases respond better to early diagnosis and treatment, resulting in greater control over morbidity and mortality. This is not always true, however, and may require clarification, particularly when there are feelings of unwarranted guilt or self-blame.

Course of Illness

The natural history of the disease (disability) is an important clue to expected course and outcome. A static condition obviously offers greater predictability for purposes of long-range planning. For example, following the acute phase, the patient with a spinal cord injury stabilizes at a certain level of physical function determined by the site or extent of lesion. The disability remains constant except for complications secondary to the established condition, such as decubitus ulcer, which responds well to medical management. It would be very unusual to experience wide deviation from the established level of function without a major technological breakthrough to bring this about.

Conversely, diseases that are known to be progressive produce changes that may interfere with established patterns of activity. The rate of progression will be of primary concern. Some diseases progress slowly over a period of years, while others advance rapidly resulting in dramatic shifts in functional capacity during a relatively short period of time.

R. was a 23-year-old-man diagnosed with a very aggressive soft-tissue tumor in his thigh with metastasis to the lungs. Amputation was not recommended because of the advanced stage of his disease. Radiotherapy and chemotherapy were given simultaneously instead. Except for occasional absences related to the chemotherapy schedule, R. continued to work for several months more as a delivery man. However, with full knowledge of his poor prognosis, he and his fiance advanced their wedding plans.

B., another young man of 23, discovered a similar mass in his jaw. Since this was found at a very early stage, B was treated for cure with surgery and adjuvant chemotherapy. He was advised to leave college only during the semester in which he had the surgery. He has since completed his B.S. and gone on to graduate school.

Other conditions are potentially reversible, either as a result of rehabilitation efforts, as in stroke, or a result of surgical intervention, as with coronary bypass operations and transplants. In these circumstances, the person may require assistance in returning to a normal state of affairs, exercising reasonable caution but not undue fear.

Finally, the issue of the degree of threat to one's life is often the first concern of the patient. Some disorders do, in fact, have a possibility of recurrence. This is true for heart disease as well as some forms of cancer. Again, a rational approach to interpreting statistical data is desirable so that unrealistic expectations in either direction are avoided. The patient who has a 10 percent chance for five-year survival may need to reprioritize his life's goals. In facing the fact that life is finite, even persons with a good prognosis for long-term survival decide to reconsider their goals, although, obviously, it is less urgent that they do so.

Course of Treatment

It is interesting to note the role an individual assumes in regard to initial and ongoing treatment. To what degree does he participate in treatment decisions? Does he act as his own advocate in exploring options? What compromises, if any, are being made? For example, in seeking relief from unrelenting pain, one may finally elect to have a neurosurgical procedure that will result in considerable morbidity. Or the person with end-stage renal disease (ESRD) may refuse a kidney transplant, resigning himself instead to hemodialysis a certain number of hours per week for the rest of his life.

Many diagnostic procedures with treatment modalities present a certain amount of risk to the patient. Individuals should be encouraged to give thoughtful consideration to each, before deciding if the risk outweighs potential benefit on a personal level. Here responses vary from overconcern with minimal risk to abdicating responsibility (''Whatever you think is best'') when a clear choice is involved.

Treatment plays a role in planning to the extent that it can be expected to interfere with ongoing activities. The specific modality, expected side effects, length of hospitalization, or frequency of follow-up treatments will need to be considered in order to avoid setting the patient up for failure. How the patient complies with the agreed upon regimen is also significant.

Most important, of course, will be residual disability, which may be either disease related or treatment related. The earlier the permanent effect is known, the better it can be planned for. For example, if a deficit is surgically induced, the counselor may be instrumental in preparing the patient preoperatively for anticipated changes in appearance or function. Follow-up sessions would focus on resolving the loss and facilitating adjustment to the disability. Unfortunately, most disabling conditions are much less predictable and planning must be also flexible enough to allow for individual response to a given environment. The physician or other health care professional frequently has the task of providing information to facilitate such planning. Care must be taken to present a sense of realism. Either undue optimism or undeserved pessimism are potentially harmful in the long run. Whether temporary or permanent, treatment side effects have signficant implications for psychosocial response in terms of body image, self image, and interference with normal activities.

Pharmacologic agents used in treatment may cause adverse side-effects that impact physical or psychological function. Certain anticancer drugs, for instance, are implicated in peripheral neuropathies and hearing impairments. In most cases, these toxic effects are reversed if the drug is withdrawn.

Imbalances in body chemistry may be manifested in changes in cognition or behavior. Uncharacteristic neurological symptoms, muscular weakness, mental confusion, depression, anxiety, or other affective states should be checked out with appropriate sources. In obtaining medical information, it is good practice for the counselor to inquire about potential drug reactions, chemical changes, or residual effects of long-term chemotherapy that may affect appearance or behavior. Not infrequently, concern extends to genetic considerations as well.

Lifestyle Information

Lifestyle information is a valuable tool in assessing adaptations to preexisting disability, in facilitating adjustment of the newly disabled, and in preventing further problems by encouraging the disabled individual to become cognizant of lifestyle in all aspects of everyday life. It may be useful in promoting a greater understanding of perceived or real losses and the changes that may result in established roles. Furthermore, as is indicated in other chapters in this book, other professionals may benefit from information that will enhance their effectiveness in working with a specific patient.

IMPLICATIONS FOR COUNSELING

Every medical condition, whether temporary or permanent, major or minor, will interfere in some way with expected developmental changes or established living patterns. The extent to which this occurs depends upon the unique characteristics of the disability, the individual's emotional response, the limits imposed on everyday activities, the strengths summoned to compensate for such imposition, and the quality of support from one's social system, including family, friends, and community.

A diagnostic category does not provide adequate information about the disabling effects of a certain condition. There can be tremendous variances intradisease and interdisease. Stolov (Stolov & Clowers, 1981) makes two very important points in this regard:

1. There is no one-to-one correlation between a disease and the spectrum of associated disability problems. The same disease can produce separate sets of disability problems in different individuals.
2. There is no one-to-one relationship between a disease and the amount of residual disability. Disability problems can be removed even though the disease is unchanged. (p. 2)

Strategy for Intervention

In earlier comments a deliberate attempt was made to generalize medical information on the premise that disabling conditions differ tremendously in cause and effect. Only after a specific diagnosis is given can one ask questions appropriate to the nature of the condition, recommended treatment options, and expected outcome including increased risk of secondary problems.

Here I intend to direct the discussion to my own clinical experience in oncology. The disease entity known as cancer may occur in any of the body systems. Most cancers are treated for cure or long-term control, while others advance rapidly to an uncontrolled stage terminating in death. All cancers are considered life-threatening. Therefore, treatment is potent, may last over a period of years, and may result in significant disability. An Adlerian approach to counseling in this particular setting has proven effective regardless of site or stage of disease. Focusing on choice, however limited, encourages a patient to consider his role in shaping this experience to counteract feelings of loss of control.

The newly diagnosed cancer patient, similar to the individual suffering a heart attack or other major trauma, experiences at least momentarily the ultimate stress, the threat of death. Since, according to Adlerian theory, the lifestyle "blooms" under stress, the counselor is provided valuable information in a relatively short period of time. Initially, maladaptive behavior may be maintained by those in contact with the patient who justify his reaction ("Poor guy, he doesn't know what hit him") or personalize the experience ("I'd probably be the same").

However, as his medical condition stabilizes, the patient consequently becomes accountable. Those same people who may have been solicitous in the beginning suddenly become intolerant of certain behaviors. At this point, the counselor is provided an opportunity to be more direct by sharing lifestyle information. The patient is encouraged to consider alternate ways to achieve worthy goals.

Early in the counseling relationship, the process of eliciting lifestyle information may have therapeutic value as well. During the medical workup, most patients welcome the chance to discuss themselves in a way that appears completely unrelated to their illness. The practitioner may occasionally digress to questions that provide an opportunity for the expression of current concern. Then, encouraging the patient to consider how other stressful situations may have been approached, serves to put the illness in perspective. The patient is supported in stepping back temporarily from an overwhelming situation and assisted in developing problem-solving skills. At the same time, the task of assembling a dependable support system begins with past experience indicating those who can be counted on for meeting different needs. Thus, the patient may experience movement from a fixed and hopeless position to one of realistic planning in concert with the disease or degree of impairment.

Specific problems that routinely surface in a hospital or clinic setting include miscommunication between the patient and the treatment team, misperception of treatment goals, noncompliance with prescribed treatment, and so on. Encouraging the patient to consider an issue within the context of his lifestyle may provide important clues to identifying the roots of conflict. Likewise, reasonable remedies may be found. For example, the patient who needs to feel in control might welcome the opportunity to participate in all aspects of his rehabilitation planning. Giving that patient the responsibility of scheduling his own treatments with the various professionals discourages the use of nonproductive behavior in achieving this hidden goal.

Many cancer patients opt for a curative surgical procedure including amputation, the rerouting of important body functions, or wide resection of an area resulting in significant functional or cosmetic deficits. Chemotherapy and radiotherapy may have similar, though often temporary, results. The potential gain does not diminish the insult to body image or eradicate feelings of loss, although sometimes this is difficult to acknowledge. Again, recurring dreams or other lifestyle information may give some hint as to the meaning of the sacrifice, making it accessible to counseling. The anticipated or perceived loss may be much greater than the actual loss, a problem sometimes resolved by simply clarifying medical information.

In presenting the treatment of choice, side effects thereof, and anticipated outcome, the physician bears the burden of reducing complex information to layman's terms. It is beneficial for the counselor to be present at the time of these discussions, or at least to be familiar enough with the specifics, in order to know if the patient's perception is accurate. Each patient handles this information in a uniquely different way, perhaps giving another clue to lifestyle. The person who feels like a martyr in other life situations will act accordingly. He'll endure the discomfort of troublesome side-effects without complaint, even though some measure of relief could be obtained if the problem were known. Another person might focus on the details of the treatment schedule, route of administration of medication, and all possible adverse reactions. One response is no better than another, just different. The question is whether or not it serves an adaptive function.

CASE HISTORY

The young business executive appeared undaunted by his cancer diagnosis. He quickly became capable of discussing his condition in a very knowledgeable manner, impressing everyone with his superb adjustment. About a year later he became very depressed and was referred at that time for counseling.

It was soon obvious that this individual had never dealt with the emotional aspect of his illness. He recited the clinical issues of his case with complete objectivity. The first two counseling sessions, when Mr. E. required a structured format compatible with depression, were devoted to gathering lifestyle information. His early recollections were remarkable for the lack of emotional involvement. Consistently an observer, he took in every detail of the mysterious behavior of adults. He seemed to focus on one or two unrelated elements, in each displaying endless curiosity. People were either in power or, conversely, powerless. One end of the continuum or the other. No in between. When father was around, he was clearly in charge; otherwise, things were delegated to mother. There was always order, precision, a sense of control.

This man's cognitive approach to situations, as reflected by his early recollections, dictated the format of the next few counseling sessions in which we focused on salvaging his job. Outstanding assignments were prioritized and a step-by-step plan devised to complete each task. Week by week we monitored his progress in this area, while slowly beginning to address the emotional component of his illness. A Gestalt technique, in which the patient is asked to ascribe feelings to a familiar object, enabled him to begin to express emotion. In one such exercise, he used the telephone on my desk to illustrate feelings of being overextended, of continuing to attempt to process each new demand, and of the mounting stress, which eventually led to burnout. He acknowledged feelings of frustration, anger, inadequacy, and helplessness in what had gotten to be an untenable position— business per usual despite concerns about his illness and the constant battle of adverse side-effects to treatment.

An overriding theme in his early recollections seemed to be "competent men are in charge." As he began to understand the insidiousness of his disease, he was gradually able to refocus his need to control from the disease itself to the situations created by the undulant course of remission and active disease. He became more adept at swaying with the tide rather than continually fighting it. Eventually, building flexibility into a self-imposed, rigid system became a challenge to him.

As a first-born, Mr. B. has an overriding sense of responsibility toward his family and a traditional view of the male role. Although he recognized the value of a reduced workload while undergoing aggressive treatment of his disease, his wife's desire to assist temporarily by returning to her former job was initially perceived as a threat. Within the context of lifestyle, he was able to examine these notions, finally reaching an arrangement with his wife that was mutually satisfying.

CONCLUDING REMARKS

A number of chapters in this text are specific to special populations. In reading these chapters, the reader will note that the basis of counseling intervention is a firm understanding of the underlying medical situation. Whether the condition is acute, stable, chronic, or progressive has far-reaching implications for the individual in psychological and social adaptation to the resultant disability.

From the moment of presenting symptoms, the patient experiences a loss of control, ranging from minor inconvenience to total disruption, over his environment. At least for some period of time, he is forced to cope with the fear of the unknown and to submit to various diagnostic procedures. Endless probing, invasion of privacy, emotional distress, and physical pain become commonplace. To the proposed treatment recommendations, he is expected to give a thoughtful, informed response when, in fact, he has at best a superficial understanding of the problem. The treatment may inflict pain, discomfort, toxic side-effects, disfigurement, and permanent disability.

The concomitant psychological reactions include feelings of helplessness, hopelessess, fear, anxiety, depression, loss of self-esteem, and body-image disturbance. How one struggles to resolve these feelings and to cope with social consequences involving role negotiation, job loss, or marital discord raises issues for counseling intervention.

Lifestyle counseling emphasizes increased awareness, consideration of strengths and weaknesses, exercising choice in regard to behavior change, and the learning of strategies conducive to meeting one's goals. The therapeutic climate of encouragement, which also defines a place for humor, conveys a concern for the individual. Intervention may be predictive, preventive, or remedial, making it an excellent choice for widespread application.

While the counselor's overriding purpose is not to master scientific or technical information, it is incumbent upon this practitioner to bring into the counseling arena factors that may impinge upon the problem at hand. At times a very general approach may be appropriate, while in other instances information specific to an individual is needed. Always, there must be an effort to separate hard facts from probabilities, allowing for the diversity of expression of the same disease in different individuals. The best source of specific medical information is the patient's physician and other professionals involved with his care. Conferences, professional journals, and reputable research further increase one's general knowledge of the medical aspects of disability.

REFERENCE

Stolov, W.C., & Clowers, M.R. (Eds.). *Handbook of severe disability*. Washington, D.C.: U.S. Department of Education, Rehabilitation Services Administration, 1981.

Chapter 9

Work Adjustment Techniques in Lifestyle Counseling

Robert A. Lassiter

We do not know enough about ourselves. We are ignorant about how we work, about where we fit in, and most of all about the enormous, imponderable system of life in which we are embedded as working parts.

—Lewis Thomas *(The Medusa and the Snail)*

Practitioners who work with individuals having a severe physical disability have searched for an integrated and systematic counseling approach to be used in work adjustment. One result of this effort to find or discover a useful model has been the application of lifestyle counseling in conjunction with a rational-emotive therapy approach.

This chapter includes the following components: (1) a definition of the work adjustment process that relates to the nature of the severe physical disability, (2) a description of work adjustment techniques, (3) some assumptions about the individual counseling approach as one major method or technique, with implications for strategies for intervention, and (4) a model for use in developing a lifestyle counseling approach combined with the rational-emotive approach, with consideration given to the limitations of such a system.

This chapter will explore the rehabilitation process for severely physically disabled people who have acquired a disabling condition as an adult, as opposed to those who have a congenital problem or who suffered a physical trauma at an early age.

THE WORK ADJUSTMENT PROCESS

The rehabilitation process consists of a planned, orderly sequence of services related to the total needs of the handicapped person. It is concerned primarily with

145

problems resulting from work rather than from the disability itself. Whether the counseling is provided by a rehabilitation counselor, a psychologist, a social worker, or a special education teacher, the process involves a face-to-face relationship between the handicapped client and the practitioner. This increases the likelihood that the client will move toward maximum work adjustment.

Who is the severely physically disabled person? Since medical factors alone are insufficient for deciding who is severely disabled and who is a likely candidate for rehabilitation and future employment, additional factors such as functional capacities, age, work experience, geographical location, and education must also be considered. A severely disabled person who has experienced paraplegia or quadriplegia, cancer, or a stroke (cerebral vascular accident) may or may not require some type of work adjustment program—there is no need for modifying or changing work behaviors when appropriate ones are either maintained or an adaptation has been achieved (Lassiter, Lassiter, Hardy, Underwood, & Cull, 1983).

Work adjustment specialists, then, are people who deal with severely physically handicapped people who have other difficulties related to work or who are, in general, highly troubled about work. Otherwise, the clients will be provided programs that are remedial or educational in nature or will be offered job placement services.

One of the problems that work adjustment specialists face in providing an effective program is the lack of a systematic approach that can assist the client in gaining insight about how his lifestyle works to his advantage and how it works to his disadvantage. The emphasis at the present time is on assisting the client to become more attuned to job preparation and learning more effective work behaviors. Also, there is a tendency to teach a client "adjustment to the facility," which may or may not lead to adjustment to the world of work.

As Neff (1977) points out in his book, *Work and Human Behavior,* work adjustment services as a part of the rehabilitation process have improved greatly over the past ten to fifteen years. The process has progressed from making estimates or guesses on the outcome of (inappropriate) paper and pencil tests, on to gross measurement of actual performance, through work samples and other more realistic assessment methods, and, now, to more valid job simulation and job tryout efforts. And yet, little emphasis is given to the training and development of staff in providing a method that would offer opportunities for counseling as a special element in the adjustment process.

Studies over the years related to whether people do well or poorly in work have led to professional and public acceptance of an important truism; that success in interpersonal skills is much more important than task- or work-related skills and that failure in work, more often than not, results from an inability to get along with peers, authority figures, and subordinates, and *not* from lack of job skills. Few practitioners in the field of work adjustment would question this assumption; however, in practice the teaching of specific skills for the client to use in interacting with others has never been set up in a clear and organized way.

The process of work adjustment requires a variety of experiences to help severely physically disabled people acquire numerous skills in order to be successful in the competitive labor market. Work adjustment helps them develop self-confidence, self-control, work tolerances, skills in interpersonal relations, understanding of the world of work, and a positive attitude toward work, which will aid in handling the day-to-day demands of a job.

The work adjustment process is neither a new term nor an entirely new program in the field of rehabilitation. However, this aspect of the rehabilitation process continues to be misunderstood by many people employed in related work and is also misinterpreted by many who are involved with the practice of counseling people with severe disabilities. As Hoffman (1972) said, "Work adjustment, a treatment process utilizing work or aspects of work to modify behavior, is also at times defined as an evaluative process. It is not an evaluative process but is as the words indicate, an adjustment or treatment process" (p. 5). Hoffman continues: "In work adjustment, the objectives are to determine the success or failure of the adjustment plan to determine when to terminate the work adjustment process" (p. 5).

Many rehabilitation facilities operate on the premise that all work is therapeutic and therefore a work adjustment program is nothing more than providing the client with some type of work activity. Others point out the need for a well-planned program that will look at the uniqueness of the individual and the variety of services required from a trained staff.

According to Wright (1980):

> For young people in work adjustment, many times the individual lacks the acceptable behaviors that are considered appropriate and this may result from the disability being acquired during adolescence. A somewhat similar process often occurs when adults become disabled by accidents, injury or through physical ailments. The condition may lead to incapacity or institutionalization and this will separate the disabled people from the usual work routine. Prolonged disablement without some kind of work adjustment program may lead people to lose their self esteem as well as the particular skills needed for the work. Work adjustment in a rehabilitation program results from alterations of both behavioral and attitudinal components of the personality pattern through the work experience. The objective is an adequate work personality (p. 283).

Work Adjustment Theory

The staff of the Minnesota Work Adjustment Project (Lofquist & Dawis, 1969), in a rather bold effort to provide the rehabilitation profession with a theory of work adjustment, states:

> Work adjustment is defined as the function of the degree of correspondence or agreement between an individual and his work environment. The individual brings to the job certain work abilities and vocational needs (preferences for specific reinforcing or rewarding conditions in jobs). The job in turn has certain ability requirements and offers opportunities for workers to gain specific reinforcers (e.g., money, social status, security). The level of correspondence between the abilities of the individual and the ability requirements of the job is referred to as *satisfactoriness*. The level of correspondence between the vocational needs (preference) of an individual and the reinforcer systems of the job is referred to as *satisfaction*. Satisfaction and satisfactoriness are both related to tenure (remaining on the job or in an occupation). If satisfactoriness is sufficiently low, the worker is fired or demoted. If satisfaction is sufficiently low, the worker will quit the job. (p. 37)

The statement of this theory or definition of work adjustment is clear and parsimonious and provides one base in the establishment of what may be called a "tentative frame of reference" (Lofquist & Dawis, 1969). And, while all definitions of work adjustment have application to the establishment of sound work adjustment programs for people, Lofquist and Dawis (1969) state that the theory can be specifically applied to adjustment to work for those people who have severe physical disabilities. Therefore, work adjustment may be seen as a function of the worker's satisfaction with the job and the satisfactoriness of the worker in the job.

The Minnesota studies also produced a number of measurement instruments for applying the theory's concepts. To measure the outcomes of work adjustment, the *Minnesota Satisfaction Questionnaire* and the *Minnesota Satisfactoriness Scale* were developed. The General Aptitude Test Battery (GATB), a standard measure of general abilities, is used to measure vocational abilities. The occupational aptitude patterns developed through the U.S. Employment Service are used to measure ability requirements. In addition, the *Minnesota Importance Questionnaire* (MIQ) was developed to measure the vocational needs of workers, and the occupational reinforcer patterns were published as a basis for determining the reinforcer systems of the job (Lofquist, Dawis, & Hendel, 1972).

The application of this Minnesota theory of work adjustment and its instruments can be helpful in terms of the whole area of counseling, the development of work personality, and may eventually lead to job placement (Bitter, 1979).

Approaches to Vocational Adjustment

Dunn (1974) has identified three primary approaches to vocational adjustment. These are verbal, situational, and environmental approaches, as discussed by Bitter in his book, *Introduction to Rehabilitation* (1979):

1. Verbal approaches can include individual counseling and group counseling. Individual counseling is intended primarily to assist with personal adjustment and group counseling is intended to help the person with problems involving interaction with others. Verbal approaches may include classroom instruction and videotape counseling.
2. Situational approaches in work adjustment provide experiential opportunities for clients and include the use of production work in a sheltered environment, community job site assignments, and behavior modification techniques.
3. Environmental manipulation involves the elimination of job site barriers and the use of prosthetics for maximizing an individual's efficiency. Barrier elimination includes eliminating architectural barriers as well as work rules or other organizational controls that make it difficult to accommodate a disabled person at work. "Job engineering" makes it possible for the physically disabled person to do the work. Prosthetic strategies that attempt to maximize the behavior efficiency of disabled persons include job performance aids like an artificial limb or some other device that enables the person to perform certain tasks.

Clearly, work adjustment, as a process employed in rehabilitation, has shifted from vocational guidance and the giving of occupational information to more specific methods found useful in learning theories. Neff (1977), in his discussions of techniques of work adjustment, states that

> . . . the problems of adjustment to work are, in some sense or other, problems of personality. Where these problems are severe they cannot be solved by the giving of occupational information or the administration of tests. Some type of reconstruction of relevant areas of the personality appear to be required. The result has been an increasingly intensive search for appropriate methods of treatment. (p. 216)

Methods that this search have produced include individual and group counseling, rehabilitation workshops that utilize work activities related to real life or simulated production standards, behavior modification, classroom instruction, modeling and imitation learning, and manipulation of a particular job as well as the work environment (Lassiter et al., 1983).

Of the two special areas of rehabilitation that are closely allied, vocational evaluation and work adjustment, it is clear that the evaluation or adjustment process is more sharply defined, and its techniques or methods are based on the results of research skills and knowledge on the part of the evaluator. However, work adjustment specialists who work with the severely disabled person are quite often at a disadvantage in efforts to provide appropriate adjustment services in this new and emerging program. They are the true mavericks in the field of rehabilitation.

INDIVIDUAL COUNSELING: A BASIC TECHNIQUE FOR WORK ADJUSTMENT

In tracing the development of work adjustment as a new professional discipline, an appreciation can be gained for the early efforts of practitioners as they searched for methods and techniques to provide work adjustment training. The technique of individual counseling has been chosen as the focus for this chapter because all methods or techniques that are found useful in work adjustment depend on an effective and strong individual counseling relationship.

The focus of the counseling relationship will be on lifestyle counseling as established by Adler, with rational-emotive therapy developed by Ellis (e.g., 1962) used as the reinforcer. Additional approaches are selected from what appears to be the best in the various doctrines, methods, or styles as outlined by others—an eclectic approach in individual counseling.

In recent times, rehabilitation counselors, psychologists, special education teachers, and professional counselors have been challenged as never before to work with a large number of clients who, for one reason or another, have not been able to adjust to the work environment. This challenge to work adjustment personnel is accompanied by diminishing resources available for staff and special services, resulting in the need for more effective and efficient ways of helping individuals make a suitable adjustment to the world of work.

Developing a Counseling Approach

In formulating a particular approach of counseling for work adjustment, it is important for the individual to consider the key ingredients that are necessary for effective counseling. The first consideration must be given to the counselor as a person; this includes his values, beliefs, needs, and other personal characteristics that permeate everything he does in his many functions as a counselor. It is important to have congruence between the counselor as a person and the counseling approach he plans to formulate.

Thus, the important first step in formulating a position or pattern to follow is for the counselor to attain a high level of awareness of his philosophical beliefs, values, needs, and so on. Without this awareness, the base of his pattern or approach is shaky. (Passons, 1975, p. 4)

The second ingredient is an awareness of all existing theories and a determination of which parts of the theories are compatible with the individual counselor and his counseling style and even the individual counselor's lifestyle.

The third area to explore in setting up an effective approach includes the processes used by other counselors to formulate a personal approach. As one becomes more aware of self and increases the ability to consider theories and various approaches of counseling, the process used to evaluate them becomes important. Shoben (1962), who has written about the counselor's theory as a personality trait, has stated

> In the psychological realm, then it is hardly surprising that the touch-stones by which we often evaluate a theory are our own experience, our previously developed ideas about the ways in which men do and should behave, and our particular complex of values associated with ourselves and our fellows as interacting and sentient organisms. (p. 618)

Shoben has related this process to the proliferation of theories of counseling and the variation in them. If there was a theory that was right for every counselor, there would not be so many to consider (Shoben, 1962).

Three prominent psychologists or counselors, Carl Rogers, Rollo May, and Abraham Maslow, have influenced the thinking of and enhanced the attraction to the lifestyle counselor as a model. Their various theories—client-centered therapy by Rogers (1951), existential psychology by May (1958, 1972), and humanistic psychology by Maslow (1954)—have been influenced by Alfred Adler (1931, 1935) and his work, either directly or indirectly. For example, there would be little or no hesitancy on the part of these men or their followers to accept the following ideas: (1) human beings are basically innately social, so their behavior comes about as a result of efforts to achieve social belonging; (2) behavior is purposeful and goal oriented in that it represents an attempt to fulfill a significant need, and usually the purpose relates to the desire to find an appropriate social position; and (3) perceptions are significant aspects of behavior, because people tend to conduct themselves according to their perceptions of the circumstances (Wright, 1980).

Let us examine the views of these men, focusing on the role they played in the formulation of each man's own theories, rather than on the way the technique is used in counseling.

Carl Rogers: Client-Centered Therapy

In looking for areas of compatibility with Adlers' concepts, it is important that we examine some of the things Rogers says that are basic to the client-centered approach. For example, the counselor will be more effective with client-centered therapy if he holds a coherent and developing set of attitudes deeply inbedded in his personal organization, a system of attitudes that is implemented by techniques and methods consistent with it. As we look further into the theory expressed by Carl Rogers, we see an emphasis on the emotional warmth of the relationship with the counselor, a relationship within which the client can perceive for the first time the hostile meaning and purpose of certain aspects of his behavior and understand why he feels negative about it. He can experience himself as a person having hostile as well as other types of feelings and do this without negative feelings because another person has been able to adopt his frame of reference to perceive with him, yet to perceive with acceptance and respect. Another aspect of the client-centered therapy approach is that the individual discovers he has within himself the capacity for weighing experiential evidence and deciding upon those things that make for long-run enhancement of self.

From various studies conducted on client-centered therapy, Rogers (1951) provides a list of things that happen to an individual in successful therapy. The person tends (1) to perceive his abilities and characteristics with more objectivity and with greater comfort, (2) to perceive all aspects of self and self in relationship with less emotion and more objectivity, (3) to perceive himself as more independent and more able to cope with life's problems, (4) to perceive himself as more able to be spontaneous and genuine, (5) to perceive himself as the evaluator of experience rather than as existing in a world where the values are inherent in and attached to the objects of this perception, and (6) to perceive himself as more integrated, less divided. In summary, Rogers says the individual client changes in three general ways: he perceives himself as a more adequate person with more worth and more possibility of meeting life; he permits more experiential data to enter his awareness and thus achieve a more realistic appraisal of self, his relationship, and his environment; and he tends to place the basis of standards within himself, recognizing that the goodness or badness of any experience or perceptual object is not something inherent in that object but is a value placed on it by himself (Rogers, 1951).

Ansbacher and Ansbacher (1956) noted that in the development of his client-centered therapy Rogers depended on his observation of the process.

> The outcome is a series of propositions which could be matched to a considerable extent with the propositions derived from Adler. . . . Just to give a few examples, Rogers refers to: one basic tendency and striving to actualize, maintain, and enhance the experiencing organism; behavior as goal-directed; the individual as an organized whole, the consistency of the self; the individually perceived world; and better interpersonal relations as the outcome of therapy. (p. 15)

Abraham Maslow: Humanistic Psychology

Abraham Maslow's "hierarchy of needs" appears to be in keeping with the Adlerian concept of dynamic forces descending from the striving for perfection to the striving for self-enhancement. The concept of a hierarchy was suggested by Maslow to Ansbacher and Ansbacher (1956) as a way to reflect Adler's theories: "While rudiments of Maslow can be found in Adler, Maslow's theory is helpful for a fuller appreciation of Adler. . . " (p. 124).

Ansbacher and Ansbacher (1956) further state

> With respect to Adler's answer to these questions, we should like to refer to Maslow much more for his essential similarity. Maslow postulates a basis for social behavior which is "instinctoid" but weak, just as social interest is innate, but needs to be nurtured. . . . Human nature carries within itself the answer to the question, How can I be good? How can I be happy? How can I be fruitful? The organism tells us what it needs and therefore what it values by sickening when deprived of these values. (p. 150)

In his book, *Motivation and Personality,* Maslow speaks of the influence of Alfred Adler on what he calls the "self-esteem needs." He says that all people in our society (with a few pathological exceptions) have a need or desire for a stable, firmly based, usually high evaluation of themselves, for self-respect, for self-esteem, and for the esteem of others.

> These needs may therefore be classified in two subsidiary sets. These are, first, the desire for strength, for achievement, for adequacy, for mastery and competence, for confidence in the face of the world, and for independence and freedom. Second, we have what we may call the desire for reputation or prestige (defining it as respect, or esteem from other people), status, fame and glory, dominance, recognition, attention, importance, dignity or appreciation. These needs have been relatively stressed by Alfred Adler and his followers and have been relatively neglected by Freud. More and more today, however, there is appearing widespread appreciation of their central importance among psychoanalysts as well as among clinical psychologists. . . . GEMEINSCHAFTSGEFUHL, a word invented by Alfred Adler in his book, *Social Interest,* is the only one available that describes well the flavor of the feeling for mankind expressed by self-actualizing subjects. (Maslow, 1954, p. 45)

Maslow goes on to say about such individuals,

> They have, for human beings in general, a deep appreciation of identifi-
> cation, sympathy, and affection in spite of the occasional anger, impa-
> tience, or disgust exhibited. Because of this they have a genuine desire
> to help the human race. It is as if they were all members of a single
> family. One's feelings toward his brothers would be on the whole
> affectionate, even if those brothers were foolish, weak, or even if they
> were sometimes nasty. They would still be more easily forgiven than
> strangers. This is what Adler called the older brotherly attitude. (p. 165)

Maslow's hierarchy of needs and his statements regarding humanistic psychology, which represent what has been called the "Third Force," are not altogether
compatible with the Adlerian view. However, many similarities exist. Ansbacher
and Ansbacher quote Maslow from a well-known paper he delivered on the subject
of trauma: "Only a deprivation which is at the same time a threat to the personality, that is, to the life goals of the individual, to his self esteem, or to his feeling
of security, will have frustrating effects" (Ansbacher & Ansbacher, 1956,
p. 293).

Rollo May: Existential Humanism

The approach closest to Adler's is existential and humanistic—a term that
describes the therapist's attitude and stance toward the client. While existentialism
tries to understand man as he exists and experiences his own world, humanism is
concerned with man's relationship with his environment.

> Existential-humanism, then, is concerned with man's relation to him-
> self—his feelings, thoughts, guilt, anguish, joys, loves—and man's
> relation with his world and others. It maintains that man, especially in
> psychotherapy, can be understood by himself alone but also in relation-
> ship to his fellow man. While existential-humanism understands man's
> essential aloneness, it also recognizes his dependence upon others.
> (Dreyfus & Nikelly, 1971, p. 13)

The task of the counselor is to try to understand both the real and apparent world
of the client—to understand the client's world through the client's eyes.

> The therapist (or counselor) demonstrates his concern for the client and
> tries to assist him in gaining a greater clarity or appreciation in order that
> he can make more effective choices. Many times clients are unable to
> verbalize their anger, guilt, love, dependence, despair, and loneliness.

The therapist, if he is seeing the world through the eyes of the client, can demonstrate an understanding and a willingness to share in these feelings without fear or judgment. Such a human relationship permits the client to explore his own feelings without trepidation. The existential-humanistic position maintains that the relationship between client and therapist is the single most important therapeutic variable. (Dreyfus & Nikelly, 1971, p. 14)

Existential-humanistic psychotherapy and Adlerian psychology agree on the importance of a human relationship, where there is a cooperation between the client and work adjustment person. As Adler stated, psychotherapy is an exercise in cooperation.

Arbuckle (1970) defines the existential-psychologist goal in therapy as

To help the individual achieve a state of acceptance, of responsibility for self, thus to be free . . . man is free—he is what he makes of himself, the outside limits and restricts (e.g., a handicapping condition), but it does not determine completely one's way of life. Existence precedes essence . . . man is not static but he is rather in a constant state of growing, evolving, becoming. He is in a state of being, but also non-being . . . existentialism sees counseling and psychotherapy as primarily human encounter . . . the stress is on today rather than yesterday or tomorrow. A real human encounter must be in terms of now, and life and living are in terms of what is, not what was or what might be. (p. 142)

Coulson, (1972) a well-known and prominent leader in the development of encounter groups with Carl Rogers in La Jolla, California, stated:

What does one actually learn in an encounter session? The client has achieved an expanded range of choice. He can be more present to people when he wishes, and more private, also, when he wishes that. He can be in charge of his life through being more aware of where he is; that is to say less compelled by his habits, with less need to defend against his experience, with greater sensitivity to the full range of feelings all people have. Individuals often wind up looking much as they did before the individual encounter, but with a difference. I know it in my own life; this time I can choose to be the way I am, and I can sense in myself the real possibility to be other than how typically I am, if I judge that to be appropriate. I am no longer compelled to be one way, one could not ask for more. (p. 95)

This can be seen as an existentialist statement and as analogous to the situation of the severely disabled person. The person who is severely physically handicapped and is working toward a new adjustment to life and to work can expect at least the opportunity to interact with other people in order to make better decisions regarding adjustment to life and to work.

Perhaps no individual is better known for his leadership in the field of existential psychology than Rollo May (e.g., 1958). May is of special interest to our discussion in this area since he studied under Adler in Vienna. In his major writings it seems clear that Adler's theories were a significant influence, even though he came to depend more on the "attitude" of another important teacher, the existentialist theologian Paul Tillich. In *Power and Innocence* (1972), May discusses power and powerlessness sounding, as O'Connell (1976) says, "like an advanced Adlerian by his cogent approach to the necessity, types and purposes of power or influence . . . but, it is the social side of power that is stressed. The desired emphasis seems to fit Adler's concept of 'social interest' '' (p. 11). In his article, "The Friends of Adler Phenomenon," O'Connell gives credit to May and other existential or humanistic leaders but examines these leaders in view of their critical comments about Adler. This article describes carefully the ways May and others were taught by and influenced by Adler—but, once taught, became their own thinkers—i.e., developed their own "style."

The following quotes from May (1972) confirm his recognition of his indebtedness and his respect for Alfred Adler:

Power and the sense of significance are intertwined. One is objective form and the other subjective form of the same experience. While power is typically extravert, significance may not be extravert at all, but may be shown (and achieved) by meditation or other introvert, subjective methods. It is nevertheless experienced by the person as a sense of power in that it helps him integrate himself and subsequently makes him more effective in his relations with others. Power is always interpersonal; if it is purely personal, we call it strength. As one watches [a child] building blocks and then knocking the construction down to build it again, one realizes that power and aggression have positive values. From there the child goes on to explore, to experiment, to master his world as best he can and as far as his level of development enables him . . . but if we assume an Adlerian notion of "striving for superiority," or else an equivalent to the appetitive behavior of animals seeking stimulations, the difficulty disappears. To Alfred Adler goes the credit of his first insisting that aggression, which he originally called "will to power," was fundamental in the human life. Adler believed that civilization itself arises out of man's need to increase his power vis-à-vis nature. This is shown particularly in Adler's changing the phrase "will to power" to "striving for superiority" and then to "striving to perfection." (p. 35)

May goes on to say "Communication leads to community—that is to understanding intimacy and the mutual valuing that was previously lacking. Alfred Adler's work, for example, is centrally based on power needs in individuals" (p. 247).

May's statements are important in viewing the nature of man:

> Therapy is concerned with helping the person experience his existence as real which includes becoming aware of his potentialities and becoming able to act on the basis of them, the significance of a commitment is not that it is simply a good thing or ethically to be advised, it is a necessary prerequisite rather for seeing truth. (1958, p. 22)

There is no question that the work adjustment staff working with severely physically handicapped people can benefit from a thorough study of an existentialist psychology since the rehabilitation concept is itself "an existentialist one."

In rehabilitation, the basic need for self-esteem is usually left for each individual to work out. Looking at counseling from an existential-humanistic viewpoint allows us to focus on what Wax (1972) calls a new dimension of rehabilitation in work adjustment. Wax reviews the two primary themes of traditional rehabilitation: achievement and interaction, which he states are necessary but may not be sufficient, and then goes on to discuss the idea of the possibility of what he calls the "third dimension" being added. With the onset of severe disability, many times the individual must be alone and face his existential aloneness. For many, being alone is synonymous with boredom, alienation, loneliness, isolation, abandonment, or exile. Wax presents four major reasons for assisting the severely physically handicapped person in becoming aware of self from an existential viewpoint:

> (1) a rich inner life may make being alone less painful, (2) inner space (or thought) may be the only area left for a feeling of freedom and autonomy for those who are dependent on others, (3) effective use of this inner space (being happy with your thoughts and feelings) offers an alternative to the hyperactivity of people who fear depression or existential despair and (4) solitude and the ability to think and ask yourself the hard questions gives us the opportunity to develop a philosophy which helps us to live what must be lived, e.g., a life of severe disability. (p. 17)

ALFRED ADLER AND LIFESTYLE COUNSELING

Now we begin to take a look at lifestyle counseling as developed by Alfred Adler. In this examination, reference is made to the theoretical framework and pattern as established in earlier chapters. But it seems important at this time to review some of the basic areas of lifestyle counseling in light of their development by Rogers, Maslow, and May.

Adler, for the sake of clarity, divided all the problems of living into three areas: problems of behavior toward others, problems of work, and problems of love. Most of Adler's writings and lectures dealt with the problems of social relations or the social interest, but he did indicate the importance of work or occupation in *What Life Should Mean to You* (1931):

> If "to make money" is the only goal and no social interest is bound up with it, there is no possible reason why he should not make money by robbing and swindling other people. If, in a less extreme attitude, only a small degree of social interest is combined with the goal, his activities will still not be of much advantage to his fellows, although he may make plenty of money. Even a mistaken way may sometimes seem to be successful in one point. If, on the other hand, an individual goes through life with the right attitude (GEMEINSCHAFTSGEFUHL) we cannot promise that he will meet immediate success. But we can promise that he will keep his courage and will not lose his self esteem. (p. 278)

It should be noted that an understanding of lifestyle counseling is not limited simply to clients who are referred for work adjustment. An awareness on the part of the work adjustment specialist's own style and how it unfolds in a person's personal and professional life on a daily basis is a significant asset.

First Step

As we have seen, the first step in assisting the client in learning about his lifestyle is to take a look at family constellation—such things as description of siblings, notions about what people in the family were like, birth order, sexual differences among siblings, their interrelationships with the client and with each other, and so forth are the kinds of data required by the work adjustment specialist.

In performing this first step, the practitioner is in a better position to help the client look at thoughts and feelings at this early period of growth so that the client can come up with some hints as to "What kind of kid was I then?" and, correspondingly, "How does that little person's way of coping affect my present ways of coping with life?"

An abbreviated form (Rule, 1974) of the family constellation questionnaire, originally developed by Dreikurs (1967), is presented in Appendix D. In using this form, the counselor must keep in mind that the client's responses are his perceptions of an early environment (whether real or fiction) that reflects his choice of reaction to the world as a youngster. The notions or conclusions that emerge from the answers to the questions will provide a clearer historical perspective of present values and techniques of coping with life, opinion of self and others—in short, the beginning of an insight into how the lifestyle is functioning. At this point it might be well to refer to the list of lifestyle examples developed by Mosak (1971). This can be used as a very general guide to the work adjustment specialist in attempting to understand what is going on with the client's lifestyle.

It is important in using the Abbreviated Form to relate the information to how the client is progressing in the work adjustment program. Since the purpose of collecting information is to alter the mistaken goals as they relate to the immediate situation, rather than to modify the basic personality and lifestyle of the client, it would be well to use what Rogers calls a client-centered approach or attitude, indicating that the practitioner is just guessing by using such questions as "Could it be that . . . " This tentative approach may better help the client get in touch with his lifestyle patterns. Even if one has studied in this field for several years and has had much practice, nothing is gained unless the client honestly responds to the practitioner's tentative statements about him. References found in this chapter can be extremely helpful to work adjustment staff as they begin to practice this approach, especially if they are using the abbreviated form of the family constellation plan and have received only minimal data and instruction in regard to interpreting the family constellation as one part of the development of the client's lifestyle.

Second Step

The second step to consider in the development of the client's lifestyle is to question the client about his earliest memories, those reminders he carries about with him of his own limits and of the meaning of circumstances in his life.

> There are no "chance memories"; out of the incalculable number of impressions which happen to an individual, he chooses to remember only those which he feels, however darkly, to have a bearing on his situation. Thus his memories represent his "story of my life"; a story he repeats to himself to warn him or to comfort him, to keep him concentrated on his goal, and to prepare him by means of past experiences so that he will meet the future with an already tested style of action. (Ansbacher & Ansbacher, 1956, p. 351)

The interpreter would do well to look at each early recollection (ER) individually, interpret each one, then try to piece together the overall flavor provided by a least three ER's and how they supplement each other (Rule, 1976). Some general guidelines for interpretation may be found in Ansbacher and Ansbacher (1956). An abbreviated form (Rule, 1974) for eliciting early recollections is presented in Appendix D.

Interpretation is based on themes or patterns that emerge from the Family Constellation Form and the ER form. What is the client currently programming himself about self, others, and life? In work adjustment, there is an opportunity to practice an overall interpretation of the data, a holistic view, integrating the family constellation with the early recollections. This is a tentative interpretation to be made with the client's assistance, and nothing is provided the client in an authoritarian way.

Nikelly and O'Connell (1971) have commented on action-oriented methods that can be helpful to clients. They suggest that the counselor emphasize the positive aspects of the client and minimize the negative ones. For instance, after the client has expressed unpleasant and disjunctive feelings about himself, the counselor can immediately state that he respects him and considers him to be a capable person who can become successful within his own limits. Also, they indicate that an effective and practical approach to lifestyle counseling is to encourage the client to interpret his own behavior and then to consider alternative solutions that might prove effective. He should search his life pattern and suggest alternative behaviors to reach his goals rather than seek for deep and hidden motives. Thus, the client's interactions are analyzed, not his subconscious psyche.

The stages of the therapeutic process do not necessarily follow the same order and often vary in emphasis and length depending upon the client. Dreyfus and Nikelly (1971) summarize the following phases, which are more or less present in all existing psychotherapies.

(1) The first stage sets the communication and establishes rapport between the counselor and the client. A trusting relationship of mutual cooperation and respect, and an agreement of objectives is established. (2) In the second stage, the client's current behavior, as he experiences it, is examined and with it his own life situation (birth order, family constellation, and early recollections) in an attempt to identify a common denominator from these characteristics. The emphasis in this stage is on investigating and uncovering. (3) During the third stage the therapist extracts from these characteristics an underlying pattern of behavior and explains it to the client. The client's fundamental approach to life is interpreted to him. (4) In the fourth stage the client is encouraged to work through his problem and to implement his insights. (p. 84)

The fourth stage is considered to be the most significant stage for eliciting behavior change or a change in fundamental goals. Of the many choices that are available for effective counseling at the fourth state, rational-emotive therapy developed by Albert Ellis appears to be one of the most useful.

ALBERT ELLIS AND RATIONAL-EMOTIVE THERAPY

On the surface, the two appear quite different—one, Adlerian, focuses, at least initially, on information gathering and history; the other, rational-emotive, emphasizes "here and now" counselor impressions and recommended behavioral changes for the client. In addition, there are major differences in methodology as well as technique. However, it appears that much of the basic philosophy and general goals of each are much more similar and convergent than they are different or divergent. As Albert Ellis (1973) founder of the rational-emotive approach states:

Rational-Emotive therapy owes a great debt to Alfred Adler . . . RET is not only a theory of personality development and change, as is individual psychology, but it is a specific methodology . . . consciously and unconsciously, Alfred Adler was certainly one of the main mentors in the formulation of RET and it is highly probable that without his pioneering work, the main elements of Rational-Emotive Therapy might never have been developed. Adler was much more tenacious in holding to the hypothesis that a person's emotional reactions and in fact his entire healthy or neurotic lifestyle, directly correlated with his basic ideas, beliefs, attitudes, or philosophies, and are in essence, cognitively created. For example, Adler stated: "It is very obvious that we are influenced not by 'facts' but by our intepretation of facts . . . everyone possesses an 'idea' about himself and the problems of life—a life pattern, a law or movement that keeps fast hold of him without his understanding it, without his being able to give any account of it." (p. 112)

One of the major objectives of this chapter is to provide suggestions for work adjustment staff to consider in emphasizing a program for clients without in any way suggesting the elimination or minimization of the positive effects of the current approaches that are used in the facilities. In fact, it appears that the combined approach of lifestyle counseling with rational-emotive training can enhance the existing ones.

Arnold Lazarus, a psychologist, and Allen Fay, a psychiatrist, have stated in their book, *I Can If I Want To:* "We firmly believe that counseling is education rather than healing. That it is growth rather than treatment" (1975, p. 20). Perhaps this new emphasis on "teaching" rather than the amorphous and easily misunderstood terms "counseling" or "therapy" can facilitate the client's adjustment to the world of work.

Rational-emotive training is a method of teaching basic principles of interpersonal relations to individuals. It specifically shows clients how to eliminate fears of failure, how to be more tolerant and less hostile, how to gain their own qualified self-acceptance, and how to achieve frustration tolerance. It differs from many therapies in that directiveness, activity, structuring, and homework assignments are employed. Such an approach may help clients function more effectively in work by actively teaching them certain basic principles of interpersonal relations that promote better self-understanding as well as increase insight into others.

Rational-emotive therapy was founded by Albert Ellis in 1955, and brought to national attention and prominence with the publication of his book, *Reason and Emotion in Psychotherapy*, in 1962. Ellis, with a background in psychoanalytic theory and its practice, became dissatisfied with the results he obtained in working with his clients, and began a long and exhaustive period of study to formulate a new and more effective approach. In this search, he turned to such men as Alfred Adler and other prominent psychologists whom he perceived as providing a teaching model rather than a medical model. Also, Ellis turned to the stoic Greek philosophers, such as Epictetus.

Epictetus observed that:

> It is not things themselves that disturb people, but their ideas about things . . . when we meet with troubles, they become anxious or depressed, let us never blame anyone but . . . our opinions about things. The uneducated person blames others when he does badly; the person whose education has begun blames himself; the already educated person blames neither another nor himself. (Nikelly & O'Connell, 1971, p. XX)

Rational-emotive counseling is based on the assumption that people become disturbed by acquiring irrational thoughts, beliefs, and philosophies. Furthermore, it is these philosophies, and not the events that happen to the individual, that truly upset him.

> When an activating event occurs in a person's life in point *A* and is followed at point *C* by disturbed consequences (such as feelings of anxiety, hostility, depression and guilt) *A* does not really cause *C*. Instead, *C* actually follows from *B* (the individual's belief system about what happens to him at *A*.) Thus, if a child fails arithmetic at point *A* and is agitated and depressed at point *C* it is not his failure that is causing

these emotional consequences; rather it is his irrational belief at point *B* that he should not have failed. That it is awful for him to have done poorly, and that he is a worthless person for failing. The child is then taught to dispute at point *D* his irrational beliefs at point *B* by persistently asking himself, "Why should not I have failed? Where is the evidence that it is awful for me to have done poorly?" etc. RET also gives him activity homework assignments such as deliberately taking the difficult subject like arithmetic to prove to himself that either he can succeed at them or that he can fail without denigrating himself as a human being, or it may even give him the homework assignment of deliberately failing at something. This results at point *E* in two main effects: A cognitive effect, whereby the child changes his basic philosophy to something like, "It is decidedly *disadvantageous* or *inconvenient* to fail arithmetic, but it is hardly awful"; and following this, a behavioral effect. (Ellis, 1973, p. 55)

The rational-emotive approach emphasizes reality testing, whereby clients learn to develop a more objective appraisal of themselves and their world through learning to identify self-defeating attitudes and beliefs. Then clients learn to diminish or eliminate them through rational self-examination methods, which include active self-questioning and purposeful action to promote living a more rational and pleasureable existence. These methods are targeted toward helping clients identify and assertively go after what they vocationally want and are capable of achieving (Knaus, 1974).

The work adjustment specialist, having gone through the process of lifestyle counseling with his client, is in a good position now to identify the main problem or problems the client is experiencing about work. The worker can discuss with the client what he hears the client telling himself, evoking from the client what is really disturbing him, showing the client how he is *demanding* rather than *desiring* certain goals, and assisting the client in challenging or disputing the client's irrational ideas concerning his career planning. Homework assignments can then be given focusing on behaviors that will lead to a more rational approach for selection of a particular job or adjustment to present employment.

According to Gandy and Rule (1983),

The RET concept of self acceptance is different from many other forms of therapy which attempt to promote people's feelings of "self esteem" or "self confidence." It encourages people not to rate themselves, their totality, their essence, or their being at all, but only to rate their specific traits, deeds, and performances. From a scientific point of view, there is no such thing as a "bad" person but only a person who performs bad acts. Generally the person also performs good acts, but it would also be scientifically untenable to describe the person as a "good" person. A human being is a person who is capable of performing both constructive and unconstructive behaviors. If human beings choose survival and happiness as their main values, they will be more likely to achieve these goals if they work to maximize their constructive behavior and to minimize their unconstructive behavior. (p. 142)

In regard to this concept, Ellis (1973) states:

Adler shows that he clearly grasped the most important idea which was later to be promulgated, and probably in somewhat clearer form, by rational-emotive therapists: namely that the value or worth of an individual cannot really be scientifically or empirically measured. It is largely a definition or tautological concept that depends upon his thinking and convincing himself that he is a "good person" or a "bad person" or is "worthwhile" or "worthless." (p. 113)

As Adler wrote: "Let us be very modest, then, in our judgment of our fellows, and above all, let us never allow ourselves to make any moral judgments, judgments concerning the moral worth of a human being" (Ansbacher & Ansbacher, 1956, p. 463).

Ellis is not widely perceived as an existentialist; however, two of his key words are "choice" and "control":

RET follows the humanistic educative model which asserts that people have a great many more choices than they tend to recognize. . . . [B]ecause of innate and acquired tendencies, we largely (though not exclusively) *control* our own destinies and particularly our emotional destinies. And we do so by our basic values or beliefs—by the way that we interpret or look at the events that occur in our lives and body actions we choose to take about these occurrences. (Ellis & Greiger, 1977, p. 12)

Arbuckle's (1970) earlier description of the existential psychologist's goal in therapy runs parallel to the basic philosophical stance taken by Ellis.

Perhaps the major difference between RET and other approaches is its strong adherence to the concept of teaching people ways to eliminate or minimize self-defeating behaviors. The teaching is authoritative but not authoritarian; in addition, it incorporates a concept of closure or graduation from therapy to a continuing self-instructional program of learning. This graduation, as with other graduations from educational programs, can be viewed as a commencement—a beginning for the person who is about to begin working. From a rehabilitation perspective, this is a beginning for clients to work toward independence now that they are equipped to deal effectively with negative thoughts leading to the basic negative feelings of anger, anxiety, depression, or guilt that they are bound to experience during work.

AN EXAMPLE

Over the past six years, I have had the opportunity to use lifestyle counseling as described in this chapter as a fundamental part of a work adjustment plan with clients in individual counseling. Encouragement or reinforcement aspects of lifestyle counseling, as noted in this chapter, have been based on the cognitive-behavioral approach found in rational-emotive therapy.

Rule (1977, 1979) has experimented with systematic uses of humor designed to encourage individuals to take less seriously the vanity inherent in their lifestyles. The use of humor is also greatly valued as a means of challenging irrational or inappropriate thoughts leading to irrational or inappropriate feelings. The following example of its effectiveness is excerpted from a personal journal that tells the story of how one person benefited from lifestyle and rational-emotive methods. It should be noted that this individual is a 57-year-old professional who was trained in both lifestyle counseling and rational-emotive therapy earlier. This part of the journal deals with the self-directed use of humor in the person's adjustment to work:

> Through lifestyle counseling, I was able to identify the overriding goal or purpose in my life: striving to be good at everything I tried in all areas of living! What a set-up for RET! I demanded that I always be a good husband, a good father, a good friend, a good worker, and so forth. My counselor earlier had suggested to me tentatively that I was striving not only to be good at what I was up to, but that I was maybe even "cleverly arranging" to be perceived as good by others. Well, maybe so, isn't that really the social interest? Just the ability to identify this overriding demandingness on my part was humorous itself—thinking how my striving for perfection or superiority was to be always good! It came across clearly that this striving for power, by being *good* at it, was a choice I made early in life and that this pattern was continuing to guide my behavior as a grown man. Fortunately, since no event in my life had occurred that blocked me entirely from this major goal, I recognized the striving for goodness was usually working to my advantage: a husband for thirty-three years—a father of four healthy adults—a few intimate friends—and, an achieving and successful person at work. But, an acute awareness of when I was *bad* at any of these tasks I was really *bad*—and,

I knew that when this happened I was *good*, very *good*, at putting myself down—that my feelings then were resulting from negative thoughts which led me to anger, guilt, anxiety and depression.

Quickly, I could almost automatically use rational-emotive techniques of humor to dispute and challenge the irrational thoughts and feelings that came when I was *bad*. When your major goal or purpose is like mine, the possibility of using RET successfully is a challenge, especially when you're worried about losing the *good* old *goodness* that goes into being a husband, a father, a friend and a worker.

I had just experienced a stroke. Since I was fortunate in having around me people who reinforced my humor, that is, family and friends, physician, nurses and other therapists—I found myself worried most about my ability to return to work, and of course returning and adjusting to my job and continuing to be *good* at it. Looking back to the early times of recovery I can remember that speaking, reading and writing were not only things that I could be *good* at, but were a major part of my work . . . I knew that I was a *good*, articulate speaker, a good reader, and a good writer—or, at least I "cleverly arranged" to be perceived by many of my colleagues at work that I was *good* at all three; the major duties of my job required me to be somewhat *good* at all three in my tenured professorship.

With aphasia resulting from the stroke, for a while, I could not do any of the three—not do them good—just not do them at all. My physician suggested that I try singing and with sheet music held above my head I began to sing without hesitancy and with no apparent problem with speech. When a visitor came, he had to endure "What Kind of Fool Am I?" and the night nurses came around to applaud—I knew that it was crazy but I liked the attention and my new unique way of speaking with song. It also occurred to me that I really was good and learning to be *good* at having a stroke!

As time passed and some speech returned, I began to read the newspaper, starting with the headline and without comprehending the subtle meaning I was reading "Doonesbury" out loud. This effort made me feel that I was being a *good* patient for my speech therapist. Because of partial paralysis of my dominant hand, my efforts to be good at writing were delayed, and I'm still working on it. One thing that I've proven is that I can re-learn to use the dictaphone for entries like this one, and, I'm able to put things well enough that the typist usually tells me that I'm *good* at this too!

Well, it's August '82, and I'm back at work now—with hesitant speech, but it's getting better. I'm reading three or four books a week, and I've just completed working with my wife on the editing of a book.

With this dictaphone and use of typewriter for limited periods of time, I am writing again. I knew it! The lifestyle is at work: I'm told that I am the "best patient that my doctors and therapists ever worked with." I'm really *good* at it. And, I'm enjoying using humor in the rational-emotive techniques. What would I have done without this stroke?

But, there is one thing I find that with practice and more practice I just can't get *good* at. I remember the first "real" book I read with comprehension: Agnes DeMille's *Reprieve: A Memoir.* [1981]. The book is about her experiencing a stroke, what it felt like at first, the agony over her inability to walk and talk, the pain that she endured because of paralysis and of course Miss DeMille's courage, which she maintained throughout the recovery. Her advice in the book is for people who have had a stroke: Be patient . . . I amuse myself here because practicing to be patient works some of the time. However, I'm reminded that this is something I'm not so *good* at; for me, it's a little like striving for humility—to try to be humble! (Lassiter, 1982)

These brief excerpts show a blending of the lifestyle approach with rational-emotive methods, similar to a confluence or a flowing or coming together of the two. And, as Ellis and Greiger (1977) indicate, "Emotional disturbance largely consists of taking life too seriously; exaggerating the significance of things" (p. 5). The following points come from a list of examples of clinical findings about the use of humor and its advantages to counseling (Ellis & Greiger, 1977):

(1) Humor can help clients laugh at themselves with their vulnerabilities and fallibilities. (2) If clarifies many of the client's self-defeating behavior in a non-threatening, acceptable manner. (3) It provides new data and potentially better solutions, often in a dramatic, forceful way. (4) It relieves the monotony and overseriousness of many repetitive and didactic points which often seem essential to effective therapy. (5) It dramatically and rudely interrupts some of the client's old, dysfunctional patterns of thought and sets the stage for using new, more effective patterns of thinking, emoting, and behaving. (6) It shows people the absurdity, realism, hilarity, and enjoyability of life. (7) It effectively punctures human grandiosity—quite a disturbance in its own right!

LIMITATIONS

The major limitation of the use of lifestyle counseling and rational-emotive therapy is the possibility that work adjustment personnel will embrace the approaches as an answer to all the problems presented in individual counseling and as a solution for the handicapped person to overcome all difficulties associated with work. Careful study of each method can lead a person to consider the combined approach as a panacea. This may be so since each system possesses principles that are easy for the teacher or counselor to put forth authoritatively. In close proximity is the notion that, in dealing with a dogma or set of rigid procedures, the work adjustment person will not recall that the guidelines are set for a base for all theories and that an eclectic approach, which is more moderate and avoids extremes, is more suitable. For example, one limitation that is usually not discussed in trying to learn one or more approaches is that whatever is chosen will work better if the individual's life and habits are considered. As Adler (1935) said: "A psychological system has an inseparable connection with the life philosophy of its formulator" (p. 12).

Another major limitation of the use of lifestyle counseling and rational-emotive training is that both approaches require that the client have the intellect and alertness to understand the basic principles, methods, and techniques that are being used. For example, a client must have the intellect to gain the insight and to become a partner with the counselor or the work adjustment person. It is clear that intelligence is required to acquire the insight of the mental pattern representing the lifestyle and it is equally clear that rational-emotive therapy appeals to people who have the ability to acquire knowledge and cognitive skills. Individuals who gain insight into a problem at work are encouraged to see that some hope for change exists and even make a genuine commitment to change, but, doing it is actually the hard part.

In addition to this more general limitation, the following specific problems may be found in employing the rational-emotive approach in a work setting. RET appears to be a relatively simple approach. Because of this simplicity, practitioners many times fail to perceive the more subtle nuances, for example, the ability to distinguish between authoritative and authoritarian. Furthermore, the program is highly verbal and requires that clients use a fairly high degree of abstract thinking. Thus, many clients with problems in a work adjustment program will not benefit.

An additional limitation may be seen in the need for strenuous training on the part of the work adjustment specialist in both lifestyle counseling and rational-emotive methods.

> Even though that combined approach will in the long run be more economical in that people who are highly troubled about work can become more effective at work and will not return again, again and again . . . bureaucracy may set some rigid guidelines that appear to be taking less time—less consuming, but in the long run . . . (Lassiter et al., 1983, p. 32).

SUMMARY

The purpose of this chapter was to relate Adlerian lifestyle to the work adjustment process. Included were a brief description of severe physical disability, a description of the various components useful to work adjustment methods and techniques, and a review of some major existential-humanistic attitudes that were directly or indirectly affected by the thinking of Alfred Adler. Consideration was also given to rational-emotive therapy to be used in the encouragement or reinforcement phase and to the linkage that exists between lifestyle counseling and rational-emotive techniques. Furthermore, an example was provided from a personal journal showing the benefits that may be derived from both approaches. Finally, the limitations that are found to exist in lifestyle counseling as well as in rational-emotive techniques were discussed.

REFERENCES

Adler, A. *What life should mean to you*. Boston: Little, Brown, 1931.

Adler, A. Prevention of neurosis. *Journal of Individual Psychology*, 1935(4) 3–12.

Ansbacher, H.L., & Ansbacher, R.R. *The individual psychology of Alfred Adler*. New York: Harper & Row, 1956.

Arbuckle, D.S. *Counseling: Philosophy, theory and practice*. Boston: Allyn & Bacon, 1970.

Bitter, J.A. *Introduction to rehabilitation*. St. Louis: C.V. Mosby, 1979.

Coulson, W.R. *Groups, gimmicks and instant gurus*. New York: Harper & Row, 1972.

DeMille, A. *Reprieve: A memoir*. Garden City, N.Y.: Doubleday, 1981.

Dreikurs, R. *Psychodynamics, psychotherapy, and counseling*. Chicago: Alfred Adler Institute, 1967.

Dunn, D.J. Adjustment Services: Individualized program planning, delivery, and monitoring. Menomonie, Wis.: Research and Training Center, University of Wisconsin-Stout 1974.

Ellis, A. *Reason and emotion in psychology*. New York: Lyle Stuart, 1962.

Ellis, A. *Humanistic psychology: The rational-emotive approach*. New York: McGraw-Hill, 1973.

Eillis, A., & Grieger, R. *Handbook of rational-emotive therapy*. New York: Springer, 1977.

Gandy, G.L., & Rule, W.R. The use of group counseling. In R. Lassiter, M. Lassiter, R. Hardy, J. Underwood, & J. Cull (Eds.), *Vocational evaluation, work adjustment, and independent living for severely disabled people*. Springfield, Ill.: Charles C Thomas, 1983.

Hoffman, P.R. Work evaluation: An overview: In R.E. Hardy and J.G. Cull (Eds.), *Vocational evaluation for rehabilitation services*. Springfield, Ill.: Charles C Thomas, 1972.

Knaus, W.J. *Rational-emotive education: A manual for elementary school teachers*. New York: Institute for Rational Living, 1974.

Lassiter, R.A. Personal journal, August 21, 1982.

Lassiter, R., Lassiter, M., Hardy, R., Underwood, J., & Cull, J. (Eds.), *Vocational evaluation, work adjustment and independent living for severely disabled people*. Springfield, Ill.: Charles C Thomas, 1983.

Lazarus, A., & Fay, A. *I can if I want to*. New York: Morrow, 1975.

Lofquist, L., & Dawis, R. *Adjustment to work*. New York: Appleton-Century-Crofts, 1969.

Lofquist, L., Dawis, R., & Hendel, D. Application of the theory of work adjustment of rehabilitation counseling. Minneapolis Industrial Relations Center, University of Minnesota. *Minnesota Studies in Vocational Rehabiliation*, XXX, Bulletin 58, 1972.

Maslow, A.H. *Motivation and personality*. New York: Harper & Row, 1954.

May, R. Contributions of existential psychotherapy. In *Existence*. New York: Simon & Schuster, 1958.

May, R. *Power and innocence*. New York: Norton, 1972.

Mosak, H.H. Lifestyle. In A.G. Nikelly (Ed.), *Techniques for behavior change*. Springfield, Ill.: Charles C Thomas, 1971.

Neff, W. *Work and human behavior*. Chicago: Aldine, 1977.

Nikelly, A.G., & O'Connell, W. Action-oriented methods. In *Techniques for behavior change*. Springfield, Ill.: Charles C Thomas, 1971.

O'Connell, W. The friends of Adler phenomenon. *Journal of Individual Psychology*, 1976, *32*, 5–13.

Passons, W.R. *Gestalt approaches in counseling*. New York: Holt, Rinehart & Winston, 1975.

Rogers, C.R. *Client-centered therapy*. Boston: Houghton Mifflin, 1951.

Rule, W.R. Abbreviated lifestyle form (unpublished), 1974.

Rule, W.R. Rehabilitation uses of Adlerian lifestyle counseling. *Rehabilitation Counseling Bulletin*, 1976, *21*, 306–316.

Rule, W.R. Increasing self-model humor. *Rational Living*, 1977, *12*(1), 7–9.

Rule, W.R. Increased internal control using humor with lifestyle awareness. *The Individual Psychologist*, 1979, *16*(3), 16–21.

Shoben, E.J., Jr. The counselor's theory as a personality trait. *American Personnel and Guidance Journal*, 1962, *40*, 617–621.

Thomas, L. *The medusa and the snail: More notes of a biology watcher*. New York: Viking Press, 1979.

Wax, J. The inner life: a new dimension of rehabilitation. *Journal of Rehabilitation*. 1972, *38*, 14–18.

Wright, G.N. *Total rehabilitation*. Boston: Little, Brown, 1980.

Chapter 10

Avocational Counseling for Lifestyle Adjustment

Warren R. Rule

Slightly over a hundred years ago, former U.S. President James A. Garfield expressed an intriguing observation:

> We may divide the whole struggle of the human race into two chapters. . . . First, the fight to get leisure; and then the second fight of civilization—what shall we do with our leisure when we get it (National Geographic Society, 1975, p. 33).

This conclusion, if even only partially true, reflects the immense importance, frequently overlooked, of leisure in our lives. Sometimes avocational counseling is used to seek an answer to this question of "what shall we do with our leisure when we get it." However, before we explore this action-orientation, some definitions and concepts need to be clarified.

"Avocational counseling," as defined here, is a broad term that relates to how individuals spend their nonworking time. The process of avocational counseling varies according to the purpose for which it is intended; there can be several different emphases. Avocational counseling can be tailored to leisure enjoyment, stress management, retirement planning, time management, lifestyle enhancement, specific self-change strategies, as well as to adjustment to disability, etc. In this chapter, the focus will be on avocational counseling for adjustment to disability and leisure satisfaction.

Much confusion surrounds the definition of concepts used to describe activity related to the passage of time. As Bolles (1978) notes, nonworking time can be broken into personal care time, sleep, house and family care, and free time. The leisure enjoyment of free time will be emphasized in this chapter because disabled individuals, particularly severely disabled individuals, are often confronted with much free time.

In considering the issue of leisure enjoyment of free time, the practitioner is faced with yet another question: just how does the concept of "leisure" fit into or relate to free time? There seems to be no one definition of leisure. It can be free time, an activity that is freely chosen, a state of mind, playfulness, the spirit with which one does anything, lifelong enjoyment, realizing self-actualization potential, etc. For the purpose of the present discussion, "leisure" refers to a freely chosen activity that one truly enjoys. As a result of engaging in this activity, a person may or may not—depending on many variables—experience additional benefits that are byproducts of the activity (e.g., a generalized flow, a spirit of engaging life, an enriched state of mind, etc.).

In an effort to put these various terms into perspective, the relationships may be expressed as follows: *avocational counseling* varies according to the broad functional goals that the individual has for all or part of his nonworking time; a person's *free time* is a slice of his nonworking time; and *leisure* is most often an enjoyable activity that is part of someone's free time. However, sometimes a byproduct of leisure activity is a leisurely attitude or spirit of satisfying playfulness that can generalize into daily living. Furthermore, for the purposes of this chapter, avocational counseling views leisure as either a means to an end or as an end in itself, depending on the purpose of the avocational counseling.

THE NEED FOR LEISURE ENJOYMENT

The need for leisure enjoyment is apparent from many perspectives. For the first time in the history of civilization, huge groups of people in the industrially advanced countries no longer have to preoccupy themselves with work as the overriding concern in their existence (Morrow, 1981). A century ago the average workweek was approximately 72 hours; today it is almost one half that, leaving a great deal of nonworking time. Compton and Eddy (1981) estimate that this comprises 225,000 hours of a person's total life space. Sad to say, many choose the path of least resistance by becoming locked into ultimately unsatisfyng activities such as obsessive television watching, frequent substance abuse, and so on. In addition, increasing numbers of individuals are doubting that the "Protestant Work Ethic" yields worthwhile dividends of happiness. The tilt of the social landscape indicates—for better or for worse—that many people indeed feel *entitled* to fun and happiness.

Trieschmann (1974) observed that "The key to coping with one's disability is to receive enough satisfaction and rewards to make life worthwhile" (p. 558). However, the process of finding leisure satisfaction can be difficult and complex for the disabled. Within the context of society's apparent preoccupation with fun, happiness, and beautiful people, the disabled individual must often contend with one of his most obvious conditions—the loss of some liberty. As Eisenberg (1977)

notes, the fact of physical restriction may well be less serious than its consequences (e.g., relationships, barriers, dependency, etc.). So, the disabled person
often has an abundance of nonworking time in addition to a somewhat restricted
range of choices in deciding what to do with this time.

COUNSELING APPROACHES FOR ENHANCING LEISURE ENJOYMENT

The counseling process for enhancing leisure enjoyment is, as McDowell
(1976) observed, more complex than simply matching a person to an activity. In
this section, we will consider procedures in the counseling process that relate to
increased leisure enjoyment for the client. The focus here will be on leisure
enjoyment that the individual can experience outside of an institutional setting;
recreational activities within an institutional setting will be deemphasized. As may
be guessed, the procedures used in the counseling process for enhancing leisure
enjoyment do not necessarily flow in a systematic, orderly fashion. However, a
pattern will generally unfold in the following sequence: exploratory discussion of
the problems associated with free time, assessment, analysis, and action.

Exploratory Discussion

Difficulties with leisure enjoyment are often expressed implicitly, rather than
explicitly. It is unusual for a client to state forthrightly, "I am experiencing
difficulty with my leisure enjoyment." The practitioner should be alert to hidden
messages that are attached to feelings, thoughts, and behavior. Several examples
are given by McDowell (1976):

1. Expressed *feelings*—about boredom, procrastination, guilt anxiety,
    obsessions, uncertainty, unsureness, flightiness, social isolation,
    and so forth.
    Affective content in client responses may include the following
    phrases—"I *hate* the thought of this coming weekend," "I feel so
    guilty being away from the kids and enjoying myself," "I'm *quite
    depressed* in my free time," "I'm always so *anxious* and *uncertain*
    when it comes to planning my days off."
2. Expressed *thoughts* and *interpretations*—about leisure involvement,
    social relationships, and behavior.
    Cognitive content in client responses may include the following
    phrases—"I don't know what to do with my time," "I'd like to
    but . . . ," "I'm bored," "I feel so obligated," "My wife and I
    don't have any common interest," "Work takes my mind off

myself,'' ''I can't stand doing nothing,'' ''Just sitting around gets on
my nerves,'' ''I'm always wasting time,'' among many others.
3. Maladaptive behavior the client wishes to alleviate—''chronic'' television watching, sleeping, or drinking. (p. 55)

As a part of the exploration process, the practitioner would want to discuss
several factors with the client. They might include how the passage of time relates
to the lifestyle tasks of life: social, occupational, and relationship to opposite sex.
Especially for the disabled, particular consideration might be given to personal
and medical care as related to free time. Along this vein, some disabled individuals
may be so preoccupied with the limitations imposed by their disabilities that they
greatly reduce their range of choices. Others may be somewhat inefficiently
spending so much effort with self-maintenance use of time that they believe
themselves to be too busy for extended leisure enjoyment. Consequently, as a part
of the process of enhancing an individual's leisure enjoyment, sometimes the
focus for some clients must shift from dealing with too much free time to carving
out individual blocks of time for leisure enjoyment.

Assessment

Having identified a perceived sensitivity to how one deals with the passage of
time, the practitioner can proceed into the phase of assessment. Assessment
generally involves a process of gathering information related to how the person is
presently functioning (i.e., thinking, feeling, or doing) or how the person would
like to function. The next phase after assessment, analysis, involves the attempt to
synthesize this information into meaningful conclusions that lead to action-
oriented goals.

The tools for assessment may be loosely categorized into two groups: standardized and nonstandardized. The standardized instruments are administered according to prescribed directions, scored uniformly, and interpreted in reference to
specific norm groups. The nonstandardized tools are less structured and are not
designed with standardized conditions in mind.

Standardized

The *Leisure Activities Blank* (LAB) was developed by McKechnie (1975). This
self-administered instrument identifies activity factors and is based on 120 recreational activities. The respondent indicates the extent to which he has been involved
in the activity in the past or to which he expects to participate in it in the future. The
norm group represents a relatively affluent segment of society, a feature which is
said to provide a ''recreation-ideal.'' However, comparisons with such a privileged group could lead to confusing inferences on the part of many clients.

The *Leisure Interest Inventory* (1969), developed by Hubert, determines preferred leisure activities based on five typologies: sociability, games, art, mobility, and immobility. This self-administering test forces choice among 80 groups of these activities.

A number of leisure assessment tools, both standardized and nonstandardized, have been developed for use with target populations. Many of these instruments are evaluated by Wehman and Schleien (1980) in terms of testing criteria such as norm referenced vs. criterion referenced, reliability, validity, ease of administration, etc. These include Davis's (1957) *Recreational Directors' Observational Report* (Psychiatric); Joswiak's (1975) *Leisure Counseling Assessment Instruments* (Developmentally Disabled); Wessel's (1976) *I Can* (TMR—Children); Knox, Hurff, and Takata's (1974) *Deaf-Blind Assessment* (Deaf-Blind, Birth-Adolescence); Williams and Fox's (1977) *Minimum Objective System* (Severely Handicapped); Cousins and Brown's (1979) *Recreational Therapy Assessment* (Nonambulatory Adult); and others.

In addition to the examples of leisure instruments selected above, a number of interest tests have been developed. These instruments, while developed primarily for vocational counseling, sometimes have helpful implications for avocational counseling and leisure satisfaction. The *Strong-Campbell Interest Inventory* (Campbell & Hansen, 1981) consists of over 300 items. In addition to including basic interest scales and general occupational scales, it shows how similar respondents' interests are to the interests of people working in a wide range of occupations. The *Kuder Preference Record–Vocational* (Kuder, 1960) consists of triads of items for which the respondent indicates the activity he would like to do the most and the one he would like to do the least. Scores are provided for the following interest clusters: outdoor, mechanical, computational, scientific, persuasive, artistic, literary, musical, social service, and clerical. Another interest inventory is the *Self-Directed Search,* developed by Holland (1972). This tool is self-administered as well as self-interpreted. The respondent determines his own scores or occupational clusters from the areas of realistic, investigative, artistic, social, enterprising, and conventional.

Nonstandardized

A number of nonstandardized tools and information-gathering assessments can be used for leisure purposes. Perhaps the most basic nonstructured technique, yet one that is easily overlooked in the practitioner's eagerness to assess the client, is simply to ask the client what he enjoys the most. Sometimes this response leads to very fruitful information.

A number of interview procedures and questionnaires exist that are designed to elicit specific information on variables related to an individual's use of leisure. Edwards (1977) has developed the Constructive Leisure Activity Survey, which is devoted to broad classifications of leisure activity. McDowell (1976) has formu-lated a somewhat more general interview process. Lewinsohn, Munoz, Youngren, and Zeiss's *A Pleasant Events Schedule* (1978), while originally developed as a treatment device for depression, has broader applicability for overall leisure. Closely related information can be obtained through the *Reinforcement Survey Schedule* (Cautela & Kastenbaum, 1967). If "values" seem to be the desired avenue of exploration, Simon, Howe, and Kirschenbaum (1972) offer many exploratory procedures. Overs and Page (1974) have developed the *Avocational Title Card Sort* as a means of assisting the individual in prioritizing preferences for activities.

Sometimes difficulties in leisure enjoyment result from broader personal issues than the inability to identify or give priority to satisfying leisure activities. In certain leisure-related problems as well as in other personal problems, Lazarus and Fay (1975) suggest encouraging the client to identify those things he really likes versus what he believes he should like. Another approach they recommend is to request that the client list the things he quit doing because he could not do them perfectly. They suggest that helpful information may also be obtained by asking an individual to identify his unrewarding habits.

Other self-monitoring procedures can be used in order to identify and explore areas of the client's daily living. One approach is to keep an hourly log of activities during the day. This may be accompanied by a subjective assessment of the emotion attached to each activity. Possibly a rating scale can be used as a means of determining the degree of satisfaction enjoyed by each activity. The recording of fantasies and daydreams can also sometimes yield fertile information about one's idealized leisure activities.

The flow of time can be regarded as having three dimensions: past, present, and future. Some leisure difficulties can be resolved by focusing on variables in only one time frame. Yet, leisure exploration can sometimes be enhanced by exploring the relationship of factors in an additional time frame or even in all three time frames (Rule & Jarrell, 1980). Sometimes, past currents of thinking, feeling, and behavior flow into the present and then the flow is redirected from present awareness to a recycled past. Possibly the flow of present awareness might be, on other occasions, channeled toward imagined future destinations. Or perhaps at times, the past currents are, for various purposes, allowed simply to flow toward future destinations, by passing present awareness.

The Adlerian lifestyle approach, discussed in previous chapters, can often yield helpful information about this relationship. The past has a large bearing on the individual's present, and because behavior seems to be goal directed, the past influences the future as well. Very significantly, the lifestyle approach can play a major role in determining a client's difficulties with leisure satisfaction and, as a result, can be useful in both the assessment and analysis phases (Rule & Stewart, 1977). By yielding information on the client's dimly conscious goals regarding self, others, and life, the lifestyle can shed light on dimensions of leisure difficulties that need further exploration and resolution. Thus the lifestyle can serve as an indicator of which assessment instruments may be useful in providing leisure information. In addition, this approach can be used as a framework for interpreting the assessment results in the next phase, analysis.

Analysis

Once the practitioner has the assessment results before him, he proceeds to study and synthesize the information. Initially the practitioner relies on his past experience and intuition in providing direction; later in the analysis, the client's reactions to the assessment information and to the practitioner's interpretations become the overriding focus.

As Neulinger (1974) notes, leisure has one and only one essential criterion, the condition of perceived freedom. In other words, the activity must be carried out freely in order to be considered a leisure experience. He further discusses other dimensions that have a bearing on leisure activities: motivation for the activity and the goal of the activity. The motivation issue entails whether or not the satisfaction gained from the activity results from engaging in the activity itself (intrinsic motivation) or from the result of some payoff from the activity (extrinsic motivation). In regard to the goal dimension, the activity with an instrumental goal may be pursued for the sake of achieving another, final goal; whereas an activity meeting a final goal represents the end result. The client's presenting difficulties with leisure would, of course, be the determining factor in selecting which activities satisfy the requisite conditions of motivation and goal orientation. For some clients, the assessment instruments express the results in terms of specific activities; other assessment procedures, as noted previously, identify broad interests that must, in turn, be converted into specific activities.

In the process of helping clients identify or experience satisfying leisure activities, the practitioner can expect to encounter varying degrees of difficulty in analyzing profiles. The assessment results can yield several areas of high interest or activity clusters that come as a delightful surprise to the clients, who then immediately take action steps. As can be imagined, the majority of leisure involvements do not proceed this smoothly. Edwards (1977) provides some ideas for analyzing the results of those individuals whose profiles are more difficult; the following is a summary of her suggestions:

1. No main interest, few "no interests," and many medium interests. The focus should be on practical activities, thereby reducing the range to consider. An activity could be found that combines as many of the client's interests as possible, because a single interest is unlikely to be satisfying enough for this kind of person.

2. Too many main interests. This seems to be a common pattern. Individuals are so enthusiastic about so many pursuits, try to do them all, and, as a result feel unfulfilled. A key seems to be prioritizing a few for the present while saving some for the future.
3. No high interests, many "no interests," very few medium interests. A not-too-unusual profile for the severely disabled. The practitioner should look for a new twist to a medium interest that the person does not know about. Volunteer work is sometimes successful. Pursuing the classified ads in the phone book can possibly give leisure direction. Individuals in this category are often reluctant to try the unknown, so the helper should be prepared to use encouragement liberally in addition to suggesting practical solutions.
4. High interest that shows up only once. These "random highs" are not confirmed by the other instruments or sources of information. The focus should be on trying to fit the random high in with another interest or pattern of interests. This may serve to reinforce a more obvious interest.
5. Atypical interests. Sometimes the instruments will not have a broad enough range. Practitioner intuition, based on a large field of experience, is important here. Sometimes those persons seeming to be in this category may be honestly lazy and not wanting to do anything during their leisure time.

Regarding the perspective of work and leisure, Bolles (1978) suggests that "the principle of alternating rhythm" be considered. He contends that leisure should complement one's work. The person should identify his oldest and most enjoyed skills. If one's work does not satisfactorily utilize these skills, the person could choose leisure activities that will. If the individual's job does satisfactorily use his skills, then the person can use his leisure time to explore and develop his newest and potentially most enjoyable skills. This principle of alternating rhythm has obvious implications for the disabled client who is no longer able to engage in his chosen work. Perhaps leisure pursuits could be selected that would employ those skills and interests that were satisfied by his previous work. In regard to related considerations, Overs, O'Conner, and Demarco (1974) offer helpful guidelines on the relationship between various activities and limitations imposed by disabilities. Bolles (1978) has also developed a helpful "leisure map" based on Holland's (previously discussed) six areas of interest.

The practitioner should be ever alert for the appearance of inconsistencies during the sharing of this analysis process with the client. Inconsistencies can appear in many forms and, when explored, can result in very valuable insights: discrepancies between client fantasies or fears of an activity and the reality of it; a high-interest area accompanied by a strong negative reaction; a low-interest area accompanied by a strong positive reaction; a discrepancy between what the client says as compared with his behavior; inconsistencies between ability and interest; discrepancies between practicality and interest; etc. Often, as Edwards (1977) asserted, emphasizing specifics might be a productive way of breaking down many of the above inconsistencies. Then the practitioner can deal with specific solutions. For instance, by learning specifically what a person expects to gain from an activity, the practitioner may be able to suggest an imaginative substitute for the person whose leisure aspirations appear to greatly exceed his abilities.

The Adlerian lifestyle approach can yield helpful information in the analysis stage. In addition to providing helpful assessment information, the lifestyle can reflect the standards of satisfaction the person uses. Furthermore, pitfalls in decision making can perhaps be avoided by an increased awareness of a client's lifestyle. For example, in trying new leisure activities, some clients may be more vulnerable than others. Failure experiences can be growth producing for some clients; for others, they can be devastating.

Action

In the final phase, reconsideration must be surely given to the goal for avocational counseling with a particular individual. If the goal for the counseling involvement is to increase leisure enjoyment, then the activities recommended as the result of exploration in the assessment and analysis phases will usually be ends in themselves. If the overriding goal for avocational counseling is for the activities to be instrumental in bringing about change in other dimensions of a person's life, then the activities may be viewed as means to an end, an end that may not be leisure related (to be discussed further below). The distinction here may determine the activities selected, how the individual will feel about and respond to the activities, and what course of action is to be taken in pursuing the activities.

The main emphasis in this chapter has been on avocational counseling for leisure satisfaction. In this approach the basic purpose is to help the individual become involved in enjoyable activities. This process often entails not only recommending activities to the client but also specifying ways and places for becoming involved with the activities. Edwards (1977) suggests maintaining a comprehensive activity file. This file, organized by major leisure categories, would include community resources, sources of leisure information, newspaper clippings, schedules, book lists, etc. By utilizing this extensive file, the practitioner is in a better position to recommend convenient alternatives for the client. Edwards suggests that activities can be organized in terms of those that a person can do alone, those to be enjoyed with significant others, and those that can be pursued with people outside of one's social network.

Occasionally, the client will need to seek out additional information on his own. Additional reading may be assigned at the library. Sometimes this client may benefit by talking to individuals who are happily engaged in the activities under consideration. Perhaps observing some of the activities can be instructive. The more responsibility the client takes for exploring and selecting the activities, the greater the chances are that the client will ultimately find them satisfying.

In the process of exploring the ways and places of leisure activities, the practitioner may need to explore with the client what activities he will deemphasize or eliminate in order to accommodate the newly chosen ones. Perhaps an overall time-management plan will be necessary so that a pleasant flow of events is achieved. Lakein (1973) offers some helpful time-management tips. This area may be particularly critical for severely disabled individuals with many self-maintenance concerns or those with huge blocks of uncommitted time.

Barriers

In the action phase of helping in which the client explores what to do and how and where to do it, the practitioner should be mindful of obvious and not-so-obvious barriers to leisure satisfaction. Edginton, Compton, and Hanson (1980) suggest consideration of the following broad categories of barriers to leisure fulfillment: attitudinal, communicative, consumptive, temporal, sociocultural, economic, health, leisure values and skills, and experiential. Inconsistent and conflicting goals can also serve as functional barriers (such as wanting security and adventure at the same time).

Two of the most sabotaging psychological barriers to leisure satisfaction are high standards and procrastination. High standards or perfectionism can easily prevent a person's enjoyment of a leisure activity. The individual may feel he has never done well enough, or he may be afraid of failure, or perhaps will expect too much of others' involvement. With the second barrier, procrastination, the person might be telling himself any one of many irrational messages (Ellis & Knaus, 1977) in order to postpone an encounter with the activity. Either one of these two barriers is apt to exist not only in a person's approach to leisure but in other dimensions of his life as well. The understanding gained from the Adlerian life-style approach may be helpful here.

Self-Management

Avocational counseling can be directed toward purposes other than leisure satisfaction. One such purpose is self-management. In this approach the goal of the enjoyable activity is instrumental in nature, i.e., the goal of the activity is secondary to or is a means to achieving another goal. This primary goal relates to self-change in a dimension of the person's life that is not necessarily directly leisure related.

Examples of this application might include the process of a recovering substance abuser quickly becoming involved in a preselected leisure activity when he finds himself weakening in his efforts to abstain from the self-defeating chemical. Another use involves a client selecting an enjoyable leisure setting or activity for the purpose of trying out risky behaviors, e.g., assertiveness, interacting with the opposite sex, etc. Also, an individual who is vulnerable to depression could, upon recognition of cues signaling the onset of a depressive state, enmesh himself in an absorbing leisure pursuit. Furthermore, a unifying leisure activity may help in solidifying a potentially disintegrating family. The unifying thread in this use of leisure is that the pleasant quality of the activity will take the rough edge off of an otherwise very difficult process.

Often in this approach, satisfying activities are viewed in terms of their relationship to the person's target behaviors for change. Activities may be judged in regard to their ability to elicit certain behaviors or in their likelihood of reinforcing certain behaviors. In this approach, the strategy is to use contingency management in order to help the individual achieve the desired behavior change; a strong emphasis is on specific goals and performance criteria. Activities, events, and experiences are thus valued for their reinforcing properties. Rimm and Masters (1979) have divided these reinforcers into five categories: material, social, activity, token, and covert. The use of pleasant activity and experiences in this manner is thus usually a part of a broader counseling strategy. Indeed, Karoly (1980) observed that "positive contingency control may well be the most versatile tool in the realm of behavior change" (p. 225). Additional reading in the use of these techniques may be found in Watson and Tharp (1977), Rimm and Masters (1979), Kanfer and Goldstein (1980), Mahoney and Thoreson (1974), Thoreson and Mahoney (1974), and Goldfried and Merbaum (1973).

Follow-up is an important final step in the action phase. The practitioner and the client should devise a procedure that indicates to what degree the client's goals were met. This may take the form of subjective ratings, logs, tallies, reports, observations, etc. Specificity in follow-up should be encouraged as much as possible. The emphasis, however, must ultimately be on the client's perceptions, because leisure satisfaction is by nature a very subjective experience.

Stress Management

Somewhat related to self-management strategies is the emerging area of stress management. Satisfying leisure activities have a definite place in an overall stress management plan for adjustment to disability.

A stressor can be viewed as "any demand on your mind or body" (Schafer, 1978, p. 27). All stressors seem to cause wear and tear. However, "pleasant" stress seems to cause less harm to the mind and body than does "unpleasant" stress. Stressors may also be few or many in a person's life. Some disabled people may suffer from too few stressors and, as a result, be understimulated, whereas other individuals may be overwhelmed with stressors at work (e.g., high-pressure sales, certain hospital work) or during "nonworking" time (e.g., mothers with small children, compulsive gamblers, active job seekers, etc.).

Another significant factor that is related to avocational counseling is the dimension of newness versus familiarity. It seems that, in general, the greater the amount of new stressors, as opposed to familiar ones, the greater will be the impact on the individual. From a somewhat different, yet related, perspective, von Beralanffy (1968), a general systems theorist, contends that systems need both maintenance and change in order to function satisfactorily. However, individuals seem to vary in the degree of needed personal balance between these and related factors. As Selye (1974) has observed, some people are stress seekers and some are stress avoiders.

From an avocational counseling perspective, then, it is sometimes helpful to explore with a disabled client what is his own "comfort zone" (Schafer, 1978) of stress. In terms of amount of stimulation for this zone, one person may require a wide range (2 to 8 on a scale ranging from 1 to 10), another individual may feel he must always be on the go (a range of 7 to 10), and a third person may get very tense at the hint of a lot of stimulation (a range of 1 to 5). This will, of course, vary among lifestyles. Perhaps the stereotypic lifestyle of "excitement seeker" would lean toward one extreme, whereas the "inadequate" lifestyle would be found near the other.

In terms of stress management and leisure activities, the practitioner may, at times, want to respect the "comfort zone" of the disabled client. At other times, particularly if secondary gains are involved with the client's comfort zone, the practitioner may want to be instrumental in expanding, raising, or lowering the limits of the zone—what is comfortable for some individuals may not necessarily be healthy for them.

SUMMARY

Avocational counseling can be used for many different purposes. In adjustment to disability, avocational counseling is often directed toward leisure satisfaction. The primary goal here is for the selected activities to be freely chosen and enjoyable in and of themselves. The issue of freedom in choosing activities is an important one for the disabled. This seems so because these individuals sometimes have plenty of "free time" while, paradoxically, having their freedom of choice of activities somewhat limited by the nature of their disabilities. The practitioner must be especially mindful of the obvious and not-so-obvious barriers to leisure satisfaction. The suggested sequence of avocational counseling phases are exploratory discussion, assessment, analysis, and action.

REFERENCES

Bolles, R.N. *The three boxes of life*. Berkeley, Calif.: Ten Speed Press, 1978.

Campbell, D.P., Hansen, J.C. Manual for the SVIB-SC11 (3rd ed.). Stanford, Calif.: Stanford University Press, 1981.

Cautela, J.R., & Kastenbaum, R. A reinforcement survey schedule for use in therapy, training, and research. *Psychological Reports,* 1967, *20,* 1115–1130.

Compton, D., & Eddy, J. Developing leisure behavior: Education, counseling, and therapeutic recreation. *Counseling and Human Development,* 1981, *13*(6), 1–16.

Cousins, B., & Brown, E. *Recreation therapy assessment,* Jacksonville, Fla.: Amelia Island JCFMR, 1979.

Davis, J. Recreational directors observation report: *Occupational therapy: Principles and practices.* Springfield, Ill.: Charles C Thomas, 1957.

Edginton, C.R., Compton, D.M., & Hanson, C.J. *Recreational leisure programming: A guide for the professional.* Philadelphia: Saunders, 1980.

Edwards, P.B. *Leisure counseling techniques.* Los Angeles, Calif.: University Publishers, 1977.

Eisenberg, M. *Psychological aspects of physical disability: A guide for the health care worker.* New York: National League for Nursing, 1977.

Ellis, A., & Knaus, W.J. *Overcoming procrastination.* New York: The Institute for Rational Living, 1977.

Goldfried, M.R., & Merbaum, M. (Eds.). *Behavior change through self-control.* New York: Holt, Rinehart & Winston, 1973.

Holland, J.L. *Professional manual for the self-directed search.* Palo Alto, Calif.: Consulting Psychologists Press, 1972.

Hubert, E. *The development of an inventory of leisure interests.* Doctoral dissertation, University of North Carolina, 1969.

Joswiak, K. *Leisure counseling program materials for the developmentally disabled.* Washington, D.C.: Hawkins and Associates, 1975.

Kanfer, F.H., & Goldstein, A.P. (Eds.). *Helping people change* (2nd ed.). New York: Pergamon Press, 1980.

Karoly, P. Operant methods. In F.H. Kanfer & A.P. Goldstein (Eds.), *Helping people change* (2nd ed.). New York: Pergamon Press, 1980.

Kuder, G.F. *Administrator's manual: Kuder preference record.* Chicago: Science Research Associates, 1960.

Lakein, A. *How to get control of time and your life.* New York: Signet, 1973.

Lazarus, A., & Fay, A. *I can if I want to:* New York: Morrow, 1975.

Lewisohn, P.M., Munoz, R.F., Youngren, M.A., & Zeiss, A.M. *Control your depression.* Englewood Cliffs, N.J.: Prentice-Hall, 1978.

Mahoney, M.J., & Thoreson, C.E. *Self-control: Power to the person.* Monterey, Calif.: Brooks/Cole, 1974.

McDowell, C. *Leisure counseling: Selected lifestyle processes.* Eugene, Ore.: Center of Leisure Studies, 1976.

McKechnie, G. *Leisure activities blank.* Palo Alto, Calif.: Consulting Psychologists Press, 1975.

Morrow, L. Essay: What is the point of working? *Time,* May 11, 1981, pp. 93–94.

National Geographic Society. *We Americans.* Washington, D.C.: National Geographic Society, 1975.

Neulinger, J. *The psychology of leisure.* Springfield, Ill.: Charles C Thomas, 1974.

Overs, R.P., O'Conner, E., & Demarco, B. *Avocational activities for the handicapped.* Springfield, Ill.: Charles C Thomas, 1974.

Overs, R.P., & Page, C.M. *Avocational title card sort.* Milwaukee, Wisc.: Curative Workshop of Milwaukee, 1974.

Rimm, D.C., & Masters, J.C. *Behavior Therapy* (2nd ed.). New York: Academic Press, 1979.

Rule, W., & Jarrell, G. Time dimensions in leisure counseling. *Journal of Leisurability*, 1980, *7*, 3-8.

Rule, W., & Stewart, M. Enhancing leisure counseling using an Adlerian technique. *Therapeutic Recreation Journal*, 1977, *11*(3), 87–93.

Schafer, W. *Stress, distress and growth*. Davis, Calif.: International Dialogue Press, 1978.

Selye, H. *Stress without distress*. New York: Signet, 1974.

Simon, S.B., Howe, L.W., & Kirschenbaum, H. *Values clarification: A handbook of practical strategies for teachers and students*. New York: Hart, 1972.

Takata, N.: *Play as exploratory learning*. Los Angeles: Sage Publishers, 1974.

Thoreson, C.E., & Mahoney, M.J. *Behavioral self control*. New York: Holt, Rinehart & Winston, 1974.

Trieschmann, R. Coping with disability: A sliding scale of goals. *Archives of Physical Medicine and Rehabilitation*, 1974, *55*, 556–560.

von Bertalanffy, L. *General systems theory*. New York: Braziller, 1968.

Watson, D.L., & Tharp, R.G. *Self-directed behavior: Self-modification for personal adjustment* (2nd ed.). Belmont, Calif.: Wadsworth, 1977.

Wehman, P., & Schleien, S. Relevant assessment in leisure skill training programs. *Therapeutic Recreation Journal*, 1980, *14*(4), 9–21.

Wessel, J. *I can physical education program*. Northbrook, Ill.: Hubbard Scientific Co., 1976.

Williams, W., & Fox, T. *Minimum objective system*. Burlington, Vt.: University of Vermont, Center on Developmental Disabilities, 1977.

Chapter 11

Neuro-Linguistic Programming Techniques and Lifestyle Adjustment to Disability

Larry Katz

Consider, if you will, that all the counseling theories you have been exposed to are as rough maps of the complicated and changing territory of human behavior. These charts, plus the counselor's own senses and behavior, point the client in a direction that will hopefully result in the reaching of agreed-upon goals.

Treated in this way, each of the maps, or models, are shown to have features that are useful, and like a jigsaw puzzle or a treasure map, models overlap and carry on from where others stop. This chapter focuses on two complementary ways of describing human behavior, the Adlerian and the more recent Neuro-Linguistic Programming (N.L.P.), which is essentially the study of the structure of subjective experience (e.g., Dilts, Grinder, Bandler, Bandler, and DeLozier, 1980). Emphasis will be on N.L.P. as a counseling tool, interwoven with Adlerian concepts when appropriate. N.L.P. has been gaining recognition as a useful communication and behavioral change model by many and varied professions since its birth in the early '70s. At that time, Richard Bandler and John Grinder, while studying communication patterns of professionals in the arts of therapy, teaching, and business found themselves evolving a new art.

The process began with the observation and study of successful people in the communication business. Patterns of verbal/nonverbal behavior were elicited and replicated in various ways. If the results obtained were similar to those obtained by the "pros," great! If the results were different, great! Questions pointing out differences were asked, probable answers tested, and the self-evolving nature of N.L.P. manifested.

What has this to do with the Adlerian lifestyle theory of behavior and your work as rehabilitation counselor, occupational therapist, etc.? Generally, this chapter is

This chapter is dedicated to my parents, Dave and Charlene, who started it all; to N.L.P.—R.B.J.G., D.H.T.T. and the rest who added water; and to those I have had the opportunity to work with, who have provided the fertilizer; and to G.V., who waited patiently to type this.

about beliefs. It is intended that your beliefs about your capacities as a professional be challenged and expanded, leading to a different quality in your interactions with other human beings and with yourself. How many of us are not limiting ourselves? Do we sit comfortably behind a desk with relaxed shoulders and a pen held gently in our hand as we do (the dreaded) paperwork? How soon can we experience a sense of ease and greater vitality in holding this book with just the necessary amount of energy? Can we remember how effective we are in working with some clients and question how we are different with those that we are not?

As pointed out in a previous chapter, what we believe others are, life is, and I am, are very basic influences on how we act. Proper contextualizing and expanding these beliefs will give us more choices in how we act, think, or feel, thus allowing us to be more effective than we are already.

INTERVENTION STRATEGIES

As your client comes into the room, you notice a different gait and posture. Creases are formed above the eyes, hands clenching, and suddenly you hear a loud voice say "It's YOUR fault!" Your eyes scan as you catch your breath, becoming even more aware of the other's rapidly moving chest and flaring nostrils.

If this situation brings back similar experiences from your history, remember your responses and the eventual outcome. If this description is unfamiliar, you have an opportunity to prepare.

Rapport

To review:

> Dreikurs systematized Adler's techniques of therapy by distinguishing four essential but overlapping stages in the therapeutic process which are applicable to all types of maladjustment. These stages do not necessarily follow the same order and often vary in emphasis and length depending upon the client. These phases are more or less present in all existing therapies. The first stage sets the pace of communication and establishes rapport between therapist and client. A trusting relationship of mutual cooperation and respect and an agreement on objectives is established. (Nikelly, 1971, p. 28)

This concept of "rapport" has been recognized as effective within the N.L.P. model. Now, how is "rapport" established, and what are your criteria for knowing when you have it? Nikelly (1971) offers the following suggestions:

The therapist sets the client at ease during the first interview by being relaxed and friendly; irrelevant or neutral comments may help to desensitize the client and lessen the tension. The therapist can further relieve the client's anxiety by explaining the purpose of the first interview: to identify the problem before agreeing upon the goals of therapy . . . [H]is facial expression should convey respect and attention as well as interest. He must not interrupt, neither must he jump to conclusions. The client must be allowed to state the problem the way he sees it, with his own opinions, and subjective impressions. (p. 30)

In N.L.P. training, these concepts are converted into specific behaviors as one practices getting into rapport with another, verbally and nonverbally. Further, specific behaviors are checked out with the other in terms of their affect. The term "mirroring" is used to describe a process of meeting the client at his model of the world. To practice, assume the posture of your client either as if you were looking in a mirror or as if the image was reversed. Change your position to match gestures and gross body movements slightly after the other person has and do this to a lesser extent and speed so you don't feel like a marionette.

You may also pace a client's behavior verbally, while you are pacing his body analogue. Qualities of speech, tone, timbre, intensity, and rate can be matched or approximated by most people. Matching a client's intensity and rate of speech can be an "instant rapport" technique with some people, and it is a useful first exercise to practice. The client's choice of words is another important area to consider, for as the client talks, certain classes of predicates will be used more often than others, or you may find particular sequences.

a. "I hope you *see* what I mean."
b. "Do you *hear* what I'm saying?"
c. "I *feel* worms *crawling* inside me."

These are examples of three different expressions of perceptual modalities: *V*isual, *A*uditory, and *K*inesthetic, other modalities include the *G*ustatory and *O*lfactory systems, though they are used much less than the V-A-K in our culture.

A verbal mirroring response would usually include a predicate in the same modality:

a. "Let's *look* at that again."
b. "Sure, what you *say rings a bell* for me."
c. "How *slowly* do you believe they *move?*"

Each of these responses match modality V-A-K, although they do not necessarily imply agreement.

As you think back to encounters with others, you may have had the experience of knowing what the other person was thinking. These experiences may have increased as you became familiar over time with certain mannerisms others exhibited in particular contexts. In N.L.P. terms, this observing, remembering, and comparing of impressions is called "calibration."

Skill in calibration can be improved in several ways. First, conscious practice, realizing that what you observe is a reflection of how the other person is accessing/processing information, deciding, motivating, angering, etc. Second, knowing what specific behavior to pay attention to; eye movements, head movements, skin color changes, lip size changes, etc., are generally unconscious behaviors that can be calibrated to identify what sensing systems (V-A-K) a person is using in relating to the environment.

Asking a person to relate one's earliest memories presents a remarkable opportunity to calibrate such specific behaviors, known as "accessing cues" in N.L.P. When does a behavior become an accessing cue? When it is associated with a pattern. If, when you ask the client to relate three early memories and each time you notice the eyes shift up and to the client's left, you may have discovered a pattern. Similarly, asking questions in different modalities will probably give you information as to what different accessing cues apply. Notice where a person's eyes move when you ask questions like:

a. V — "What *color* was your first bike?"
b. A — "What does your doorbell *sound* like?"
c. K — "How *cold* was the lake?"

Other questions can be used in the early memory phase of information collecting that are specific to sensory modality:

a. V — "Who do you *see* when you remember that?"
b. A — "How did they *sound*?"
c. K — "What did you *feel*?"

Other accessing cues, changes in tonality, muscle tension, squinting, and blinking can also be associated with patterns of thinking in specific systems.

Testing your observations is important, and you may do this in a rapport-enhancing way as you elicit what systems the person was using. Try mirroring posture and voice qualities when you ask "I'm curious, what were you aware of just then?" The response, if oriented in one system or another, with specific predicates, will tell you how the person is representing the experience; meanwhile, you can compare the nonverbal behaviors that you observed while calibrating. You may then act as if the person is using a particular system when the individual is exhibiting the same nonverbal behavior. If, for example in responding to a question, the person's eyes shift upwards and the description is of a visual nature, you may tentatively decide that a person is accessing visual information when this individual is silent and the eyes are shifted upwards. Whether the images are of remembered scenes or from one's imagination is yet to be determined. However, this specific information can be determined.

With practice, the process of determining what systems a person is operating from can be done quickly. Also, the information can be used to pace smoothly what your client is experiencing by feeding back your tested observations. The technique of pacing the experience of the other person with statements that are verifiable seems to make statements that are ambiguous more easily accepted. This acceptance makes your task easier when you decide to *lead* your client to a different state of "being" (happy, sad, confused, wonder, etc.) or to a different mode of accessing. A practitioner does this when asking a client to "look at it from my point of view," or "step in my shoes," etc. An example of this is illustrated below:

Verbal	*Nonverbal*
"You are standing in my office, saying it's MY	(Stand up/mirroring)
fault, and I want to know what you *feel* to be my	(Look down)
fault. If you could put yourself in my shoes, seeing	(Look up)
you standing there angry, you might ask yourself,	(Softer tone)
'What is being talked about?' So, stand there	(Sit down)
or sit down and tell me what's going on."	

Sometimes, you may wish to lead a client out of a state of "depression" or a state in which the client seems unable to think or answer questions. In such a case, reflecting back your observations may be useless if the individual is not able to process what you say. N.L.P. refers to this as a "stuck" state, and there is room for a good deal of creativity in breaking it. This may be done by asking the client to stand up, walk, change breathing, look up (is it a coincidence that when things are positive we say they are looking up?), or sing "The Star-Spangled Banner," or by gently lifting the client's chin so he can see your smiling face, etc. From the few suggestions offered, you may notice the emphasis on physical, or active behavior, rather than increased effort in talking. Once the "stuck" state has changed to a more receptive one, mirror, pace, and lead with your behavior as expressed through words, gestures, and touch. The next question becomes obvious: where do we *lead* our client to? And this is the next important phase.

Information Gathering

At this point, it is helpful to refer again to how Dreikurs systematized Adler's work:

In the second stage, the client's current behavior, as he experiences it, is examined and with it, his whole life situation (birth order, family atmosphere, early recollections) in an attempt to identify a common denominator from these characteristics. The emphasis in this phase is on investigating and uncovering. (Nikelly, 1971, p. 30)

In N.L.P. training, gathering information about a client's present state and desired state is emphasized as 90 percent of the work. For in the accurate gathering of data, expressed in terms of goals and outcomes, many clients are able to show insight or put the pieces together in a meaningful way for themselves. A useful tool for this is called The Meta-Model. As described by Dilts (1981):

The Meta-Model provides an identification of linguistic patterns which could become problematic in the course of communication and a series of responses through which two individuals may use to insure more complete communication. Attention to non-verbal gestures and behavior and to context will also greatly enhance the unambiguous transference of information. (p. 12)

A few examples of linguistic patterns that can prevent accurate understanding are:

Statement	Response
a. *Deletions*—"It's your fault."	"*What* is my fault?"
b. *Lack of Referential Index*—"They say so."	"*Who* are they?"
c. *Comparative Deletion*—"It's better not to say."	"Better for who?"
d. *Unspecified Verbs*—"They scare me."	"Scare you how?"

Words like "tension," "frustration," "satisfaction" (nominalizations), "can't," "shouldn't," "always," "never" (modal operators of possibility and necessity), "good," "bad," "crazy," and lost performatives (i.e., "Who says it's good, bad, etc.") represent other meta-model violations.

You may wonder if it's possible to talk without linguistic violations. Stop wondering! We violate *all* the time we talk or write. The value of the meta-model is in the use we as professionals make of it to identify those "common denominators," to use Dreikurs' terms, that limit the choices our clients have on the level of language and communication.

Lankton, in his book *Practical Magic* (1980), illustrates many meta-model violations and the hierarchy with which it would be useful to challenge a statement such as this: "I can't find what I need to get love from any of these angry wombats and it's just making me crazy."

Now the speaker is in a spot. First, he presupposes that wombats exist, then that they are angry (mind reading), and worse, that they are making him crazy (causal modeling). The bleakest of assumptions on this highest logical level leads to further complications: at the next level we find that there are not any (universal quantifiers) wombats that are other than angry and that the speaker can't (modal operator) find what he needs to stop them. All of the wombats are the same, too (generaliza-tion). At the more mundane level, the statement implies that the speaker is having a rough time trying to find (unspecified verb) what the "something" is that he needs to get love (Nominalization). All in all, it is a real tough jam. (p. 54)

Armed with the ability, knowledge, and sensory acuity to gain rapport and gather useful information, how do you decide what information you need? If you are in a strange city, and only know that the bus station is on 12th and 0 Streets (your destination) then you need to know where you are presently in order to determine the appropriate direction.

As an example, the previously discussed early memories provide many oppor-tunities for the practitioner to identify and to test patterns of accessing cues (eye movements, posture, etc.), meta-model violations, as well as the basic goals a person has incorporated, and the typical manner of behaving to achieve those goals. Now, the client comes to you with a problem; if you are sure that you understand it, given the context (where, when, how, with whom, etc.), and how the person appears (a calibrated impression), then you need to know what the client wants for the outcome, or *desired state*. A basic presupposition that has proven useful is for the practitioner to obtain a statement of what the client wants in positive terms. This approach saves time and lessens confusion. Moreover, outcome-of-the-outcome questions usually elicit positive frames.

Client	*Counselor*
"I want to lose 50 lbs."	"What would that get you?"
"I don't want to feel anxious."	"How would you feel if you weren't?"
"I want to quit smoking."	"How would you be if you quit?"

After eliciting a statment in positive terms, you may get a representation of what the client's desired state is and the resources the client thinks are necessary with the following questions:

What do you need to be able to do that?
How would I know if you were that way?
Pretend as if you could, and show me your being _____ (happy, confident, sexy, mature, etc.)

Remember, the best evidence is behavioral, so if you are not sure what a client wants, have the client demonstrate, if possible.

INTERVENTIONS

John works in a behavioral training program and has been there for one year. For the last month, he has arrived late, sometimes by as much as three hours. Although I had no plan as to what to try, I asked John to sit and I matched his speed as we sat together. He looked listless. "John," I said, "I want to . . ." and then a belch escaped me, quite loud. The effect on John was startling, he straightened up and laughed uproariously. As he was laughing, I touched his shoulder, taking away my finger as he was getting control of himself. Afterwards, he was somewhat more alert, and as he looked at me, I touched his shoulder at the same place and with the same pressure. He continued to look at me curiously. I expected, from N.L.P. training, that the touch (anchor) would act as a stimulus to trigger his laughing. It did not. So, I opened my mouth as if a belch would again erupt, and John immediately reacted in the same "joyful" manner as before. I continued holding my finger on his shoulder. After he calmed down, we talked about his tardiness.

The discussion proceeded as follows: "When the alarm goes on I turn it off and think (eyes upright) that nothing will be any different, and I (eyes downcast) don't feel like getting up. So I don't." "Well, John, when you turn off the alarm you can't see how things will be, we never know what will happen, and how curious could you feel (I dropped my left hand down so his eyes went down-right) knowing that? Somewhat, maybe."

I guessed then from the way John looked, that he was "stuck" when the alarm rang, that he did not feel as if he had energy. So I said, "John, when the alarm goes off tomorrow it could sound like (and I touched his shoulder and opened my mouth) this." John again laughed as before, and through gulps of laughter, he said, "O.K." I also told him to be at one of our other contracts that he had not worked before. After he agreed to this I asked him what would happen, when, next day, his alarm sounded. He laughed and said "I'll turn it off."

John has been on time for the last six weeks. While he was at the other work site, I telephoned a supervisor there and asked him to question John about what he remembered when he woke up. The supervisor reported that John laughed while saying it was like any other day.

This is really an example of using a high energy resource state (laughing) and combining it with what was once a signal for accessing a low energy state (alarm clock). These signals, which are discreetly paired with behavior, are called "anchors." In the case above, a kinesthetic (touch on the shoulder), a visual (opening the mouth), and an auditory (belch) were all paired with John's alarm clock.

Anchoring is done all the time. We do it unconsciously, and many times this lack of awareness is not useful. For example, what happens if I consistently have clients sit in a particular chair in my office while they relate problems? The chair, my office, or I might become paired with the relating of problems and the physiological byproducts such as ulcers, rashes, headaches, fever, etc.

Another N.L.P. intervention technique is to change history. This includes having a person reexperience minor problems in the past with the anchored resource (identified by the client, it could be assertiveness, confidence, etc.) that was needed for a different outcome. The next step is projecting into the future the same types of situations with the satisfactory resource unanchored.

Dissociation is another intervention technique. This is an example, with one client who became angry at the sound of another person's voice. I asked the client to take a remembered time and run the person's voice "backwards." This was done for a few remembered times, and again, projected into the future in fantasy. The person has had fewer instances of immediate anger, although association with the other person over time can still lead to arguments. For a more thorough description of techniques, consult Bandler and Grinder (1975, 1979), Farelly and Brandsma (1975), and McMaster and Grinder (1980).

CONCLUDING REMARKS

N.L.P., like any other discipline or art, requires practice, competent teaching, and an open mind. Some people who have taken training have dropped out or have been turned off by what they perceive as a highly manipulative form of helping. Others, myself at times, have become discouraged by the perceived failure of some technique or other. And still others become despondent when they can't seem to remember how they communicated before they got into N.L.P. These descriptions are of a few of the traps that have been recognized, and for each trap there are at least five ways out. Remember, N.L.P. is a "tool," a self-sharpening and evolving one, to be sure! Still, it is a tool to be applied by people in conjunction with their present philosophies, methods, and values. When something doesn't work, try something else. The old maxim "If at first you don't succeed, try and try again," is missing the words "something else."

The intent of this chapter was to challenge and expand beliefs. N.L.P., in my opinion, focuses on the development of its user in terms of awareness, skill in observing, flexibility of behavior, and sense of playfulness and humor. When I "work" with someone there is a feeling of playfulness lurking someplace, and my beliefs about being serious, honest, straightforward have all become expanded so that I can still choose to be like that or I can be humorous, authoritative, brotherly, fatherly and sometimes, motherly.

And if that doesn't work I'll try something else, or ask others what they would do or fantasize about persons who could succeed and what they would try or . . .

194   LIFESTYLE COUNSELING FOR ADJUSTMENT TO DISABILITY

REFERENCES

Bandler, R., & Grinder, J. *The structure of magic I*, Palo Alto, Calif.: Science & Behavior Books, 1975.

Bandler, R., & Grinder, J. *Frogs and princes*. Mohab, Utah: Real People Press, 1979.

Dilts, R. *Neuro-linguistic programming (training manual)*. Santa Cruz, Calif.: Division of Training and Research, 1981.

Dilts, R., Grinder, J., Bandler, R., Bandler, L., & DeLozier, J. *Neuro-linguistic programming: The study of the structure of subjective experience* (Vol. 1). Cupertino, Calif.: Meta Publications, 1980.

Farrelly, F., & Brandsma, J. *Provocative therapy*. Cupertino, Calif.: Meta Publications, 1975.

Lankton, S. *Practical magic*. Cupertino, Calif.: Meta Publications, 1980.

McMaster, M., & Grinder, J. *Precision: A new approach to communication*. Beverly Hills, Calif.: Precision Models, 1980.

Nikelly, A.G. (Ed.) *Techniques for behavior change*. Springfield, Ill.: Charles C Thomas, 1971.

Chapter 12

Lifestyle Counseling for Independent Living

Martha Hughes Lassiter

The lifestyle approach to counseling as developed by Alfred Adler can also be viewed in the context of skill development in independent living. These are skills that are crucial to all well-functioning persons but may be more difficult for a severely disabled person to develop. Included in these very important competencies are the knowledges and practices that go into the tenure of control over one's life: skills in problem solving and decision making: skills in understanding self and interacting beneficially with other people; and skills involved in accepting oneself, including one's disabilities, and, beyond acceptance, in appreciating one's own special uniqueness and potential for living.

In order to explore the application of the lifestyle approach to independent living, background material is presented to describe the independent living movement, its inception and implementation by practice and by law, as a growing force in society. To this information about independent living is added some examples of persons who are severely disabled and attempting to live independently and who are in the process of developing further the skills that enable them to be as self-reliant as possible or feasible.

Further, the use of the lifestyle approach to counseling is described as a tool that may be of special use to the development of skills of independent living. Special strategies for intervention or change are presented in the context of the activities of a center for independent living.

INDEPENDENT LIVING: BACKGROUND AND PRESENT STATUS

Independent living, according to Frieden, Widmer, and Richards (1983)

as it relates to severely disabled people, means making decisions which affect one's own life and being active in the mainstream of community

> life. Goals of independence for severely disabled people are potentially
> the same as those for anyone else. . . . However, severely disabled
> people are often prevented from reaching these goals by physical,
> psychological, social, and environmental barriers. (p. 254)

Again, independent living can be defined as the control over one's life, based on
the choice of acceptable options that minimize reliance on others in making
decisions (Shinnick, Hoffman, & Burdy, 1983, p. 264).

Begun in the early 1970s by a group of disabled persons who were determined to
penetrate and overcome the artificial barriers that were preventing their being in
control of their personal destinies, the movement has grown dramatically in
succeeding years. It is impossible to separate happenings in a specific field, i.e.,
legislation affecting persons with disabilities in 1973 and in 1978, from the
societal influence that spawned them. Ranking high in importance were the civil
rights laws of the '50s and the implementation of those laws in the '60s and '70s.
More visibility of racial minorities led to more visibilities of other minorities:
women and the disabled. The understanding of the importance of self-esteem and
control of one's life for racial minorities began to extend to the minorities who
were disabled.

The 1973 Rehabilitation Act, Section 504, acted to prevent discrimination
against "otherwise qualified handicapped" people. In the same year, Public Law
94-142 insisted on the rights of all disabled children to the age of 21 to be educated
and in the "least restrictive" setting appropriate. For the first time, the issue of
"mainstreaming" began to be discussed pro and con. The movement of disabled
people into the mainstream of American life continued as group homes and
halfway houses were developed to accommodate the kind of disabled persons who
no longer needed the severe restrictions of life in an institution. The 1978
amendments to the Rehabilitation Act resulted in the availability of federal grants
for federal-state funding with a 90/10 ratio. This set in motion the development of
the independent living centers.

The independent living center is one of three basic types of independent living
programs identified by Frieden (1980): (1) the Independent Living Center, a
nonresidential program controlled by consumers providing services for relocation,
personal care attendants, peer counseling, advocacy, and other services specific to
the center; (2) the Independent Living Residential Program, an alternative type of
housing, controlled by consumers, with attendant care, peer counseling, transportation services, and other services specific to the program; and (3) the Independent
Living Transitional Program, which provides independent living skills training
pertinent to activities of daily living, housing, and other services specific to the
program. Each of these three programs provides services that are supportive to the
disabled person who is concerned with a greater amount of personal control and
consumer control or heavy consumer involvement.

For further clarification, a number of terms are defined according to their specific meanings in the context of the independent living movement.

Consumer—The severely disabled person concerned with being independent and autonomous.

Peer counseling—Counseling by a disabled person who has attained disability-related experiences, knowledge, and coping skills and assists other disabled individuals in coping with their disability-related experiences. (Eighth Institute on Rehabilitation Issues, 1980)

Service provider—A person providing direct services to the trainee; examples are the physical therapist, personal care attendant, person providing transportation, etc.

Advocacy—"Action by individuals or groups on behalf of one or more disabled persons to insure their rights and interests" (Wright, 1980, p. 740).

Personal care attendant—An attendant who provides whatever personal care is necessary for the consumer; it is crucial that the consumer provides the parameters.

At the present time, approximately 200 independent living programs are operating in the country, with probably every state represented by the time of this publication. Equally dramatic may be the rise of consciousness of the American public to a greater understanding of disabled persons as more like than unlike, as persons more capable than incapable, and more visible than invisible.

The kinds of skills being learned are the ones Carl Rogers talked about in *On Becoming a Person* (1961). They are skills that can be thought of on a continuum —skills that are a lifelong challenge. The skill development in independent living is not limited to a particular group of disabled persons. However, it is both cognitive and affective in nature and is most appropriate for persons whose most severe disability is physical. For the purposes of this chapter, the disabled persons will be understood to be within the normal range mentally and emotionally.

Earlier the statement was made that the crucial skills leading to independence and autonomy may be more difficult for a severely disabled person to develop. Logic might lead one to believe that this is almost always true. After all, the severely disabled person must have help and may, in the case of congenitally affected persons, have always had to depend on a certain amount of help. Certainly, society is more understanding of a person who is blind being guided or a person with severe arthritis being fed than it is of a nondisabled person depending on others.

A specific example may raise further questions about the complex set of circumstances that may lead a person to be more independent—or more dependent. Mr. B. was in his mid-50s. He had a progressive disease that was destroying his vision. Since he was in his 40s, he had moved through the stages of loss of vision. Finally, in spite of medical intervention, the remainder of vision was gone and he was totally blind. His comment over many months following this event was, "As long as I could see the curb, I was all right." The counselor worked with Mr. B. to help him to work through the adjustment to being totally blind. After two years, Mr. B. seemed little closer to adjustment, seemingly unable to proceed from the grief and loss stage. The counselor consulted with a counselor who had worked with Mr. B. eight years prior to his losing total vision. The first counselor reported that Mr. B. had always complained bitterly about his progressive loss of vision, apparently not able to move beyond the attitude of "if only it hadn't happened to me."

A theory was generated that perhaps the disability was a factor influencing Mr. B.'s inability to move ahead with his life, but the more important factors might lie elsewhere. The counselor worked out a new plan with the client's full cooperation and began to collect the data necessary to help the client discover his life goals as set out by the lifestyle approach. Family constellation (only child) and very early recollection provided information reinforced by the client's feeling of self as a powerless person to whom everything happened: "a Victim" (Mosak, 1971). It is clear in this particular case that the development of the lifestyle came many years before the disability. And the proposition might be raised realistically that as long as Mr. B. held on to self-pity and resignation and preferred the rewards offered that behavior, the adjustment process would not proceed.

LIFESTYLE COUNSELING AS A TOOL FOR IL SKILLS

The discovery of the lifestyle may be an invaluable tool in discovering the *real* problem that the severely disabled person may be grappling with. As in all counseling situations, the presenting problem, which, in the case of the consumer of IL, may be described as making adjustments to blindness, deafness, spinal cord injury, or a debilitating disease, may be severely complicated by other serious problems including a lifestyle that may have been at times a self-defeating and negative influence.

Skill development in independent living has been defined here as those skills that are incorporated into the well-functioning, independent person who has a degree of control over the events in his or her life. They are the same skills that enable that person to penetrate barriers. These are the kind of skills that may very well be the top priority skill training items in a counseling setting in an independent living center.

In the independent living center, skill development is most likely to be a goal of the peer counseling sessions. The type of peer counseling session most appropriate for the lifestyle approach is probably group counseling. Lifestyle counseling can be time consuming in its demands for information gathering and reflecting by the client, and the group approach, by using a partnership method, would provide the means for the time required. The partnership method also provides built-in support through the partners' commitment to each other.

The peer counselor in the independent living center is a peer of the persons involved in the center, i.e., he or she is also severely disabled. The peer counselor is required to have coping skills and to have attained a satisfactory adjustment to disability. The peer counselor may or may not have a preparation for counseling grounded in academic theory and practice usually associated with counseling the disabled person. For this reason, an instructor with the necessary experience in lifestyle counseling may be invited to work with the group as a helping person in the early stages: information gathering and information exchanging.

It is important to point out that, although not necessarily prepared by the traditional university course work, the peer counselor nonetheless is expected to go through a training course. This course may be quite intensive, including supervision paired with experiential on-the-job training. A part of this training could well be an experience by the peer counselor of discovering his or her personal lifestyle with the help of someone trained in the discipline.

The group setting may be especially helpful in the process of encouragement, a "very powerful motivating and therapeutic device" (Nikelly & Dinkmeyer, 1976, p. 97). It is practicable to think that the special ties that can form in a group who share many problems can be the most secure setting for working toward an understanding of self and developing insight into methods of change.

It is important to note that the use of lifestyle counseling in the context of the independent living center is a use of the approach as a learning device, an educational tool. In this setting, the premise is that a severely disabled person with serious adjustment problems would be provided more appropriate therapeutic techniques by a professional counselor.

Lassiter (1974) describes an activity schedule for group counseling in rehabilitation settings that combines the use of group work and individual conferences. This could provide a workable guide for use in the independent living center. In addition, Lassiter notes that "this pattern of organization of small group work in rehabilitation will require modification by the practitioner to meet the reality of (the) particular work situation" (p. 56).

An activity schedule in an independent living center might consist of one week for choosing the group members, limiting the group to two or three partnerships (four to six persons), and four weeks for the information gathering period, with the group meeting together two hours per week and the partners meeting with each other privately another two hours per week. This might be followed with one week for individual conferences with the peer counselor. By this stage, it is expected that the group members will have explored their own individual lifestyles and now be prepared to look at their life goals as they apply to their earlier stated goals of independence and autonomy.

CASE EXAMPLE

An example of how this might work can be seen in the case of Ms. J. When she was 35 years old, Ms. J., who had been a recreation therapist in a small city, was injured in an automobile accident. The physical involvement resulted in a partial paralysis of one leg and considerable loss of vision. She was able to move around with the aid of a walker. Ten years later, Ms. J. was living in a "home for adults" where she shared a room with three other women.

When Ms. J. came to the independent living center she always clutched a heavy bag, explaining that she had to keep her valuables with her. Living in her present circumstances, sharing a room with others, she was afraid of having her valuables stolen. She had good reason to be concerned since she had lost a bracelet she cherished and believed it had been stolen.

Rather than complain about the theft, Ms. J. had begun to collect the items she felt she could not bear to lose and carry them around with her. She brought the bag with her to each group or individual session. By the counselor's exploring her family constellation and early recollections, Ms. J. was able to gain some insight into some of the barriers that were interfering with her own needs for independence. From an early age, Ms. J. had valued cheerfulness and being pleasant in all circumstances; with help, Ms. J. was able to recognize a major lifestyle goal as being a "Pleaser" (Mosak, 1976). She never wanted to be disliked by anyone, even someone who would steal from her. With additional reflection and with the encouragement of the group who were involved in exploring, in a tentative fashion, new behaviors of their own, Ms. J. began to try to practice expressing her feelings more honestly.

As an intelligent person who had been independent and had been able to cope with problem solving fairly well when she was physically well, her situation as a severely disabled person had worked, in conjunction with her need to please, to her severe disadvantage. Understanding her new insights and coupling that with a wry sense of humor, Ms. J. began to practice some new assertive behaviors. She was encouraged by her peers at the independent living center. At this writing, she is still carrying the heavy bag wherever she goes but is talking about buying a chest with a large padlock.

SUMMARY

This chapter has provided some practical information in exploring the lifestyle approach to counseling in the context of skill development for independent living. It has stressed the limitations of the approach described as appropriate to the person whose major disability is physical. It has pointed out by the use of examples how one's personal lifestyle may interfere with the goal of independent living: the achievement of skills that allow the severely disabled person to be independent. In addition, it has provided the description of one setting where the physically disabled person may benefit by the lifestyle approach to counseling.

REFERENCES

Eighth Institute on Rehabilitation Issues, Conference on Peer Counseling, position paper. Chicago, 1980.

Frieden, L. Independent living models. *Rehabilitation Literature,* 1980, *41,* 7–8.

Frieden, L., Widmer, M.L., & Richards, L. The independent living program movement. In R. Lassiter, M. Lassiter, R. Hardy, J. Underwood, & J. Cull (Eds.), *Vocational evaluation, work adjustment and independent living for severely disabled people,* Springfield, Ill.: Charles C Thomas, 1983.

Lassiter, R.A. Group counseling with people who are mentally handicapped. In R. Hardy & J. Cull (Eds.), *Group counseling and therapy techniques in special settings,* Springfield, Ill.: Charles C Thomas, 1974.

Mosak, H.H. Lifestyle. In A.G. Nikelly (Ed.), *Techniques for behavior change,* Springfield, Ill.: Charles C Thomas, 1971.

Nikelly, A.G. and Dinkmeyer, D. The process of encouragement. In A.G. Nikelly (Ed.), *Techniques for behavior change,* Springfield, Ill.: Charles C Thomas, 1976.

Rogers, C.R. *On becoming a person,* Boston: Houghton Mifflin, 1961.

Shinnick, M.S., Hoffman, S., & Burdy, N. Guidelines for the development of independent living services in rehabilitation facilities. In R. Lassiter, M. Lassiter, R. Hardy, J. Underwood, & J. Cull (Eds.), *Vocational evaluation, work adjustment and independent living for severely disabled people,* Springfield, Ill.: Charles C Thomas, 1983.

Wright, G.N. *Total rehabilitation,* Boston: Little, Brown, 1980.

Part IV

Interventions for Specific Disabilities

Chapter 13

Lifestyle Intervention for Physical Therapists

Rita M. Riani

Try to remember a time in your life when you needed help because of a physical difficulty. Most of us can call to mind some time when we were dependent on someone else for assistance of some nature. Perhaps after breaking a leg, we found ourselves unable to open doors because both hands were holding the crutches that made it possible to walk. For some of us, recurrent back pain makes it difficult to perform routine daily activities or make it into work everyday. Think of the inconvenience many of us have experienced from just a simple cut on one finger of our dominant hand. These examples may seem minor, but the point is that most of us can recall some of the feelings that arise related to any condition, no matter how minor, that limits our control over our bodies and renders us to some degree dependent. These feelings could include anger, frustration, anxiety, fear, and depression.

Coupled with pain, it is easy to see how a physical limitation, especially when permanent or severe, could have a drastic impact on the emotion and mental health of any "normal" individual. Add to these feelings the conditions often associated with an extended period of recovery and rehabilitation following the onset of a disabling condition. Whether one is hospitalized or at home, there is often further loss of control over one's immediate environment, thus increasing feelings of dependency, social isolation, loss of privacy, and a significant reduction in choices available on a day-to-day basis. Although it may not be possible to help someone to avoid all of these situations completely, physical therapists, like other health providers in the rehabilitation field, can do quite a bit to lessen the degree of the emotional reactions and situational problems mentioned. This goal can be accomplished only when we recognize and acknowledge the strength of the link between the emotional, psychological, and physical sides of all individuals, ourselves included. When this is accomplished, patients can truly be approached holistically; by taking into account feelings and thoughts, the process of physical rehabilitation will hopefully be enhanced.

As is well known, the curriculum in physical therapy is geared predominantly toward teaching evaluative and treatment techniques, providing a strong theoretical basis on which to build. Of equal importance, and an area in desperate need of attention in many curricula, is the physical therapist's ability to enter into and communicate effectively in interpersonal relationships. It is my contention that physical therapists who are able to relate genuinely in human relationships, listen attentively, provide warm encouragement, confront effectively, and provide accurate feedback will positively affect outcome and increase the chances of long-term, successful rehabilitation. With a strong sense of self and well developed interpersonal communication skills, therapists will be better able to cultivate self-responsibility, problem-solving skills, and decision-making abilities in the patients they treat, thus speeding the recovery process and enhancing rehabilitative efforts. Utilizing the lifestyle approach to understanding and modifying human behavior, it may be possible for therapists in all settings to gain an awareness not only of personal behaviors, but also the patterns of behavior of their patients in the context of an overall life pattern, thus enabling them to structure treatment plans and approaches individually, according to each patient's needs.

THE ROLE OF THE PHYSICAL THERAPIST

As part of a multidisciplinary health care team, the physical therapist is responsible for helping patients reach their maximum level of functional independence following the onset of a disease, injury, or accident. Ideally, the goal is for patients to be able to resume those activities, both vocational and avocational, that previously made life meaningful for them. When this is not possible because of the nature and/or degree of the disability, the physical therapist may be involved in the exploration of and training in new skills that will enable patients to become as active as possible and to reclaim roles as contributing members of society.

The scope of operation of physical therapy is extremely varied. Frequently, therapists are employed in acute general hospitals, home health agencies, children's rehabilitation centers, school settings, private practice, universities, rehabilitation centers for adults, independent and transitional living centers, and nursing homes. In addition to the various settings physical therapists can work in, they may also develop specialized skills in areas such as long-term rehabilitation, orthopedics, pediatrics, neurology, cardiopulmonary care, cardiac rehabilitation, burn therapy, cancer rehabilitation, hand therapy, prosthetics/orthotics, and geriatrics. The patients they treat may have experienced any of a multitude of acute or chronic disability or disease states. In acute care settings early rehabilitation is often aimed at improving or maintaining physical status, early mobility skills training, instruction in activities of daily living, patient education, pain reduction, wound care, and prevention of further disability and/or deformity. In these settings patients are typically seen for shorter periods of time than in long-term rehabilitation settings, and acute medical care is often the main priority.

In contrast, long-term rehabilitation patients may be followed by the same therapist, daily, for as long as several months. Treatment sessions can range from 15 minutes to several hours. The goals in these settings are usually directly or indirectly related to gaining independence in areas such as self-care skills, activities of daily living, functional mobility, vocational and avocational skills, and other independent living skills. In these settings treatments are often conducted in individual as well as group sessions, and it is not uncommon for patients to develop very close relationships with their therapists as well as other patients on the rehabilitation unit. For this reason, and simply because patients often spend a large portion of their waking hours in contact with their therapists, the quality of the patient/therapist relationship can potentially have great impact on rehabilitation outcome.

One of the physical therapist's first responsibilities is to perform a thorough evaluation and identify deficits or abnormalities in specific areas, and to document this information objectively. These areas can include joint range of motion, strength, sensation, tone, mobility, activities of daily living, balance, coordination, mental status, reflexes, etc. A physical therapy treatment program is then planned based on both the findings of the evaluation and the specific short- and long-term goals set mutually by the patient and therapist. A successful outcome will in great part be dependent on the quality of the physical therapy program outlined, the competence of the therapist in implementing specific techniques, and the motivation of the patient to participate in the program. Perhaps just as important is the therapist's ability to interact with that patient in a supportive, honest, yet challenging, manner. As in other helping situations, the therapist must be able to build a relationship based on mutual respect, trust, and understanding.

If the atmosphere is one of trust, the therapist may be free to provide feedback in a nonthreatening manner, within the context of the physical therapy treatment program, about specific observed behaviors that may be causing problems or limiting progress. If patients are able to gain an awareness of the consequences of their actions, they may then begin to develop strategies aimed at utilizing more productive behavior. In this manner they may become better able to react to the demands of life, less as a result of prior conditioning and more based on independent choice.

For the purpose of this chapter, I will limit my discussion to those patients requiring long-term rehabilitation or facing permanent disability states. These disabilities could be incurred as a result of problems including, but not limited to, arthritis, amputation, spinal cord injury, traumatic brain injury, cerebrovascular accident (stroke), and other neurological disorders.

IMPLICATIONS FOR LIFESTYLE ADJUSTMENT

In spite of the fact that the physical therapist may treat patients with a wide variety of diagnoses in varied physical settings, there is one characteristic that most cases have in common. The physical therapist usually treats people who, as a result of a disabling condition, have experienced some degree of disruption in their lives and whose ability to function in their usual manner has been compromised in some way. They are all people faced with stressful life situations and daily challenges that each will view from a unique perspective and respond to in his or her own individual way.

Attitude

The beliefs one has adopted regarding self, life, and others may directly influence the degree of success realized during the course of the rehabilitation process. One's attitudes about issues such as disability, dependency, loss of control, and failure could significantly affect the way an individual participates in a rehabilitation program and its eventual outcome.

Another way that one's basic attitudes can be significant to the overall probability of successful long-term rehabilitation is the degree to which those attitudes or the resulting lifestyle contributed to the presence of the disabling condition. Often, the presenting problem for which a physical therapist is treating an individual is a direct result of a trauma that occurred from circumstances that were completely beyond the individual's control. On the other hand, there are also many people with disabilities caused by conditions either directly or indirectly related to their manner of living and/or personality type. Examples include the various stress-related diseases, diseases related to poor dietary habits, alcohol-related diseases, or accidents and injuries incurred as a result of risk-taking behaviors. If one believes that the attitudes that individuals develop about life, self, and others will affect the choices they make in life and their behavior both now and in the future, then perhaps changes can be accomplished, when desired, by confronting these notions and choosing new, more rewarding behaviors.

As we have noted, Adlerian theory postulates that people move through life with certain patterns of behavior. These patterns are largely based on the individual's subjectively determined goals in life that were developed in early childhood. In reference to his early years, Adler said, "It was not so much my childhood experiences in themselves that were important; rather the manner in which I judged and assimilated them" (Ansbacher & Ansbacher, 1956, p. 200). Dreikurs (1953) summarizes Adler's view of the influences of heredity and environment in his statement that

> the growing child experiences both of them—and draws his conclu-
> sion. . . . He experiences his environment equally by the pleasant and

unpleasant consequences of his behavior. Therefore, the child himself integrates all his experiences, may they come from within or without. His interpretations of them gives them their significance for his actions and development. (p. 35).

Adlerians believe that our goals in life are formulated as a result of interactions with the significant people in our first social setting, usually the family, and that they will strongly influence the manner in which we choose to gain significance in an overall life plan. Adler believed this mental frame of reference, or lifestyle, guides people through life, influencing how they respond to situations and interactions with others. The lifestyles people develop help them choose behaviors that they find are successful in evoking desired responses from others. They also keep them moving toward their self-selected goals in life. In many cases, these goals are not consciously known to the individual. They often become more apparent, especially to others, during stressful situations such as the onset of a disability or initiation of a rehabilitation program. These chosen attitudes can work much to one's advantage in some circumstances and also to one's disadvantage in others. Behaviors selected as successful when interacting at home may prove very unsatisfactory for success in the office or workplace. What may have worked well for years for the client as an able-bodied citizen may now create problems following the onset of a serious disability and the subsequent rehabilitation process.

Ansbacher and Ansbacher (1956) define the term "social interest" as "the innate aptitude through which the individual becomes responsive to reality" (p. 133). Patients with what Adler would refer to as high social interest will be those people who believe they can achieve success and do so by setting goals for themselves. In these cases, the physical therapist may offer guidance, suggest specific techniques and exercises, monitor progress, and provide feedback throughout the recovery process. Success is likely because the individual has adopted a positive attitude about life, self, and others. Challenges are approached in a success-oriented manner. Other patients may be less success oriented and tend to look at life and its challenges in a more negative light. These people may have more difficulty setting goals for themselves and may need much encouragement along the way. It is for these patients in particular that the quality of the therapeutic relationship will be most important. If the physical therapist can relate to these patients sincerely, demonstrate positive attitudes, allow the opportunity for early successful experiences, and structure the program to minimize failure, even the most discouraged patients will begin to gain satisfaction from accomplishments and redirect themselves toward new, more positive and productive goals. Gaining a lifestyle awareness may help patients to identify those times when behaviors are working to their disadvantage and, therefore, provide the opportunity for change.

Image

Another more specific aspect of the self that can have a strong influence on one's attitudes and interactions is the physical self. This is the image one presents based on physical characteristics, appearance, and one's perception of them. Dreikurs (1953) states that "in most accounts of the connection between the physical structure and character, the physical factor generally, though not always, takes precedence" (p. 34). In support of this premise, Feldenkrais (1977) states that "a person's physical build and his ability to move are probably more important to his self-image than anything else" (p. 34).

Obviously, much information is available about others from the way they move, their posture, body build, and body language. It would be difficult to deny the importance today's American society assigns to attributes such as youth and beauty. This fact can create strong pressures to maintain certain appearances in order to gain positive reinforcement from those around us. The pressures can be so great that individuals may begin to measure their own self-worth based on the physical characteristics they possess. Barker, Wright and Gonick (1946) have stated that persons who live in cultures where social distinctions are made on the basis of age, sex, race, stature, beauty, or physical normality will behave, upon observing their own physique, in accordance with their evaluation of these criteria.

Barker, Wright, Myerson, and Gonick (1953) described the somatopsychological reaction, a relation dealing with "those variations in physique that affect the psychological situation of a person by influencing the effectiveness of his body as a tool for actions or by serving as a stimulus to himself and others." Wright (1960) states that

> the somatopsychological relationship involves social-psychological factors: that is, conditions that depend upon the interaction between the person and others. Much of the psychology of the individual is, in fact, a social psychology, for the way in which one feels and behaves about many things depends in greater or smaller measure upon one's relationship to other persons. (p. 3)

The nature of society's response and one's perception of that response will in large part depend on the value placed upon the trait in question and will determine how that particular trait will affect an individual's place and feelings of significance in a group. Included here may be any of the genetically bestowed characteristics such as body structure, eye color, sex, hair color, race, etc. Very significantly, the same concept is true for traits that are acquired later in life, such as a physically disabling condition. The values that a person holds to be important for maintaining a place of significance in the world will have a great impact on the way that person responds to both the physical disability and the rehabilitation process that follows.

Consider the individual whose overriding goal is to be independent and self-sufficient, who suffers a cervical fracture resulting in a high level spinal cord injury and quadriplegia. Or the college track star whose self-worth, and social influence, is measured by athletic accomplishments, who suffers the loss of a leg in an automobile accident. It is not simply the disabling trait that an individual will be responding to but also the implications that it will have on one's ability to continue to move successfully toward one's goals in life.

Wright (1960) states that

> We are sure that there are far fewer psychological experiences peculiar to persons with physical disabilities than an offhand guess might indicate. Even in the case of sensory loss, as in blindness or deafness, the psychological significance of the deprivation has to do in large measure with such matters as the threat of social isolation, the struggle for independence, acceptance of personal limitations and so on—experiences with which many if not all humans are conversant. (p. 3)

Generally, in our culture, regardless of the disability, the tendency is to assign the disabled person a position of inferior status. This, to an individual striving constantly for a position of superiority could prove to be a devastating experience because all humans seek superiority in the sense of striving to perfect one's unique ideal of self-in-relation-to-others. Wright (1960) states that

> Physical limitations per se may produce suffering and frustration, but the limitations imposed by the evaluative attitudes toward physique cut deeper and spread far wider; they affect the person's feelings about himself as a whole. One of man's basic strivings is for acceptance by the group, for being important in the lives of others, and for having others count positively in his life. As long as physical disability is linked with shame and inferiority, realistic acceptance of one's position and one's self is precluded. (p. 14)

However, not every person who acquires a disability will react negatively to that condition. There are those who would view this circumstance as a major life challenge and channel all of their resources into compensating for the deficit. Dreikurs (1967) stated that "by courage and training, disabilities may be so compensated they even become great abilities. When correctly encountered (note the conditional and not the automatic result!) a disability becomes a stimulus that impels towards a higher achievement" (p. 175).

Growth and Change

The concept of the creative power of the individual is an important one to understand when encountering patients in a therapeutic environment. Every person develops a unique, individual lifestyle; no two are the same. Even when exposed to the same environment, two people will usually respond differently to similar stimuli. Dreikurs (1967) discusses this dynamic aspect of personality development and states that it is the individual "who determines by himself what significance the forces have which affect him from within and without" (p. 173). It is this dynamic aspect of the process that makes it important to remain aware that categorizing lifestyle types and expected behaviors can be very helpful. But in many cases, all this process can offer are general probabilities based on commonly observed trends. Each individual must continue to be seen as unique and be given the opportunity to accept or reject the feedback offered by the therapist. Only when the patient is an active participant in the interpretation and reorientation process will growth and change be meaningful.

STRATEGIES FOR INTERVENTION

As is the case with other members of the rehabilitation team, the physical therapist has the opportunity to observe an individual's behavior during treatment sessions and can begin to identify typical responses to specific situations including stages of recovery, the demands of the environment, the structure of the physical therapy program, or the individual approach of the physical therapist involved. As a result, the therapist may be able to identify recurring trends and attitudes evident in a patient's specific behavior and begin to evaluate how these behaviors are either enhancing or limiting the individual's progress or movement through the process of physical rehabilitation.

General

Having a general understanding of a patient's mental frame of reference can assist a therapist in choosing the most appropriate approach to be taken with each individual. For example, patients who are heavily invested in being the "best," or number one, may react negatively to a therapist who continually points out areas of deficiency. When working with patients who believe they are helpless, and that others should rescue them out of trouble situations, a therapist might initially use a very structured program, encouraging responsibility-taking behavior and problem solving. Utilizing general lifestyle guidelines, the physical therapist could potentially tailor the treatment approach selected for each individual based on physical therapy goals as well as the patient's individual lifestyle, thus increasing the probability of success.

An additional advantage to knowing how patients usually cope is being able to predict responses to future situations based on lifestyle information and past behavior. As a patient progresses through the rehabilitation process, there will certainly be landmark events that a physical therapist may be able to predict as potentially stressful. These could include the arrival of a prosthesis, the first home visit or weekend pass, the patient's first realization that a disability will be permanent, an important family conference, the decision to order a wheelchair or other orthotic/assistive device, the loss of a significant relationship (boyfriend, girlfriend, spouse, etc.), or discharge planning. Again, various approaches could be used regarding patient participation in the activity, the way in which information is presented, who provides the information, and the support systems available for the patient following the event.

Often patients who rely on control for significance will want to be kept informed of their prognosis at all times and play a major role in any decision-making activity. Other patients may realize certain secondary gains for their newly acquired dependent role. This type of patient may attempt to manipulate the system to maintain that role as long as possible. With this knowledge, and in order to encourage self-responsibility, the physical therapist can manage significant events in the physical therapy program in a more structured, contract-oriented manner. This can help to minimize problems encountered in implementing a physical therapy program. The patient and family can also become better prepared to avoid potential pitfalls in the future when faced with similar situations.

Choosing the appropriate approach not only serves to enhance productive behaviors but can also be helpful in facilitating an understanding on the patient's part of the motives associated with the behaviors seen. This process may allow the person more freedom to identify those behaviors that are consistently troublesome. The door is now open for change, and problem behaviors such as self-depreciation, lack of motivation, dependent behavior, irresponsibility, hostility, or lack of cooperation can be more readily modified, thus enhancing the rehabilitation process.

The advisability of including other family members in all stages of the physical therapy program cannot be overemphasized. Their personal attitudes and interactions with the patient have not only had a profound impact on the patient in the past, but may also determine the eventual success or failure of the rehabilitation program in the future. Family members, or significant others, must be kept appropriately informed regarding the patient's progress and status. They must participate actively in all educational and therapeutic activities and they must be included in the goal-setting and decision-making process. In this way, all involved parties will be working toward mutually agreed-upon goals. Plans will less often be knowingly or unknowingly undermined, and many hours of frustration over unattained goals may be saved.

Using the data on an individual's family constellation, ordinal position, and early recollections, one experienced in interpreting lifestyle inventories could identify an individual's overriding goal or goals in life. This approach can provide information to identify the general attitudes that have been adopted to cope with the stresses of life.

Although the information collected might prove to be of value to a physical therapist, it would be highly impractical for therapists in a rehabilitation setting to attempt to perform complete lifestyle inventories routinely on their patients. In addition to the very real time constraints that many physical therapists are quite familiar with, most would not have sufficient training or background to collect and interpret lifestyle information adequately. However, general knowledge of a patient's characteristic patterns of behavior, attitudes influencing their mental framework, and values chosen on which to measure their self-worth can be very valuable to a physical therapist.

This type of information could be extremely helpful when planning treatment approaches, goal setting, decision making, and program modification. When assessing a patient's benefit or lack of benefit from a therapeutic program, initiation and participation in activities, responsibility-taking behaviors, coopera- tion, and overall motivation, an awareness of the basic themes that may be influencing the general direction of movement toward or away from functional independence could be an advantage to the therapist. In the presence of behaviors or symptoms that are thought to be affecting the program adversely, an awareness of these underlying themes can be helpful in modifying these behaviors more effectively and enhancing the rehabilitation process.

Often the information that is valuable in identifying lifestyle patterns is already known to the physical therapist, or at least pieces of the puzzle have become obvious. All that may be needed is to organize and analyze it in a lifestyle context, looking for an overall theme or pattern of movement. When this is done success- fully, interactions with patients in a physical therapy program can become much more meaningful, rewarding, and productive.

Specific

Lombardi (1973) has identified eight ways to obtain lifestyle information about a person. In a rehabilitation setting, it is likely that different team members would gather information using several of these areas. Although it is not probable that all disciplines will use each of the areas, it is quite likely that there will be some overlap in the areas used to obtain information about patients throughout the rehabilitation process. Several of these are techniques that the physical therapist would already be utilizing in gathering information and would, therefore, not require any additional procedures.

The first area is case history data. Physical therapists routinely gather initial information about their patients from many sources. Certainly, much information is obtained from the medical record. This can include background information on the individual's life history as well as diagnostic and progress reports from other providers on the health care team. Conversations with family members, teachers, friends, and community agency personnel can also be helpful. This type of information is gathered from sources other than the patient.

The second area is what Lombardi calls psychological interviewing. For the physical therapist this would involve talking to the patient. Here the physical therapist and the patient get to know each other. In addition to laying the foundation for a meaningful relationship, the physical therapist can use the initial interview or evaluation sessions to obtain much data from which lifestyle inferences may be made. Questions can be asked about the patient's family constellation and social milieu. Determining prior responsibilities and present rehabilitative goals can offer much insight into the patient's expectations. It may be possible to predict how the patient might face future challenges, based on the knowledge of how challenges have been faced in the past. Although the physical therapist will be able to begin to formulate ideas about what a patient's lifestyle patterns might be, during these early meetings it is also important to allow patients time to make the transition to the rehabilitation unit. Hopefully, patients, and their families, will be well informed prior to transfer, but they must certainly be given the opportunity to learn about the rehabilitation process, the services available to them, and their potential for improvement before inappropriate judgments or labels are made or applied.

The third area is expressive behavior. Here the therapist listens to what the patient says and, at the same time, closely observes the patient. Overall appearance, posture, and nonverbal communication can provide important information about a person's attitudes. The observant therapist will at times be able to identify discrepancies between what a patient says and the messages sent with body language and actual performance. Looking at these signs in a lifestyle context and openly, yet gently, confronting the patient about them can help identify the motives behind behaviors and let him see how these may be blocking progress.

Information on family constellation includes birth order variables as well as the dynamics of the family and/or social unit that the patient has functioned in and will be returning to after discharge. In addition to asking questions, the therapist will be able to collect much helpful information by observing the patient interact with family members in both therapeutic and nontherapeutic situations. Determining who holds the major responsibilities in the family, who is dependent on whom, how they have handled stressful situations in the past, and how they interact with each other can provide valuable data to the physical therapist. Are goals the same for all involved? Do interactions move them closer toward these goals or are there conflicting forces present? Answers to these questions will help the therapist to see the patient as a whole and provide information with which to effectively plan a comprehensive treatment approach.

Early recollections would be an area that a physical therapist may or may not choose to utilize. If used, probably identification of the one earliest recollection would be the most beneficial. Early recollections are said to "provide a brief picture of how an individual views himself, other people, and life in general, what he strives for in life, and what he anticipates as likely to occur in life" (Gushurst, 1971, p. 33). In addition, Gushurst (1971) described them as likely "indices of contemporary attitudes and desires" (p. 33). Obviously, looking at one or two early recollections would not provide information detailed enough on which to draw definite conclusions. They may, though, provide one more bit of information that a physical therapist could use along with the other data collected to be able to informally "size up" a patient and formulate some meaningful lifestyle conclusions. Guidelines for interpretation are discussed in Chapter 9.

Grouping, for the physical therapist, would involve observing the patient interacting with family members, the therapist, and other staff members. It could also include interactions with other patients in exercise groups, other therapeutic groups such as community dining or educational classes, or leisure activities held on and off the unit. Observing behaviors in these settings could help to reinforce or refute the therapist's tentative conclusions based on behaviors seen in individual settings. Are there patterns of behavior emerging? Is behavior consistent with stated goals? Are there behaviors that seem to be working to the patient's disadvantage in a therapeutic environment? Are the patient's responses fairly consistent when observed in different settings such as therapy, on the unit, and with the family?

Lastly, therapists may benefit from attempting to gain an understanding of any symptomatic behaviors present. Symptoms or symptomatic behaviors, like all other behavior, are consistent with lifestyle beliefs and "become part of an overall strategy dictated by the dominant goal, fitting into it in many different ways and serving many purposes" (Shulman, 1973, p. 124). Often it is these behaviors, rather than lack of potential to improve, that will frustrate progress. Much insight can be gained by observing them in light of what the patient has to gain, or what the purpose is behind maintaining these behaviors.

Symptoms can serve many purposes that may be extremely significant for a physical therapy program and its success. As described by Shulman (1973), symptoms act to safeguard self-esteem. They can help patients to avoid or postpone having to assume responsibility, or they can ensure against having to make commitments or take difficult action. Sometimes symptoms are maintained to obtain secondary gains (i.e., sympathy, service, attention). Desires for these gains may have always been strong, but now the disabling condition may provide the first real chance to cash in on them. Shulman states that the "symptoms used for this purpose work better if they have some dramatic quality which compels the attention of this observer'' (p. 127), as is often the case with long-term rehabilitation patients (i.e. spinal cord injuries, amputations, paralysis resulting from stroke, etc.). Knowing what the patient is gaining from these behaviors, and how that fits into an overall life plan can help the physical therapist deal with them effectively in the context of a therapeutic program.

Patterns of Behavior

Mosak (1971) has identified fourteen lifestyle themes, each influencing the way an individual may face life's challenges. Understandably, these themes might also influence how an individual responds to the onset of a disabling condition and the demands faced in a rehabilitative physical therapy program. The information presented in this section is designed to provide brief, simplified examples of several patterns of behavior, described in an Adlerian context to illustrate how a general knowledge of lifestyle themes could be a useful adjunct to a physical therapist in planning treatment approaches and programs.

The "Getter"

There are those whose overriding goal is to manipulate life and those around them by putting others into their service. Such a person has been called a "getter." The methods used to carry out this style of life may be active or passive and can include charm, shyness, temper, or intimidation. In a rehabilitation setting, these individuals may attempt to elicit help from family, staff, and other patients. This can cause major conflicts when the expectations of the staff or family are based on patients initiating and taking responsibility for their own self-care activities to the extent that they are able. Behaviors that would undermine active participation in a rehabilitation program could result from the mistaken notion that self-worth can only be attained when one is in control of everyone in the environment. These individuals could tend to view life as very unfair for denying them what they feel they are entitled to—either the service they are attempting to elicit from others or the life free of a disability that is no longer theirs. A therapist that was unaware of this tendency could easily become frustrated when professional and personal expectations that the patient would assume responsibility for self-care activities in a therapeutic manner were not realized. It could also be a very frustrating experience for this type of patient to be surrounded by a rehabilitation team whose major goal was not to be put into service by the patients they treat but rather to instruct them in ways to perform tasks on their own.

For example, Mary is an elderly, retired female who has spent much of her life getting other people into her service, including her children, grandchildren, and friends. She might have a difficult time adjusting to the day-to-day demands for independence that are expected in a physical therapy program. This adjustment is made that much harder when Mary sees herself in need of even more help because of the disability she has incurred. She could become confused regarding the staff's insistence that she begin to do things for herself or she might become angry and resentful when the assistance she expects and demands is not given. This type of patient can be heard to complain that the staff is not doing the job that they are getting paid to do because they will not help her or that her family would offer more help if they really loved her. A more positive and less conflicting means of obtaining control is seen in the patients who are so nice that people want to do things for them. These patients will often be very popular with the staff and can usually manipulate people into doing things for them because "Mr. Smith is such a sweet man, I didn't mind." Obviously, progress toward independence would be slow in either case.

For patients such as this, it is very important that explanations be provided in a clear and objective manner. If they can gain an understanding of the entire process of rehabilitation and the need for them to participate fully at each level, performance of routine daily activities can be made more meaningful. It may also be helpful to have these patients attempt to provide assistance to patients who are at a lower functional level than they are. This, at times, has proven to be a very enlightening and rewarding experience for some patients.

The "Driver"

The "driver" is a person who is constantly in motion toward self-set goals. This type of person is often overambitious and seldom allows time out for the luxury of a rest. On a daily basis, the physical therapist often sees this person as very work oriented, although there may be an associated lack of satisfaction gained from tasks accomplished. In therapy, people who are drivers may strive to be the best, perform the most exercises, work the hardest, and have been known to deny fatigue. Such individuals can be very pleasant to work with because of the obvious cooperation and self-motivation, and may upon request to do 10 situps, actually do 25. They will initiate activity on their own, assume responsibility for their own care, and maintain an attitude of independence in working toward all physical therapy goals. Believe it or not, problems can also arise with this type of patient.

Take, for example, the 52-year-old female executive who routinely works 10 to 12 hours a day, eats on the run, may drink several martinis at lunch, and gets no exercise all week except for Saturday afternoons when she tries to compete on the tennis court with her 18-year-old daughter. She has lived unknowingly for several years with hypertension and is now in the rehabilitation unit following a recent CVA. This patient may approach the physical therapy program with all the determination that was previously channeled into her professional life. Because her standards for herself are so high, she may have difficulty setting and appreciating small, short-term goals, losing sight of the fact that full recovery cannot be made in one week, no matter how hard one works. She may strongly dislike limits being set for her by the physical therapist and may ignore requests to gradually increase the level of activity for maximum benefit and medical safety. If there are cardiac precautions present as well, this patient may often work past the point the therapist feels is safe. In the presense of mobility limitations secondary to balance and/or coordination deficits, this patient may resist the recommendations of the physical therapist to request supervision before transferring from the bed or wheelchair or walking and will often resist the use of assistive devices (e.g., walkers, canes, braces, crutches).

In this case, a major concern for the staff can be safety. It is necessary to explain very logically, providing as much objective information as possible, the reasons for the requested behaviors, although this may have to be repeated several times. It is also very helpful for other staff and the patient's family to be aware of what the patient's daily status is and what activities are safe for the patient to be performing alone, and to provide positive reinforcement for staying within the guidelines of the outlined program.

It is always best for this patient to work on setting daily and weekly short-term goals. Other desirable strategies are for practitioners to be aware of their own goals as physical therapists, to have as much information as possible concerning status and prognosis, and to be part of all planning sessions with family and staff to the extent that is possible. All of these strategies can work to a patient's advantage where there is a good prognosis for recovery and the patient is able to see progress on a regular basis and reach a fairly high level of functional independence. On the other hand, this person can become devastated by a severe disability when there is little hope for recovery and the patient continues to set unrealistic goals. This can cause the patient to give up completely with a sense of hopelessness and extreme frustration.

The "Controller"

The "controller" is a person who wants to be in a position of control at all times and strongly resists relinquishing control to others. Different ways to implement this are to control feelings, limit spontaneity, and say what is thought to be the right thing. All of these behaviors will maximize control over one's surroundings, and allow as little chance as possible of control over one's life by others. Patients with this type of lifestyle are often at an immediate disadvantage in facing a disability, especially in the early stages. The circumstances requiring their hospitalization are often unexpected and usually beyond their control. These patients suddenly find themselves in situations where their days are not well organized, tests are ordered and performed unexpectedly and often with little explanation, their food is preselected, their schedules are set by others, and rarely is their input requested. To add to the problem this type of patient may not readily discuss personal feelings and may internalize much of the frustration felt. The frustration, coupled with the forced dependent role, may be expressed by hostility toward the staff, rebellion against the system, or a strong attempt to regain control by following the rules and regaining independence.

The physical therapist that is aware of such a patient's private logic could lessen the conflict in many ways. Initially, the patient could be given as much control over the physical therapy program as possible, first in goal setting and then later in treatment planning and discharge planning. Even if initially this control is possible only to the extent that the patient chooses between two possible alternatives, it would be beneficial. If attempts are made to give patients certain degrees of control over their environments, these plans should be taken seriously by all staff. For example, once this patient has taken part in setting his daily schedule, the therapist should make every effort to make as few changes in that schedule as possible. When changes are necessary, the therapist should notify the patient ahead of time and provide reasons for the change. Whenever possible, choices could be offered regarding the type of exercises to be done and the patient given the opportunity, at least partially, to structure the time spent in physical therapy, choosing which activities will be done first, last, etc.

The lifestyle of the "controller" could work to a person's advantage because of a preference for orderliness, organization, and a strong desire to be again in control. These factors could make one an excellent student in a rehabilitation setting. Problems could arise, however, when the lack of control and inability to care for one's own daily needs without the assistance of others results in defiance, aggression, or withdrawal, all of which could obviously undermine success if the physical therapist was not aware of the underlying reasons for the behaviors seen and unable to provide support and encouragement.

The "Victim"

People who have adopted the role of "victim" and all of the behaviors that go along with it may find that a serious disabling state may be just enough to afford them the sympathy, pity, or attention they seek from those around them. They will often display self-pity for their terrible fate. Such patients can be very difficult to deal with in physical therapy settings.

When patients are able to receive secondary gains from the significant people in their lives as a result of a disabling condition, it is often difficult to elicit self-motivation toward the goal of improving their functional level. You are eliminating the condition that affords them power. These patients are often willing to accept the dependency imposed on them by their condition if the payoffs they receive are adequate. It is common for them to be somewhat of a frustration to the staff because, in spite of the evidence of physical potential to improve, little significant progress is seen. Very often, just at the point when the staff realizes that the patient is not significantly invested in the program and begins to discuss discharge, minor gains are made. Physical therapists and other rehabilitation staff will then often give the patient the benefit of the doubt and treatment will be extended. Unfortunately, this miraculous recovery does not continue and the staff finds itself once again in the same position facing the same problems with little change having occurred in the patient's functional status.

These patients can be approached in a very supportive manner with much positive reinforcement offered for responsibility-taking behaviors. Treatment programs can be presented in mutually agreed upon contract form. Daily progress can be documented on flow sheets and charts. All professional and supportive staff will need to be kept apprised of patient versus staff responsibilities to decrease the ability of the patient to manipulate unknowing staff. In the end, the physical therapist must be willing to accept the patient's goals as the ultimate determiner of outcome, no matter how divergent they are from the physical therapist's values or goals. In fact, unless the underlying purpose of this behavior can be brought to the attention of these patients, and they choose to try new behaviors in place of the old ones, there will probably be a discrepancy between the therapist's goals and the patient's behavior up until the time of discharge.

The "Baby"

There is another lifestyle type characterized as the "baby." This person claims his place in life by using charm, cuteness, and the exploitation of others. These people have usually had someone around that would step in and take responsibility for them whenever a new or challenging situation arose. They often feel helpless when faced with new experiences and have the expectation that others should bail them out whenever necessary. As a rule, they have developed excellent social skills and they use them to manipulate people into their service.

In a physical therapy program, it may be difficult to motivate such individuals to assume and initiate responsibility for themselves and their program. They may have the idea that they are not capable of caring for themselves independently or overcoming the obstacles posed by the disability. Encouraging individuals like this to push to the limits of their potential can be very difficult. Another roadblock may be faced in attempting to elicit the assistance of the family or significant others in trying to motivate this patient toward increased levels of responsibility and independence. It may be that the very family dynamics that have played a major role in developing and/or reinforcing this type of lifestyle will also encourage continuing these behaviors in the face of a disability. Unless the patient and/or family can gain insight into the purposes behind these behaviors, understand when they are not helpful, and make an attempt to alter these patterns, it is not likely that any major change will occur. The circumstances could seriously limit the ultimate success of the physical therapy program.

It is again possible that the physical therapist, with an awareness of lifestyle interpretation and a meaningful relationship with the patient, could play a key role in presenting "here and now" information regarding specific behaviors observed during therapy sessions. This may help the patient understand how the life goals that have been adopted may be contributing to the difficulty or success experienced in coping with the newly acquired disability state as well as the demands of the rehabilitation process and physical therapy program. If there is a genuine desire on the patient's part to adopt more productive behaviors, the therapist can structure therapy sessions to encourage problem-solving and responsibility-taking behaviors, provide experiences that are success oriented, and continue to offer regular, honest feedback concerning status and progress.

CASE STUDY I

Mattie was a 67-year-old widow who had been transferred to the rehabilitation unit following bilateral below-knee amputations. She had not experienced any significant complications from surgery and had a good prognosis for functional recovery. In physical therapy she was found to be pleasant and cooperative, though quiet and somewhat depressed. She had significant difficulty in setting goals for herself in rehabilitation and gave up easily when challenged with new tasks. She often needed coaxing from the evening nursing staff to carry out functional activities, and although she assisted with her self-care, she rarely initiated activities in therapy or on the unit. The physical therapist working with Mattie was pleased with her physical recovery and positive responses to the therapeutic exercise program but there had also been some frustration on the therapist's part in not being able to get Mattie to assume responsibility for her own program and play a more active role in the decision-making process concerning her future plans.

In looking at Mattie's background, we find that she was the second born of three children, with an older sister and a younger brother. During her childhood, her mother usually worked all day, leaving her older sister to assume responsibility for most of the housework, the two younger children, and a disabled father. Mattie married young, her husband being an older, very domineering man. They lived a comfortable, happy life and raised two children. Mattie's major responsibilities during her married life were home care and caring for the children. She stated that she always remembers being taken care of, first by her sister, then—not surprisingly—by her husband. After her husband's death she relied heavily on her sister and children for support. Because both children lived out of town, Mattie planned to go to live with her sister and brother-in-law when discharged from the rehabilitation unit.

Knowing these few basic facts about Mattie's background may have given the physical therapist enough insight early in the program to recognize Mattie's behaviors in physical therapy as part of an overall life pattern. The therapist could then have structured the program to emphasize successful experiences and minimize manipulative (although primarily at a dimly conscious level) behavior. Responsibility-taking behaviors could have been encouraged by using daily goal setting, with flow sheets and charts to document activity and visualize progress. Activities could have been divided developmentally into simple singular units, and positive reinforcement provided for accomplishments and evidence of problem-solving behaviors. Recognizing and initiating this process early may have made the first several weeks spent in rehabilitation somewhat less frustrating and much more productive.

CASE STUDY II

Edward was a 59-year-old male admitted to the rehabilitation unit following the onset of a stroke. He is a local business executive who has a history of hypertension and had a heart attack three years ago. His major problems from a physical therapy standpoint were ataxia, causing him to have poor balance and poor coordination of all extremities, double vision, dizziness, and high blood pressure. The chart indicated that he had made significant progress in the acute care setting and had a good prognosis for continued improvement. Reports also indicate that Edward had a very supportive family (wife and three grown children) and was very anxious to get started in the rehabilitation program.

On evaluation in physical therapy, Edward was found to be very pleasant and extremely cooperative, although very unwilling to admit to his physical limitations. He was very self motivated as far as performing exercises on his own both in the physical therapy department and on the unit. However, he became easily angered at himself when faced with a task he was unable to perform correctly the first time, constantly saying "I should be able to do this." He was so anxious to do well that he often began a task too quickly with no forethought for safety precautions. When performing exercises, he often pushed himself too hard, doing many more repetitions than requested, and usually had to be asked to take rests. Because of his poor balance, he had continuously been instructed to ask for supervision, but was often found walking alone and performing his activities of daily living unsafely.

Edward had trouble setting short-term goals, wanting to perform the most difficult tasks first, then becoming extremely angry when he was unable to do so. Problems arose several weeks into the rehabilitation program after Edward had fallen many times as the result of his unwillingness to request help and heed the staff's concern for his safety.

In this case, we find that Edward was the first-born son of five children, who had lived his entire personal and professional life striving toward extremely high self-set standards. He had always had difficulty accepting any weakness in himself and was very task oriented in performing any job he set his mind to.

Edward's behaviors worked both to his advantage and disadvantage in his physical therapy program, as is the case with most individual lifestyle characteristics. On the positive side, he was extremely self-motivated to participate in all therapeutic activities. He initiated tasks often and worked very reliably on his own. He readily assumed responsibility for his program and took full advantage of tasks mastered. On the less positive side, from the therapist's point of view, was Edward's unwillingness to admit to deficits, thereby making it difficult for him to see the need to work on more basic skills leading up to higher level functional tasks. This also created a safety problem because he was not willing to admit that he needed assistance to perform what he considered very basic activities. In addition to being unable to prevent several dangerous falls, the physical therapist also had difficulty getting Edward to limit his physical exertion—even in the presence of fatigue and an elevated blood pressure.

An early recognition of some of Edward's attitudes could have been beneficial to the therapist in planning and initiating all phases of the physical therapy program. First, the therapist could have decided to take special care during the initial goal-setting session to break down each long-term goal, outlining the specific steps necessary to reach that goal. The therapist could also have spent additional time explaining the rationale behind each step and the therapeutic activities involved, emphasizing the need to work in a sequential fashion mastering more basic skills as a prerequisite for higher level skills. The therapist could have made a special effort to allow Edward to maintain as much control as possible over the elements of the physical therapy program. Contracts, either formal or informal, could have been introduced into the program, before problems arose, to establish a commitment and set guidelines for expected behaviors from all parties. Early orientation of the patient's family would certainly have been beneficial in providing them the opportunity to reinforce issues described above, such as safety and patience.

Often, this type of patient is anxious to return to the responsibilities at home and work. Reassurances from family members that all is well, in addition to allowing the patient to continue to be involved in activities such as money management, child care, etc., can help the patient worry less and maintain a feeling of self-worth. Patients such as this can be offered as much information as possible regarding the disability state, possible stages of recovery, and potential and/or alternative outcome possibilities. This information may help them to see their recovery process in perspective and be better able to set appropriate standards or goals for themselves within reasonable time limitations. This is not to say that patients should not be given the opportunity to "break the rules" of expected recovery. Categorization of patients should never limit opportunity.

LIMITATIONS

In view of the role of the physical therapist as described earlier, it is obvious that there would be several drawbacks to performing a complete lifestyle inventory on every patient treated. First of all, it is often the case that during the initial sessions, the therapist may intuitively size up some of the patient's behaviors in therapy and automatically structure plans to suit that individual's needs. If this process is successful and the patient continues to benefit from the treatment program, it would not appear necessary to pursue these issues further.

Because patients often present with complex and severe problems, physical evaluations may take several days and extended treatment sessions may be needed to perform the necessary exercises. In these cases, obviously it would be impractical for the physical therapist to spend up to several hours performing a formal lifestyle investigation. Focusing on the other previously discussed avenues of lifestyle consistency would be more practical.

Another limitation of this approach is that patients could be stereotyped as a result of the labeling process. This system of evaluating behavior utilizes many categories and terms to describe people. This could become a problem when (1) labels are given to people prematurely or inappropriately; (2) labels are applied with no attempt to modify behavior, thus restricting patient's growth; or (3) intellectual categorization and structured labeling is used by the therapist to avoid entering into an authentic relationship with a patient.

CONCLUSION

The Adlerian approach to interpreting lifestyles can be an extremely effective way to help people become aware of their basic motivating goals and the way these goals may be influencing their movement through life's experiences. In the course of regular counseling, people can be helped to see how the behaviors and responses they choose in life may be largely a function of the decisions they made in childhood based on their early experiences. With this awareness, they may alter the opinions they have formed and be free to choose behaviors and responses that will be more successful.

The physical therapist, as well as the patient, can benefit from a general exploration of lifestyle theory. With the information to be gained in a lifestyle evaluation, one could observe how one's own lifestyle influences responses to life, both personally and professionally. With this higher level of awareness, a better understanding could be gained about one's negative reactions and personal biases and better preparation acquired to function in a therapeutic milieu as an honest, open, helping professional.

We cannot truly be effective with our patients as long as we separate their psychological frame of reference from their physical being and attempt to treat one apart from the other. Until we see ourselves first and then our patients as holistic beings who must be approached in a holistic fashion, we will not only do ourselves and our patients a major disservice, but we will be constantly frustrated by our lack of success.

Good mental health implies having an understanding of our own basic feelings, values and thoughts. Only when we are comfortable with and feel good about ourselves, can we expect to develop genuine helping relationships with the patients we treat.

REFERENCES

Ansbacher, H.L., & Ansbacher, R.R. *The individual psychology of Alfred Adler*. New York: Harper & Row, 1956.

Barker, R.G., Wright, B.A., & Gonick, M.R. Adjustment to physical handicap and illness. *Social Science Research Council Bulletin, 55*, 1946.

Barker, R.G., Wright, B.A., Myerson, L., & Gonick, M.R. Adjustment to physical handicap and illness: A survey of the social psychology of physique and disability (2nd ed.). *Social Science Research Council Bulletin, 55*, 1953.

Dreikurs, R. *Fundamentals of Adlerian psychology*. Chicago: Alfred Adler Institute, 1953.

Dreikurs, R. *Psychodynamics, psychotherapy and counseling*. Chicago: Alfred Adler Institute, 1967.

Feldenkrais, M. *Awareness through movement*. New York: Harper & Row, 1977.

Gushurst, R.S. The technique, utility and validity of life style analysis. In J.M. Whiteley (Ed.), *The counseling psychologist* (Vol. 3). St. Louis: The American Psychological Association, 1971.

Lombardi, D.N. Eight avenues of life style consistency. *The Individual Psychologist*, 1973, *10*(2), 5–9.

Mosak, H.H. Lifestyle. In A.G. Nikelly (Ed.), *Techniques for behavior change*. Springfield, Ill.: Charles C Thomas, 1971.

Shulman, B.H. *Contributions to individual psychology*. Chicago: Alfred Adler Institute, 1973

Wright, B.A. *Physical disability: A psychological approach*. New York: Harper & Row, 1960.

Chapter 14

Lifestyle Intervention Strategies and Psychiatric Disabilities

Joe Bauserman and *J. I. Wainwright*

We were introduced to the teachings of Alfred Adler and the concept of the life-style in a seminar taught by Dr. Moe Rule. This was a powerful learning experience that influenced our thinking in important ways. No longer could we view the client as an isolated being or as the object of our technique. The patterns of living found in the lifestyle led us into interactional and systems theories and forced us to examine our own lifestyles and how they interacted with our clients. In the seminar, we did lifestyle assessments on each other under the watchful eye of our teacher, and we explored our own craziness with his support. It is fair to say that the style of this chapter is in keeping with the styles that were identified in the seminar, stubborn divergence being a shared trait. We have expressed ourselves in our own words and with our own ideas, if we can own ideas that are so heavily influenced by many people, not the least of whom are Adler and Rule. Our failure to use traditional terms and structure is not a repudiation of any person or idea, but rather an affirmation of our unique styles. Also sacrificed on the altar of style are impersonal and bipersonal pronouns, not because we are misogynists but because we happen to be men, and we are writing about ourselves and our work.

GUERRILLA CHOREOGRAPHY: COUNSELING IN THE REAL WORLD

It is always enlightening to read the theoretical and clinical wisdom of the superstars of our profession. Their brilliant conceptualizations and incisive inter-ventions are inspirational, and they become motivating ideals. In our grandiose moments we can dream of a time in the future when we shall typify the ideal counselor and receive our just reward, the one-year waiting list.

Early forays into the world of part-time private practice have sensitized us to an unanticipated but much beloved phenomenon, the placebo effect. The client who seeks out a particular counselor for assistance expects that particular counselor to be helpful, and as a result seems to be getting better before the first words are spoken. This phenomenon stands in contradistinction to our experiences as clinical supervisors and practitioners in community mental health centers. Here we stand as outposts on the frontier of the mental health delivery system. We are last resorts, forced choices, more often than not. We receive our clients by way of court orders, arm twisting, indigence, state hospitals, and default. We work with those clients who are pronounced as cured or untreatable by private programs when their insurance money runs out. Fortunately, within this population are many people who are motivated to work on their problems, and who are often surprised to find that they get much better.

Generally, we work with the unwilling, the unmotivated, the resistant, the uneducated, and the severely disturbed. We have come to think of this as the "real world." Working with the placebo-inebriated private client seems somehow supernatural, too easy and rewarding to be "real." A large number of our clients have no confidence in themselves, in the counseling process, and least of all in us. It is to these clients, whose apparent goal is to join us in failure, that we devote and dedicate this chapter. They have taught us the art of guerrilla choreography.

A guerrilla is defined by *Webster's New Collegiate Dictionary* (1981, p. 505) as "one who engages in irregular warfare, especially as a member of an independent unit carrying out harassment and sabotage." If the warlike metaphor is abhorrent to the reader, it is important to understand that these clients present paradoxical goals. The client's left brain says, "I want to change." The client as an organism, through poetry and pantomime, says more loudly, "I will not change." Our war is with the organismic imperative. Our objective is the latent force within every client toward growth and change.

Choreography is defined as "the composition and arrangement of dances"(*Webster's New Collegiate Dictionary*, 1981, p. 195). This is a metaphor frequently used by systems therapists when referring to the seemingly predictable, dancelike patterns that individuals demonstrate within the emotional systems in which they live. The integration of these strange semantic bedfellows serves to soften the warfare in which the counselor engages. His goal is to alter, through harassment and sabotage if necessary, the self-defeating dances, or patterns, of the individual in his life space.

In response to the anticipated ire of the psychotherapeutic ethicist who condemns the overtly manipulative tone of this approach, we can only say that all approaches, from Rogers' client-centered counseling (1951) to Haley's strategic therapy (1976), are manipulative in varying degrees; however, only a few deal openly with the process. In a community mental health center, given the realities of small staffs, difficult cases, large caseloads, and time constraints, it seems efficacious to dispense with idealistic pretensions of nonmanipulation. We plead guilty. This metaphorically insidious approach is born of desperation, the offspring of a stubborn will to succeed against forces that feel indomitable at times.

THE WHIP AND CHAIR: RITUALS OF COOPERATION

In beginning to work with clients having severe problems of living, the counselor must immediately engage his most powerful adversary: the client's state of fear. The client's behavioral response to fear may be more fight than flight, and the client may appear more threatening than threatened, but fear is the ultimate enemy to a successful therapeutic relationship. We believe that these individuals tend to react to novel life experiences with fear, and that they have unique styles of coping with this fear in an interpersonal context. Counseling is one of the most threatening interpersonal contexts for any individual to confront.

Out of graduate school and armed with our gentle, relationship-building skills, we found that we had high attrition rates. We learned over time that a large percentage of these cases responded much better when we were strong, active, and directive, an approach we had imagined to be counterproductive. This surprising finding, antithetical to our training and our natures, led us to theorize about the reason. The whip and chair approach to therapy is our response.

The metaphor of the whip and chair was selected because these devices give the animal trainer only the illusion of power. At any time the animals could, if they chose, tear the trainer apart. The whip and chair have impact only because the animals (and the trainer) believe they do. It is a symbolic ritual having deep significance to the participants because it enables them to work together cooperatively. Divested of ritual magic, the whip and chair lose potency and the cooperation collapses. We realize that the reader may find the words whip and chair to be offensively aggressive, and that the metaphor would be more congenial if the archetypal animal trainer had used a harmonica and an umbrella. However, we believe it is a useful image because to us it exemplifies cooperation as a consequence of ritual.

This type of cooperation, whether between lion trainer and lion or counselor and client, is capable of occurring in certain specific contexts that are laden with symbols and rituals. Each client will respond cooperatively to a counselor who can create the ritual best suited to the client's unique method of coping with the experience of fear in a novel interpersonal context.

The state of fear and excitation, fight or flight, is natural to all animals. This state precludes affiliation and cooperation. We would posit that the client, through distress or immaturity, brings this state to the first visit. The counselor, whether by empathy or good sense, shares it to a degree.

The counselor's first task is to create an interpersonal environment that is conducive to the attenuation of the fear state. This is often a unique experience in the client's life, and we believe that this experience potentiates bonding, the prerequisite of a cooperative, working relationship. The degree to which a client and counselor can affiliate is one of the key variables in predicting therapeutic success.

The experienced counselor must have a number of whip and chair rituals at his disposal in order to work with a diverse population. He must be able to assess the client's unique approach to the goal of self-protection, which translates as "not changing." The client needs the illusion of security and the counselor must attempt to provide it.

Ideally, reflective listening works and more active, controlling styles are unnecessary. Often, however, reflection leads to silence, which leads to anxiety, which leads to withdrawal. We have found that analogical communication is a powerful tool in working toward the goal of affiliation. We try to assess our clients at first sight as to whether they respond best to more or less eye contact, closer or more distant spatial relations, soft or firm voice tone, slow or fast pacing, mirroring or complementing body posture, stillness or frequent gesturing.

Just as the whip and chair provide the trainer with symbolic leadership in cooperative work with animals, the counselor's sensitivity and physical tools allow him to develop the specific behavioral analog for symbolic leadership in the counseling process. The counselor can experiment with all of the variables until he arrives at the proper combination most suitable for the individual client. The client gives the counselor feedback behaviorally and in the verbal material produced. This assessment process can go on for some time, leading to subtle adjustments and creating the optimal interpersonal context.

The counselor's physical and verbal tools, from the innate to the technical, are his whip and chair. They enable him to present the illusion of confidence, self-control, and mastery in the context he has created. This should elicit cooperation from a client who is capable of cooperating in his own unique ways.

To characterize this process in reverse, the client brings to the first visit a fantasy of what a counselor is and a fantasy of what counseling should be. It is the counselor's job to actualize these fantasies while at the same time operating in a manner consistent with his own beliefs about these abstractions. The conceptualization of the client's fantasies is largely an inferential process utilizing analogical data from the client's style of presentation, the actual content of the client's description of problems and goals, symbolic interpretation of the client's verbal content by the counselor, and thoughts and feelings in the counselor that derive from interaction with the client.

Just as the guerrilla warrior must appear to be indigenous to the countryside in which he is fighting, so must the counselor appear to be indigenous to the client's notion of counseling terrain. In working with a rural mental health population it may be as inappropriate to wear a tailored three-piece suit as to wear blue jeans. Animal metaphors certainly have more applicability than metaphors from physics or biology. Suggesting to a rural couple that their son sounds like a porcupine, scared and prickly, will help them more than talking about impermeable membranes. Space that resembles living rooms rather than treatment rooms may be more congenial to the client's inner state. It helps to be associated with a program that stresses quality of care rather than management information systems.

This call for flexibility is not meant to suggest that a counselor can be or ought to be all things to all people, but that he must be sensitive to what it is people are looking for. It may be that the client idea of a counselor is a six-foot-two 60-year-old grandfather, who has been married for 35 years, has a Ph.D., and is on the vestry of his church. The counselor can be sensitive to the gaps between himself and the client's ideal, and can be open to identifying and talking about these gaps when they are obstacles. Through this process the counselor can become the client's idea of what a counselor should be. An obese counselor can still help a client with overeating, but there is a multiplicity of interacting variables to consider.

The counselor must use his "self"(which should ideally be the sum of all of the appropriate personal tools he can identify and utilize at any given moment) in such a way that he and the client create an effective counseling environment. Each is entering a relationship and a process that are not without perils. The client faces fear of rejection, criticism, humiliation, decompensation, and a host of other threats unique to him. The counselor faces fear of failure, rejection, client suicide, and supervisory criticism, as both the client and the upcoming relationship are largely unknown.

The client has numerous means of protecting himself against such threats, but there is also a way of gaining a relationship with him. It is the counselor's first job to find this special approach. Just as the animal trainer would not use a whip and chair to organize a flea circus or M & Ms to work with lions, the counselor must find the tools to create an illusion so that the client is able to cooperate with him. The tools and the context are different for every client, but we must believe that there exists a functional ritual to elicit a therapeutic relationship with any client.

We are reminded of days long past and the dances with the boys on one side of the room and the girls on the other. We had to decide on the best approach to dance with a particular girl. Some responded very favorably to the direct approach: walk confidently to them maintaining eye contact and ask them to dance. Many others were shy and while they might dance once, there was unlikely to be much further contact. It was necessary to happen to be at the punchbowl at the same time so that shy conversation, perhaps on several occasions, could precede the first dance—all this before a good dancing relationship could develop. Counselors are simultaneously dancer and choreographer. Clients are simultaneously teacher and student, teaching the counselor what steps they know, what they have an aptitude to learn, and what dances they have no need or desire to learn. The first step in teaching a partner to dance is gaining a partner. We used to dance a lot because we approached the shy girls timidly and the assertive girls boldly. The key is in making distinctions.

UNDERSTANDING THE PROSPECTIVE PARTNER

The first important information about the client comes at the initial contact. If the client is not self referred, it is helpful to know who referred the client and the nature of the relationship with the referral resource. If the person making the referral calls us, we have to consider the client's personal investment in counseling. Is the person calling an overfunctioner or does the client elicit caretaking or project incompetence? It helps to know the referral resources. We need to know if the client is coming for himself or for someone else, the degree to which counseling is freely voluntary on the client's part. We are attentive to how the client relates over the phone, over a continuum that runs from obsequious to hostile. How verbal is the client? How articulate? How abstract? What examples does the client use to describe the presenting problem? Does the client ask questions about the agency or about counseling? Does the client prescribe his own treatment?

The relationship begins in the client's head before there is any contact, but it becomes interactional during the first telephone contact. We are sensitive to how we react to the client. Do we feel like helping, or do we feel rejecting? Do we have to question the client or does the client control the conversation? Are we looking forward to seeing the client or are we planning ways to tell our supervisor that we have too many cases and that this one should go to someone else? Do we schedule the client at the earliest possible hour or do we find logical but tenuous reasons why the earliest possible appointment time is two weeks away? By utilizing the data given by the client and our own subjective experience (relative to previous similar reactions) we can begin to generate some very tentative ideas about the client's unique contextual needs.

The first meeting is rich in information. The client's physical appearance, mannerisms, eye contact, tone of voice, and choice of words are all important variables in considering how the client relates to new experiences in general and the counseling process in particular. Close attention to verbal content can inform the counselor of the client's preferred sensory modality, as discussed by Grinder and Bandler (1976), and can be useful in developing joining strategies. Behavioral data such as choice of seating, body posture, and movements are early indicators of the client's readiness to work with the counselor.

Early interaction with the client will generate numerous hypotheses. Does the client get right into his concerns or does he talk about the weather? Does the client sit passively and wait to be drawn out or does he initiate the interaction? Does the client treat the relationship as collaborative or is he looking to the counselor to find his problem and fix it? These are all important lifestyle cues as to how the counselor needs to operate. Questions such as "What brings you here?" and "How do you feel about being here?" can reveal information on many levels.

In addition, the subjective experience of the counselor is a powerful source of data. Understanding our own countertransference responses, insofar as we are capable, has helped us to avoid making repeated mistakes.

Even in these early moments of the relationship there will be evidence of emergent interactional vectors, dynamic patterns of movement unique to the client-counselor dyad. Overt cues such as body posture (closed or open, back or forward), tone of voice, quantity of verbal communication, verbal content, amount of eye contact, and choice of seating can alert the counselor as to the likelihood of the client being a pursuer or a distancer in the relationship. Subtle cues such as the counselor's internal experience, natural body posture, and vocal response may also be making a statement about the client's operating style.

A client who sits in the corner with eyes averted and head turned, who uses a very soft voice, and volunteers no information is communicating with the counselor from an extreme emotional distance. The inexperienced counselor might react to this by aggressively pursuing the client, giving perhaps a sales pitch on the wonders of psychotherapy, rather than slowly and gently working on the client's profound fear and mistrust. This can best be accomplished by speaking softly, mirroring the client's body language or adopting a somewhat open body posture, pacing the session slowly, and communicating succinctly and concretely. At the other extreme is the client who is highly verbal and emotionally animated, sharing highly personal information immediately, and who may be very interested in the counselor as a person (''Are you married? Do you live around here?''). This client can evoke distancing behavior in the counselor, analogically rejecting to the client, and can exacerbate the client's pattern of aggressive pursuit. A more effective approach is to move physically closer to the client (leaning toward), slow the pace somewhat, and define the counseling process by focusing the client on relevant issues or history.

The counselor needs to present metacommunication that is receptive and accepting and verbal material that serves to define counseling and counselors. With difficult clients who are disturbing because of distance, pursuit, or seemingly unpredictable oscillations, the counselor must be careful in managing his countertransference lest he develop a rationale that excludes the client from treatment. It is always enlightening to hear our colleagues talk about their clients who were too resistant, unready for treatment, or improperly referred. More often than not we find evidence of unacknowledged, acted out countertransference. We also cringe to think of all of our early cases that did not work out for these apparent reasons. We are now much more congenial with the notion that we fail to connect with these clients out of ignorance and our inadequate skills.

The client's conceptualization of the problem can be very revealing. It says a great deal about what is important to him, what he is free to acknowledge, what he prefers to keep secret, and what is outside of his awareness. Over half of the marital cases at our centers initially present themselves as having problems with a child. It seems easier for many clients to experience depression than to address interpersonal impotence. Others may express fear of imminent decompensation when all evidence would indicate that they are doing fairly well. It will be important initially for the counselor to join the client in the client's perception of the problem even if reframing operations begin simultaneously. The problem the client chooses to discuss communicates about the client's openness, insight, capacity for abstraction, and readiness to work on the difficulty.

Previous efforts to solve the problem reveal cognitive and behavioral patterns in the client's lifestyle. The extremes are represented by clients on one end who utilize escalating "more of the same" (change) paradigms (Watzlawick, Weakland, & Fisch, 1974) and clients on the other end who have "tried everything and nothing works." The first clients are rigidly perseverative and tend to have trouble with creative problem solving. The second group needs immediate gratification and cannot persist with a course in the absence of significant rewards. The counselor can learn about imbedded expectations of counseling (from "Don't try to change me" to "I want results from you today") and can plan his approach to counseling accordingly. He may need to consider a strategic approach to the perseverator and a commitment to a certain number of sessions from the "results now" client.

In developing the most comprehensive understanding of the client that he possibly can, the counselor should undertake a thorough history. Counselors are often instructed in school to view clients holistically and then are not given a model of holistic assessment. A developmental history and a three-generational overview of the client's family can uncover an abundance of data that can be organized systematically. The counselor can get a sense of the client's strengths and weaknesses based on genetic factors. By studying the client's substance use the counselor can begin to understand the client biochemically, considering nutrition (especially sugar use), alcohol, licit and illicit drugs, eating patterns, and endocrine dysfunction. A medical history can reveal malfunctioning organs or organ systems and physical responses to stress. Identity issues can be inferred from successes and failures with appropriate developmental tasks. Interpersonal issues emerge in learning about important dyadic relationships in the client's life (spouse, parents, children). Systemic operations can be understood in light of the most intense triangular relationships that occur during times of stress. These triangles tend to operate in predictable emotional systems such as family, school, or work, and these systems must be assessed for structural and functional factors (Bowen, 1978). Hidden patterns often appear in viewing the multigenerational history of the family.

Societal forces must be considered in understanding both the genesis and stability of the client's difficulties. Economic problems are omnipresent, though frequently not identified, in current mental health caseloads. A job layoff is obvious, but minor shifts in family finance can lead to chronic apprehension that translates into systemic and psychic distress. There are also apparent forces beyond our comprehension that affect client functioning. Counselors must be open to cyclical patterns in the client's life and explanations about these patterns ("my period," "I always feel like this when there is a full moon," "February is always a bad month for me"). Suffice it to say that we are working primarily with unknowns and a failure to be open to the scientifically unlikely can lead to selective blindness. For example, one day we may find out that much of our information comes from pheromones. Surely, all current theories, from social learning to psychodynamics, are at best crude metaphors.

We realize that no single training program prepares counselors (or psychiatrists, social workers, or psychologists) for outpatient work with the profoundly disabled. Professionals must consider themselves responsible for their own educations, and this goes on forever. It is necessary to have a working knowledge of human development; psychopathology; neurophysiology; basic medicine; psychopharmacology; developmental disabilities; psychodynamics; personality assessment; intellectual assessment; intervention strategies with individuals, couples, families, and groups; crisis intervention; social skills training; teaching; ethics; and self-awareness. Obviously, no professional has all of these skills in depth but, just as the assessment above is an ideal, there are worthy goals to aspire to. Our clients deserve the best possible understanding.

The sum total of the counselor's assessment of the uniqueness of the client in the client-counselor relationship must be translated into interpersonal behaviors that resonate with that uniqueness. We call these behaviors joining strategies.

JOINING

One of the most jolting cultural events in our early teens was the Sadie Hawkins dance. On these occasions the roles were reversed and the girls asked the boys to dance. At other dances we had a sense of control over whom we danced with. Even if she turned out to be our ninth choice, she was the one we most wanted to dance with at that moment, and the dance was very enjoyable. At Sadie Hawkins dances, narcissism in the boys would run rampant as they regressed under the hungry gaze of a much-to-be-avoided dance partner. Those of us who maintained a shred of superego in these moments had a behavioral ideal: to dance as if we enjoyed it while at the same time discouraging chronic selection. This was tricky but we drew on our experiences with artful girls who had the same attitude toward us.

We have a more difficult task at our centers. We must dance with each partner as if we want to keep dancing regularly. Whether the much-to-be-avoided partner is called a pedophile, a rapist, or a child abuser, we must be able to transcend our revulsion at their behavior and find a connection on a person-to-person level. Sometimes this is easy but it is frequently easier to find the person "untreatable" or "resistant."

Both client and counselor start with a perception of the other as having negative power. For the client, the counselor is someone who can injure him. The client is someone who could abandon the counselor or advertise his inadequacy by not getting better. Obviously, the one responsible for acting as if he is not threatened is the counselor. It is helpful if he thinks of the client as someone who is threatened and has unique needs from counseling.

This problem is compounded if the counselor has a constricted image of the client (e.g., wifebeater) that makes the client aversive. By conceptualizing such clients as frightened and desperate and operating out of a fight or flight paradigm, image problems can be mitigated. Wife or child abusers are clearly lashing out at loved ones out of panic and desperation (fight). Child molesters have withdrawn from adult sexual relations to the manipulation of children (flight). Reading through the behavior to the person inside, it is difficult not to feel compassion and caring, even if mixed with revulsion and hostility. Good supervision can help the counselor with the countertransference problems that are unavoidable in working with this population. The counselor must be able to view every client with richness and complexity—because the client is who he is, he could only have done what he has done. It is the counselor's job to have the curiosity and objectivity to see beyond behavior that to him is intolerable or absurd and view the patterns in the client's life that made such behavior unavoidable for him.

Joining strategies can be organized along a continuum from actively passive to actively directive. Some strategies are useful with all clients, e.g., a relaxed and open body posture establishes visual openness and should be used unless it seems important to mirror the body posture of the client, often an important strategy with the more mistrustful clients. The counselor should use language that is understandable to the client but at the same time fits with the counselor that is in the client's head. In general, the counselor should bring to the interaction sights and sounds that allow the client to relax to the point at which cooperation is possible.

The most actively passive strategies are appropriate with the most mistrustful clients, people who are often called schizophrenic, paranoid, or schizoid. These clients have profound affiliation problems in their lives and typically present themselves to the counselor as terse, vague, sometimes bizarre, distant, and having no responsibility for their manifest difficulties. The counselor must focus on his metacommunication with these clients as they tend to be highly visual and acutely sensitive to mixed messages. They are quick to discard the verbal (which may not even be heard) in favor of the analogical. It is helpful to mirror the body language of these clients, perhaps moving toward slightly greater openness. The counselor must accept the client's perceptions and go at the client's pace (slowly) initially. The actual joining process for a client like this may go on for many weeks or even months. These clients will need a great deal of reassurance and specificity as time goes by, and they will present the counselor with trust rituals that he must negotiate from time to time.

Trust rituals often involve the framework of counseling, such as arrival and departure times, billing procedures, and chart security. If the counselor decides that the relationship is either unreachable or would take too long (some programs have specific time limits), he may need to move directly to the intervention phase.

For other clients, interpersonal security is enhanced by the counselor's ability and willingness to define himself in the relationship, both personally and professionally. Clients who tend to be more interpersonally aggressive are likely to test the limits of the relationship and the tolerance of the counselor. Such behavior as being late or not showing up for appointments, angry outbursts directed at the counselor, or abuse of agency support staff seem to demonstrate a need for limits in the relationship.

It is the counselor's job to accept the client as a person and make a renewed commitment to working together while at the same time defining certain behaviors as unacceptable. The counselor may find it necessary on many occasions to define what he will do and what he will not do in the relationship with the client. These clients are used to double messages as a rule, such as tolerance on a behavioral level and rejection on an emotional level, so the congruent communication of the counselor is reassuring even as it limits.

The counselor can proceed to more passive or more directive positions with the client as individual needs dictate. It is important to be sensitive to body language with these clients as their provocative behavior is likely to elicit closed, self-protective posture in the counselor unless he maintains openness consciously. These clients are wary and have their own type of trust rituals, but they will bond in a therapeutic relationship if they determine that the relationship can contain their impulses and that the counselor is not frightened of these impulses.

The most directive strategies are employed with clients who are ostensibly unjoinable. Apparently unaffiliative clients are often called psychopaths, sociopaths, and antisocial personalities. One must understand that consistent refusal to affiliate is a form of affiliation, one marked by oppositional, resistive vectors on the client's part. The counselor must join the client in such a way that the client's opposition works in behalf of the goal of counseling, but in these instances the joining and the intervention are inseparable, a combination that will be dealt with below in the intervention section.

Many clients absolutely insist on a directive counselor, either inferentially by their unruly behavior or by simply demanding structure and authority. It would be desirable if we could, as we were taught, return the responsibility to the client, but this is not always possible. Parents who have been profoundly neglectful of their children or couples who have fist fights every time they disagree often have a limited capacity to accept responsibility and exercise significant changes in a willful fashion. They may need powerful external constraints, what we call the "hovering superego." This superego may consist of a protective service worker who drops in from time to time unannounced, the local magistrate or special justice, the sheriff's department, the employer, or the counselor.

The counselor can assess, instruct, and follow up consistently, and this distasteful police work may be the very best that can be done under the circumstances. Many families prone to incest and violence tend to have multigenerational and contextual factors that make the strongest structural interventions relatively meaningless.

A client must be joined within a philosophical context defined by the client's world view, what Adler called the "apperceptive schema" (Ansbacher & Ansbacher, 1956). Guerrilla-like, the counselor must operate in a manner consonant with the client's conception of the counseling field. This requires adopting, within obvious limits, the language of the client, to the point of using favorite colloquialisms. This means employing the client's rhythm initially, starting off slowly and easily both physically and verbally for clients with slower paces. This may mean gesturing in an animated fashion and speaking in more staccato bursts with clients who are uptempo. It helps to think that the client is doing his dance and the counselor must learn the steps and the rhythm and then dance as if he has danced that way all of his life. This is an affiliation dance, and the degree to which the counselor can imagine and then produce the dance has great bearing on the future of treatment.

There is a danger at the joining stage that the counselor becomes exclusively dancer and loses the perspective and differentiation required to be simultaneously the choreographer. This is the countertransference phenomenon, as the participant observer loses the observing capacity and becomes exclusively participant without being aware of this process. Treatment is interrupted as the counselor becomes lost in either positive or negative feelings toward the client.

The dance teacher who falls in love with his student loses the evaluative eye that sees flaws and also loses the interpersonal freedom to express and change the flaws. All counselors must struggle with clients whom they enjoy so much that the desire to sustain a positive relationship supersedes effective treatment. These clients never seem to be "ready for termination."

Dance teachers also must contend with students who are so inordinately clumsy (or covertly hostile) that they are forever stomping the teacher's feet or kicking the teacher's shins. It is difficult for the teacher to maintain perspective when the strongest desire is to inflict serious bodily harm upon the student. So it is with counselors who must contend with clients who are hostile, threatening, damaging to property, boring, or so ostensibly repugnant that they arouse anger and rejection in the counselor. Most counselors have useful defenses such as rationalization, intellectualization, projection, or displacement that enable them to get rid of these clients with no sense of being either the agent of the client's departure or having colluded in failure.

Countertransference is an aspect of the work that is unavoidable to the self-aware counselor and requires constant attention. Strong feelings toward the client can also motivate the counselor in a positive way to grow and change. We began our community work as young graduates clinging confidently (counterphobically) to our narrow visions of human behavior and counseling technique. It is finally entertaining to reminisce about efforts to dispute the irrational beliefs of clients who would be called florid hysterics by our psychiatrist friends. These sessions, which seemed to go on for days, found us pursuing these eternally elusive clients through a labyrinth of cognitions. Less entertaining are memories of passive, reflective relationship-oriented work with clients who would be called borderline personality disorders. It was in these hours that we first learned what it meant for someone to "eat your lunch." Motivation, and sometimes inspiration, can be by-products of despair. We learned that a rigid, one-size-fits-all approach to these clients portended a poor success rate. We were doing the tango while our clients waltzed out of the building. We also had counseling experiences isomorphic to punk rock "slam dancing." There are clients that we just don't dance with while we are teaching them. We have to devise instructions that work from a safe distance. We enjoy dancing but student and teacher both must survive the lessons.

CHOREOGRAPHY: LEADING THE LEADER

In junior high school we used to have dances once a month when the boys' and girls' physical education classes would meet together. This was an eagerly awaited heterosexual event in our repressed lives. The chance to have close physical contact with a large number of girls was the obvious goal, but the ritual by which this took place was the dance. The particular dance that allowed the most sustained contact was cleverly named the "slow dance." Weeks of mental preparation went into selecting the perfect partner and gracefully executing the "slow dance." Partners varied widely in terms of dancing knowledge, and the "slow dance" varied from a waltz that moved all around the gym to a rhythmic snuggling that often took place in a corner and was interrupted by one of the coaches. Partner selection was motivated by lust or affection and had much more to do with appearance and personality than dance steps. The heaven that was known as the "slow dance" lasted from two to three minutes and occurred perhaps five times during a one-hour dance. Making the absolute best of this time was our fervent hope. Cotillion trained, it was our moral responsibility and great pleasure to try to leave each partner with the feeling that the two of us had danced as one. This required us to follow our partner's style at the start and attempt to influence their steps in the direction of the epitome of slow dancing, the moving waltz. This was tricky business.

Some girls had had partners, often linemen from the football team, who had inflicted brutal punishment to their feet. It was difficult to get these girls to move at all, as most of their movement was designed to keep their feet as far away from ours as possible. This led to an awkward leaning and deprived us of physical closeness. It was necessary to lean with them for awhile and at the same time demonstrate sufficient coordination that they would begin to feel safe. Other partners were afraid of close contact and it was necessary to hold them at arms length so that they could enjoy the dance. We would attempt to move a slight amount closer during each dance with grandiose expectations of dance number twelve three months down the road. This took patience, but a lot of junior high girls were very shy and the benefits were well worth the effort.

There were girls who didn't know how to dance at all. Some would want to be taught and would learn quickly. Others were not well coordinated and had to be taught step by step, very concretely and very slowly. Still others insisted on pretending as if they could dance and it was necessary to make sense of their apparently random movements and join them with the idea of shaping their steps over time. They weren't much fun but sometimes there were operating variables that made such an ordeal well worth the time and energy. Some girls would grab hold very closely and very tightly. This presented different problems in that we had closeness but no room to dance and there was the threat of the puritanical coaches and their wrath, which was reserved for offending boys regardless of who initiated the violation. Dancing with these girls required that we firmly hold them in a position that enabled us to dance without stumbling or getting in trouble. We also had to see to it that our excitation did not cause us to forget that we were dancing. In each instance we were responding to the unique needs of the partner, often giving them the illusion of leadership in order to develop a leading style that would achieve the goal of cooperative, mutually rewarding dancing.

INTERVENTION STRATEGIES

The Unreachable Client

Some clients are so upset and frightened that they isolate themselves from human contact, which is viewed as toxic, often for good reason, given the families many come from. Establishing a relationship with these people is the only way to get any helpful information to them. These clients are often called schizophrenic, paranoid, or schizoid. They trust very slowly, a bit at a time, if they come to trust at all. They cannot be joined in authoritative fashion, although some will follow instructions in a zombie-like way.

Most of the work with these clients takes place on a metacommunicative level. It is necessary to sustain the joining operations as long as it takes to create a relationship bridge that has the capacity for carrying information both ways. The counselor may have a deep understanding of the client and some very helpful insights or ideas; however, the client must be able to hear him. With these clients the intervention of choice is family counseling, but without the family, the slow work of joining becomes the intervention.

Case Study

Gail, a 34-year-old woman, was brought to the center in a catatonic state. Since the age of 16 she had been hospitalized 11 times for a total of 15 years. She had been home from the hospital for six weeks and had become progressively withdrawn, and, in keeping with her pattern, increasingly unwilling to take her medication. Her father brought a file of hospital reports that detailed the history of her problems and he had a totally pessimistic attitude about her efforts to stay out of a hospital.

While arrangements for involuntary hospitalization were being made, Gail was taken to the counselor's office. This was their first contact with each other. She sat stiffly in her chair, staring down at her knees. She was very tense, almost rigid. She showed no response to questions. The counselor sat close to Gail, directly in front of her. He told her that he would stay with her until it was time for her to go to the hospital and that he was available if at any time she wanted to talk. The counselor assumed her body posture and breathing pattern, the only bits of information available. He sustained this process for about twenty minutes and then unclenched his fists slowly (hers were clenched tightly). She then relaxed her hands perceptibly. The counselor gradually moved back in his seat and took a more relaxed position. Gail followed. The counselor then asked Gail if she was ready to talk. She looked at the counselor, said "I want to kill my father," and began to sob. After she cried she was able to speak more and agreed to go to the hospital as a voluntary patient. The counselor arranged for a three-day stay for her so that she could resume her medication. He also set up a return visit for her and her family on the day of discharge. Family counseling led to significant changes, and she has now been out of the hospital for five years, although she is still dependent upon her family for her support.

The Involuntary Client

Working in outpatient mental health, the counselor is often confronted with the involuntary client. Sometimes treatment is court ordered, sometimes the coercion is more subtle, such as the hovering attention of the protective service worker, but always the client is only aware on a conscious level of being with the counselor unwillingly. The client tends to relate negatively to the need for counseling and to the competence and character of the counselor.

The client tends to demonstrate oppositional and resistant patterns that protect self and simultaneously establish distance and nonaffiliation in the counseling relationship. Digital information from the client tends to be vague and superficial. Analogical information tends to be self protective and/or threatening.

If the client is a family, the presenting problem is often beclouded or denied, thereby making treatment irrelevant. Countertransference reactions (in the global sense) in the counselor can include confusion, feelings of rejection, fear, hostility, and frustration.

The first order of business for the counselor is managing the countertransference. It is very easy to avoid working with the involuntary client for a variety of presumably sound rationalizations: the client is not ready for treatment, this is an inappropriate referral, there is no need for treatment, etc. The counselor's style of avoidance can manifest itself here in a powerful way. Some counselors passively acquiesce to the client's perception of the situation. They may make arrangements for the client to appear at the center with no treatment being offered in order to comply with the order. Other counselors launch into an immediate attack on the client's resistance and denial, which tends to elicit more resistance and denial and destroy any chance of developing a therapeutic relationship. There are counselors who work with the client on the level that the client presents, providing the illusion of compliance by client and counselor. All are successfully avoiding treatment. Nothing is done in any of these situations to alter the client's pattern of opposition and resistance.

The counselor who can manage his reaction to the client can begin a thorough assessment of the situation, one which includes the context of the referral. The behavior of the client is so much a part of the client's relationship to the referral resource that it is essential to understand the character and motivation of the person or agency referring. It is also important to ascertain insofar as possible the degree to which the client has a lifelong pattern of opposition and nonaffiliation. To approach such a client with the goal of establishing a therapeutic relationship is both admirable for its hopefulness and ridiculous for its grandiosity. With clients called sociopaths or antisocial personalities the relationship approach is, sad to say, usually a waste of time. The client's goal is to defeat the efforts of any perceived authority figure, an unavoidable identification. Planning and intervening in strategic fashion, a simultaneous joining/intervening strategy is the most effective approach. Paradoxical approaches are worth a try with these clients and, if all else fails, another external superego does not hurt them. An example serves to illustrate.

Case Study

Buck, a 23-year-old mechanic, was court ordered to treatment as a condition of his parole. He had spent five of the previous six years in some type of correctional facility for a series of crimes including two arsons, rape, burglary, and assault. He had had individual counseling on five different occasions and records indicated no success. All records had been reviewed and the counselor had talked to the probation officer prior to the first meeting. Buck's family was fragmented and both parents lived out of state.

The counselor wore a tie and used a note pad to heighten the authority figure image. He indicated to Buck that he had been mistreated for the past six years. He told Buck that there was no doubt that he had a very serious psychiatric illness that compelled him to commit crimes repeatedly in order that he be placed in prison to be punished. He further indicated that Buck's condition was deeply rooted and untreatable and that he need not worry too much about the court-ordered treatment because he would be back in jail within two months. He said that one brief visit per month would meet the requirements of the court order and that more contact would be a waste of time. Buck returned once a month for twelve months to tell the counselor, with undisguised disdain, how well he was doing. The probation officer indicated that Buck was working full-time and had stayed out of trouble. He asked the counselor what he had done, because Buck looked forward to his counseling visits.

Many times, the involuntary client does not need such an extreme approach and only needs to learn to trust the counselor as a helper rather than an officer of the court. These clients, once trust has been established, can be treated in a conventional fashion.

The Acting Out Client

One of the most dramatic, extravagant client groups the counselor works with is the acting out client or family. They will come running to the office following or in the midst of suicidal gestures, affairs, alcohol binges, or runaways. What is enjoyable about this group is their action-oriented approach to life. What is frightening is what seems to be their relative comfort living on the thin edge of life and death or here today and gone tomorrow. Otherwise harmless and certainly natural feelings can turn into firecrackers and bombs as the client struggles to manage anxiety and protect self, often at the expense of another person.

Typically, these personalities are brittle, rigid, isolated, and distant. Their goal is survival of the self or family unit. Feelings, which may be totally out of their awareness, energize their behavior. Their lives may appear very disorganized and disorienting to the counselor. When viewing the family, the counselor may be struck by an amazing lack of cohesiveness or conversely by sticky interactions. They may relate more in accordance with prescribed roles (husband, mother, etc.) than out of a mature sense of self. Status and power are invariably issues. Safety, security, and control are the goals. Hierarchical boundaries tend to be rigid or blurred.

Effecting changes is problematic for the counselor who was taught to ask his individual clients gently about their feelings or who was trained to ask the family to communicate and negotiate a problem. The individual client will not have any apparent feelings, or the feeling his behavior expresses, which is obvious to those around him, will be vehemently denied. The family typically cannot negotiate constructively, either because their relationship foundations are too weak or because the interpersonal hazards of talking with each other are too high.

The counselor who tries to pursue these clients with these strategies is apt to leave the session feeling frustrated, angry, inadequate, and confused. Or the counselor may end the session exhausted, having spent 45 minutes trying to cork the runaway anxiety he inadvertently stimulated when he softly asked, "How do you feel about that?" He suddenly and unexpectedly finds himself trying to sweep back the ocean with a broom, and the stage is set for the client to now act out with the counselor by not showing up for appointments, not paying his bill, disappearing from treatment, or trying to kill himself.

What is often more useful and helpful with this group of clients is an active, directive, firm, no-nonsense approach that communicates safety, security, and protection. The counselor can pay particular attention to hierarchy, structure, and communication pathways, both within the family and the helping relationship. All that is needed with some families is a deeper, stronger voice tone. With others, we may have to arrange the seating, give firm directives, and even risk a confrontation. Of course, it helps to be a larger person should the counselor want to risk the latter. Responding to the context of a strong leader, people will react favorably to the unexpected and surprising. Caught off guard and presented with a forced choice, the only reasonable response they can make is to cooperate in constructive, useful ways.

Case Study

Jake and Donna were a married couple in their middle 30s who lived together with their 14-year-old son, Scott. Jake and Donna had ninth grade educations, Jake worked as a pinball machine salesman/mechanic, and Scott was in the ninth grade. Donna made the initial contact stating that she had found a marijuana pipe in Scott's room and that he refused to go to school. In addition, Scott's grades were dropping, he was frequently running away from home, usually to a nearby uncle's house, and he had recently scratched his face with a knife saying he did not want to live. Donna denied there were any marital problems.

A social history revealed a low socioeconomic family system characterized by many marriages, divorces, remarriages, alcoholism, physical abuse, withdrawing, and even disappearance in the face of interpersonal stress. Jake and Donna's marital history included a separation when Scott was two years old, with Donna moving 2500 miles away and suspending all contact with Jake and Scott for ten years. Following Donna's separation, Jake began drinking, became depressed, and did not work for 13 months. He and Scott lived with his mother. Jake obtained a divorce and Scott was told his mother was dead. However, Jake and Donna remarried when she unexpectedly returned. The family had not talked about her ten-year absence. The hypothesis generated by the counselor was that Scott's behavior expressed his goal to help his parents stay together by drawing attention to himself and withdrawing from that relationship.

Jake was alternately uninvolved with Scott or playful with him as a peer and overly cautious with Donna lest she leave him again. Donna was in the middle, overinvolved with Scott and feeling guilty about her ten-year "disappearance."

The interventions were delivered in stages beginning with reframing the marriage as extremely strong, stable, and in no danger of another separation. They were obviously meant for each other if they were drawn back together from opposite sides of the continent after ten years apart. This intervention drew on their motivation to not have marital problems, gave them a professional opinion that they wished to hear, and gave them the security they needed with each other to acknowledge and express their feelings about the missing link in their lives. It also made Scott's goal and the behaviors that suggested the goal unnecessary. But the parents' concern over his face scratching naturally remained; in addition, his running away and his school refusal persisted.

The counselor, building his relationship with Scott, joined him by expressing his anger to his mother for him. With encouragement and an air of playfulness, Scott did the same. Now that the counselor had Scott's confidence, he took a no-nonsense approach (modeling for Jake) to the face scratching, reframed the knife incident as a suicide gesture (death frightened Scott), and finally asked Scott for a decision as to whether to kill himself or not. Scott was told that any job worth doing (a reference to his school work) was worth doing well and if he chose to kill himself, a sloppy job would not be tolerated. He responded that he had no intention of killing himself or ever trying (so to speak) again.

Building on the success of this intervention the counselor took a similar position in regard to the runaways. Again Scott was given a forced choice of running away and staying away, living on roots, berries, wild squirrels, and discriminating between the edible and poisonous mushrooms, or staying home and eating his mother's cooking. The choice was his and his decision to stay implied he would now take nurturance from his mother rather than fight her, and that, receiving this nurturance, he would not need to run away again.

Now that Donna was back into the role of nurturer with Scott, the counselor gave Jake the job of ensuring that Scott went to school by directing Donna to dissociate herself from this problem and giving Jake permission to be powerful with him. Scott was given an alarm clock and the job of getting himself up and ready for school. Jake was told he could physically carry Scott to school if he refused. The communication pathways were changed here, and the counselor's authority was transferred to Jake while reinvolving him with his son. Scott responded, and the family wished to terminate.

The Resistant Client

Resistance is not a very helpful term, but we use it because it is commonly accepted. The client is doing what he does and we must understand it and develop an approach that is suitable. When counselors use the word "resistance" they seem to mean that the clients won't do what they want them to do when they want them to do it. It's as if they take the client's natural behavior as a personal affront. We do acknowledge that resistance can be a helpful reductionism if it is used to describe two people dancing in different ways, each of whom wants the other to dance like he does.

Many clients are referred to the center for treatment that they believe is unneeded. Often these cases start off as an allegedly emotionally disturbed child, and the counselor believes that family counseling is the only approach that will help significantly. Parents whose unconscious goal is to avoid their own issues do not wish to participate at all and will come in only if it is the only way the child will be seen. Other clients are referred by other professionals for treatment, but the clients do not believe that their problems could possibly be psychological in nature. They appear because they were told to come and they follow orders, but at best only a small part of the self is open to counseling. These people, for one reason or another, are unable to imagine that they could be psychologically involved in whatever the problem is.

Efforts to work with these clients tend to be straightforward at first. The counselor explores the situation with the client or family and then places the problem in a context that justifies the counseling approach. This is often enough to overcome the client's resistance and conventional treatment can begin. Other clients are less open to the psychological or contextual formulations and must be persuaded, either overtly or covertly. Sometimes these clients will agree to counseling on a trial basis to see if it helps. It is a good idea for the counselor to negotiate a commitment to a certain number of visits from these clients so that he has a chance to be effective. Their lack of investment in the process makes them likely to withdraw at the slightest provocation, and sometimes the provocative event is the counselor making progress that disturbs their equilibrium. These clients tend to be inordinately invested in their own world view and are unlikely to challenge their assumptions about life. It is the counselor's job to help them look at things differently or at least do some things differently.

Sometimes an authoritative approach will work, whereby the counselor simply tells the client or family what he believes is going on and what needs to be done. These people may never agree with him but everything works out if they will do what they are instructed to do. Once they see change, they will be satisfied, if not convinced.

If straightforward approaches do not work it is necessary to resort to more strategic techniques. For example, a worthwhile approach may be to work on restructuring the marital relationship by allowing the parents to focus on the child as "the problem." Eliciting their cooperation as a parenting team allows many marital issues to be worked on via the parenting. Interventions such as prescribing the symptom, directed play, paradox, or therapeutic double binds may be necessary (Haley, 1976; Madanes, 1981; Watzlawick et al., 1974).

Case Study

Nancy was a 49-year-old widow with two sons in their mid-20s. She was referred by a local physician who believed that she had a rather serious depression, a notion she did not share. He had been treating her for two years for medical complaints such as fatigue, sleep trouble, and migraine headaches. She had steadfastly refused to take an antidepressant or to seek counseling. The physician called the counselor to discuss her case. He described a lonely, isolated woman whose life consisted of work (as an accountant) and television. He described her sons as immature and irresponsible, and said that she was repeatedly rescuing them from financial problems. They apparently came to her only when they needed something.

The physician expressed frustration and powerlessness in his efforts to help this woman. He said she insisted there was a medical problem that he had not found that was causing all of her difficulty. Numerous medical tests had been unremarkable. The physician agreed to insist that Nancy come to the counselor to take a "test for depression." He said that she would probably agree to one visit.

The physician and counselor agreed that part of Nancy's problem was a disability of abstraction, that she narrowed her focus to specifics and could not assume holistic perspectives. They further agreed that, because so much of her life was painful and governed by forces she could not control, she had an unconscious goal of maintaining the illusion of an orderly universe through her insistence on a specific medical etiology for her symptoms. It seemed that she needed to be in control, and that all she could control at the time were the numbers at work and her belief system. The counselor told the physician that he would assume that he only had one visit with Nancy and would attempt to make the best of it.

Nancy arrived at the center on time and was given an MMPI, in keeping with her style of wanting to deal with specifics. After the test she was interviewed by the counselor in great detail regarding the specifics of her lifestyle: habits, diet, sleep pattern, hobbies, workday, leisure time, relationships. He took copious notes. History revealed that Nancy arose early, arrived at work early without breakfast, and began her day with the first of some 25 cups of coffee and 50 to 60 cigarettes. Her diet consisted of a pastry in the morning, a sandwich at lunch, and often a piece of pie for dinner. She worked alone, came directly home, and spent the evenings alone watching TV. Weekends consisted of housework and TV. Her sons appeared from time to time in need of money or lodging.

The counselor then told Nancy that he wanted to teach her an exercise that would enable her to relax when insomnia troubled her. She readily agreed to this. The counselor took Nancy through systematic muscle relaxation and then used visual imagery (accountants being highly visual). She was able to achieve a deep state of relaxation. The counselor then told Nancy while she was in a deeply relaxed state that he wanted her to imagine herself returning home from work on a Friday evening at dusk. He suggested that as she entered her dark house the only light would be her television, but that the picture would be fuzzy and the sound tinny. He told her that the Gong Show was on and that by the light of the TV she could see her dining room table, which was covered with dozens of cups of coffee, some empty and others with coffee in them. In the cups were cigarette butts and there were also ashtrays filled with smoldering cigarettes. He told her that she could see a plate of food consisting of a partially eaten sweet roll and a piece of pie and that the food was covered with roaches. Also on the table he said she would find a note from her son asking her to leave 100 dollars in her mailbox in the morning so that he could go to the beach. The counselor then told Nancy that it was time for her to go and that she should call her physician in two weeks to get the test results.

The counselor attempted to deal with Nancy's problems of perspective by giving her a holistic visual picture that summarized her lifestyle. He also made the image as sordid as possible for impact. He used the intervention after gaining Nancy's cooperation in a number of specific tasks that she could control. He made no effort to persuade her of any psychological problems and dismissed her while the image was very fresh. He delayed her next contact with the physician to give time for some change to take place.

Nancy called her doctor three weeks later and apologized for not calling the week before. She said she had been very busy. She told him that she had been making some changes in her life and was feeling a lot better. She had stopped smoking and was down to 2 or 3 cups of coffee per day. She had completely changed her diet. She had returned to her church and was becoming socially involved there. She had started to sell Avon products in her spare time and was enjoying meeting new people and making extra money, which she was planning to spend on a trip. She had told her sons that she loved them but that they would have to be self supporting thereafter. Contacts with the physician dropped from monthly to yearly checkups.

APOLOGIA

In further keeping with our own styles we have selected the word "apologia" for our final heading. "Apologia," according to *Webster's New Collegiate Dictionary* (1981, p. 53), "implies not admission of guilt or regret but a desire to clear the grounds for some course." Without "'guilt or regret'" we are recommending that counselors begin to consider the myriad possibilities of counselor behaviors open to them in the client-counselor environment. We are concerned that too many of the counselors and students that we have contact with are bound to a tightly circumscribed theory and technique that renders them helpless with huge segments of the general outpatient psychiatric population. We understand and heartily endorse the need to "'understand'" the client in some fashion and the need for thoughtful, ethical counselor conduct. This can evolve into a type of security blanket that restricts counselors in their roles as change agents with difficult cases. We are tired of hearing the easy explanation that failure to change in the client is attributable to some defect in the client rather than counselor rigidity or ignorance. We would like "'to clear the grounds'" for the "'course'" of counselor openness to the client, to himself, and to the vital new ideas that are coming from many different fields.

Our field has long been dominated by the medical model, a linear, mechanistic way of thinking that would attribute client dysfunction to some internally correctable "'cause.'" We only wish things were this simple. In the last 30 years the systems model has proposed to explicate client problems as events that occur within an emotional, interactional context having numerous antecedents, consequents, feedback loops, and circular phemomena within systems of systems of systems. These ideas are very helpful but don't always explain specific problems or help the counselor know what to do. We have found that the exclusive generalizable factor in the counselor's experience of the two-person client-counselor system is confusion. In one-to-one contact (we are frequently unable to secure family involvement), to make contextual sense of the severely disturbed client, who is typically a poor reporter, is an exercise that begs confusion. We have also found that we can conclude apparently successful treatment without understanding the client or why things changed. We do not believe that this is a result of stupidity or laziness but it reflects rather an appreciation for the complexity of these lives and the preponderance of unknowable variables.

When man attempts to deal with confusion he resorts to reductionistic explanatory metaphors. Between the explanatory metaphor of linear causality (which we believe does not explain enough) and the notion of circular, systemic causality (which is in varying degrees unknowable), we have focused on the illusion of dyadic interaction. We say illusion because there is always much more going on than two people interacting, whether one believes in a transference model or a systems model. Dyadic interaction is the metaphysical bridge that we use to traverse the gap from linear to circular, and we find that it aids us with our confusion. Of course, each of these explanations is a reductionism regardless of how simple or how comprehensive. The client is unknowable, we are ignorant, and our future together is unpredictable whenever the broadest possible perspective is taken.

Operating from that optimistic point, we are advocating a heuristic, pragmatic approach to counseling. It is heuristic in the sense that counselor behavior is oriented to discovering more and more about the client and uses each new discovery to generate more behavior promoting more discoveries. It is pragmatic in that truth is treated as a process, an unfolding illusion, and ideas are useful insofar as they have practical consequences. We believe that this approach maximizes understanding of the client through exploration and maximizes change through initiative. Unfortunately, it does not eradicate confusion. Our approach, like our field, is at this time more artifice than science.

We believe that a heuristic, pragmatic approach has two distinct advantages. The first is that the pragmatist will try something to see if it works rather than reject it at first sight because it does not appear to fit with his current theory. In this sense it can be a morphogenetic theory, becoming more and more complex over time. The private practitioner or pure theorist can afford to work in his own way and refer mismatched clients to someone else. The public practitioner must evolve a more complex theory in order to deal with the wide variety of clients he confronts, so he must be open to all ideas that may work.

The second advantage is that a pragmatic approach forces the counselor to take good care of himself. He is relying on self rather than rigid technique. If the counselor is his own tool, he is being irresponsible and incompetent if he does not maintain his own physical and mental health. Rigid purists, whether idealistic in terms of ''helping,'' ''thinking,'' or ''not manipulating,'' are in much greater danger of burning out, losing sight of the art of what is practical and reasonable.

This approach is, of course, not lacking in disadvantages. First, there is the danger of the counselor becoming technique oriented to the extent that his approach loses any semblance of a coherent theory. We believe that a healthy tension must exist between pragmatism and idealism, both within the individual counselor and within the field. The byproduct of this dialectic is theory grounded in realism, or technique guided by rationale.

Second, when we act there is always the danger of acting out. Although it may be construed as such by some, this chapter is not a paean to countertransference run amok. The counselor who is sensitive to himself, sensitive to his client in the interaction, and open to supervision can minimize the damage to the client of his emotional responses and behavioral excesses. It has been painful to learn how much of our previous behavior, believed to be in the service of the client, has been in the service of the self.

There is a particular danger in public outpatient work because of the severity of disabilities that are encountered. The interaction between a determined counselor and the abstractions of incest, violence, and psychosis is evocative of a tenacity that can drift into pugnacity or despair. We firmly believe that two hours a week of individual and group supervision is an absolute minimum to protect counselor and client from the intensity of the therapeutic interaction. We also recommend counseling for counselors.

There is a third problem that is omnipresent in our work. This has to do with the value positions a counselor must make decisions about. It is easy to use a strategic approach outside of client awareness in order to do away with child abuse or spouse abuse or incest. Many other areas of client problems are not so clear. Should counselors ever be agents of social control, as in the second case study ("Buck")? We believe there are many instances when they should. Should a counselor covertly disrupt a client's lifestyle, as in the fourth case example ("Nancy")? We believe that in this instance it was appropriate, but we have refrained in many other cases. Should a counselor lie to the client in the interest of change, such as telling a story about himself that is not true? We believe that such stories are useful therapeutic metaphors if otherwise harmless within the context of treatment, but as a rule we believe the counselor should speak the truth. These issues just add to the already profound confusion.

Outpatient work is very exciting. It has occurred to us that the nature of the work may attract more aggressive, action-oriented counselors for whom a heuristic, pragmatic approach is natural. In this chapter we have not attempted to cover intervention in any depth, for this is well beyond the chapter's scope. We have tried to evoke an attitude about outpatient counseling. The training and personal growth of the counselor should be a lifetime process, and he should be open to new discoveries within himself, within his clients, and within the literature. He should never see himself as a finished product but as an evolving process. He must nourish his curiosity, his independence of thought and action, and his openness to growth and change. The guerrilla choreographer is above all heuristic, because he learns, and pragmatic, because he works.

REFERENCES

Ansbacher, H.L., & Ansbacher, R.R. (Eds.). *The individual psychology of Alfred Adler.* New York: Harper & Row, 1956.

Bowen, M. *Family therapy in clinical practice.* New York: Jason Aronson, 1978.

Grinder, J., & Bandler, R. *The structure of magic II.* Palo Alto, Calif.: Science & Behavior Books, 1976.

Haley, J. *Problem solving therapy.* San Francisco: Jossey-Bass, 1976.

Madanes, C. *Strategic family therapy.* San Francisco: Jossey-Bass, 1981.

Rogers, C.R. *Client-centered therapy.* Boston: Houghton Mifflin, 1951.

Watzlawick, P., Weakland, J., & Fisch, R. *Change: Principles of problem formation and problem resolution.* New York: Norton, 1974.

Webster's new collegiate dictionary. Springfield, Mass.: G. & C Merriam, 1981.

SUGGESTED READINGS

Ansbacher, H., & Ansbacher, R. (Eds.). *The individual psychology of Alfred Adler.* New York: Harper & Row, 1956.

Balint, A., & Balint, M. On transference and countertransference. *International Journal of Psycho-Analysis,* 1939, *18,* 170–189.

Bandler, R., & Grinder, J. *Patterns of the hypnotic techniques of Milton Erickson, M.D.* (Vol. I). Cupertino, Calif.: Meta Publications, 1975.

Bandler, R., & Grinder, J. *The structure of magic.* Palo Alto, Calif.: Science & Behavior Books, 1975.

Bateson, G., Jackson, D.D., Haley, J., & Weakland, J.H. Toward a theory of schizophrenia. In D.D. Jackson (Ed.), *Communication, family and marriage* (Vol. 1). Palo Alto, Calif.: Science & Behavior Books, 1968.

Bateson, G. *Steps to an ecology of mind.* New York: Ballantine Books, 1972.

Berger, M. (Ed.). *Beyond the double bind.* New York: Brunner/Mazel, 1978.

Bion, W. *Second thoughts.* New York: Jason Aronson, 1967.

Bion, W. *Seven servants.* New York: Jason Aronson, 1977.

Bowen, M. *Family therapy in clinical practice.* New York: Jason Aronson, 1978.

Fromm-Reichmann, F. *Principles of intensive psychotherapy.* Chicago: University of Chicago Press, 1950.

Grinder, J., & Bandler, R. *The structure of magic II.* Palo Alto, Calif.: Science & Behavior Books, 1976.

Grinder, J., DeLozier, J., & Bandler, R. *Patterns of the hypnotic techniques of Milton H. Erickson, M.D.* (Vol. 2). Cupertino, Calif.: Meta Publications, 1977.

Haley, J. *Problem solving therapy.* Washington, D.C.: Jossey-Bass, 1976.

Haley, J. *Uncommon therapy.* New York: Norton, 1973.

Jackson, D. (Ed.). *Communication, family, and marriage.* Palo Alto, Calif.: Science & Behavior Books, 1968.

Jackson, D. (Ed.). *Therapy, communication, and change.* Palo Alto, Calif.: Science & Behavior Books, 1968.

Laing, R., & Esterson, A. *Sanity, madness and the family.* London: Tavistock, 1964.

Langs, R. The therapeutic relationship and deviations in technique. *International Journal of Psychoanalytic Psychotherapy,* 1975, *4,* 106–141.

Langs, R. The interactional dimension of countertransference. In L. Epstein & A.H. Feiner (Eds.), *Countertransference.* New York: Jason Aronson, 1979.

Little, M. Countertransference and the patient's response to it. *International Journal of Psycho-Analysis,* 1951, *32,* 32–40.

Madanes, C. *Strategic family therapy.* Washington, D.C.: Jossey-Bass, 1981.

Minuchin, S. *Families and family therapy.* Cambridge, Mass.: Harvard University Press, 1974.

Neill, J.R., & Kniskern, D.P. (Eds.). *From psyche to system, the evolving therapy of Carl Whitaker.* New York: Guilford Press, 1982.

Palazzoli, M.S., Cecchin, G., Prata, G., & Boscolo, L. *Paradox and counterparadox.* New York: Jason Aronson, 1978.

Racker, H. The meanings and uses of countertransference. *Psychoanalytic Quarterly,* 1957, *26,* 303–357.

Rogers, C.R. *Client-centered therapy.* Boston: Houghton Mifflin, 1951.

Scheflen, A. Communicational concepts of schizophrenia. In M.M. Berger (Ed.), *Beyond the double bind*. New York: Brunner/Mazel, 1978.

Scheflen, A. *How behavior means*. New York: Jason Aronson, 1974.

Searles, H. The patient as therapist to his analyst. In P. Giovacchini (Ed.), *Tactics and techniques in psychoanalytic therapy* (Vol. II). New York: Jason Aronson, 1975.

Searles, H. The countertransference with the borderline patient. In J. LeBoit & A. Cupponi (Eds.), *Advances in psychotherapy of the borderline patient*. New York: Jason Aronson, 1979.

Searles, H. *Countertransference and related subjects*. New York: International Universities Press, 1979.

Skynner, R. *Systems of family and marital psychotherapy*. New York: Brunner/Mazel, 1976.

Stierlin, H. *Psychoanalysis and family therapy*. New York: Jason Aronson, 1977.

Sullivan, H.S. *The interpersonal theory of psychiatry*. New York: Norton, 1953.

Tauber, E.D. Countertransference reexamined. In L. Epstein & A.H. Feiner (Eds.), *Countertransference*. New York: Jason Aronson, 1979.

von Bertalanffy, L. General system theory and psychiatry. In S. Arieti (Ed.), *American handbook of psychiatry*. New York: Basic Books, 1966.

Watzlawick, P., Weakland, J., & Fisch, R. *Change: Principles of problem formation and problem resolution*. New York: W.W. Norton, 1974.

Weeks, G., & L'Abate, L. *Paradoxical psychotherapy: Theory and practice with individuals, couples, and families*. New York: Brunner/Mazel, 1982.

Whitaker, C., Feldes, R., & Warkentin, J. Countertransference in the family treatment of schizophrenia. In I. Boszormenyi-Nagy & J. Framo (Eds.), *Intensive family therapy*. New York: Harper & Row, 1965.

Winnicott, O.W. Hate in the countertransference. *International Journal of Psycho-Analysis*, 1949, 30, 69–75.

Zuk, G., & Boszormenyi-Nagy, I. *Family therapy and disturbed families*. Palo Alto, Calif.: Science & Behavior Books, 1967.

Zukav, G. *The dancing wu li masters: An overview of the new physics*. New York: Morrow, 1979.

Chapter 15

Lifestyle Approaches with the Mentally Retarded

Patricia Muller Weiss and Kathleen Phayer Sadler

Genius, in truth means little more than the faculty of perceiving in an unhabitual way.

—William James (*The Principles of Psychology*)

It is hoped that this chapter will help the reader view individuals who are mentally retarded in a little less habitual way.

THE NATURE OF MENTAL RETARDATION

Mental retardation occurs in approximately 3 percent of the population, i.e., those who fall more than 2 standard deviations below the mean on the normal intelligence curve (Kirk, 1972). A more expansive definition, one most frequently used in the field, defines mental retardation as "significantly subaverage general intellectual functioning existing concurrently with deficits in adaptive behavior, and manifested during the developmental period" (American Association on Mental Deficiency, 1973).

The inclusion of adaptive behavior as an indicator provides a more accurate description of the individual's abilities and deficits. Deficits can range from none to severe among persons having the same or similar intelligence test results. Adaptive behavior encompasses how or what the individual performs in the areas of daily living, social, educational, and vocational skills. The degree to which the individual is able to perform in these life areas may be termed the functional skill levels.

For purposes of definition, the mentally retarded population may be divided into the following levels, which include both intellectual performance (Coleman, Butcher, & Carson, 1980) and functional skills:

1. Mild retardation—Minimal impact on functioning having mainly educational or academic deficits, with some social deficits, and may or may not include vocational deficits. Require special educational assistance, but may otherwise function independently. IQ range 52-67.
2. Moderate retardation—More pronounced deficits with few academic skills, vocational skill deficits, social deficits, and some activities of daily living deficits. Usually require special educational assistance as well as assistance in acquiring or handling daily living skills. May require sheltered vocational and residential experience. IQ range 36-51.
3. Severe/profound retardation—Marked deficits in all skill areas, which may include a need for continuing care, supervision, and sheltered living and vocational environments. IQ range below 35.

Attention to functional skills helps to prevent arbitrary classification and, in fact, may yield some surprising results. An individual classified as severely retarded through intellectual testing, may function proficiently in some skill areas. It is therefore important for the practitioner to assess functional skill levels as well as IQ scores.

Since most mentally retarded individuals live and function within the community, they are also faced with the three basic life tasks of work, love, and friendship that Adler proposed we all face (Ansbacher & Ansbacher, 1956).

MENTAL RETARDATION AND LIFESTYLE DEVELOPMENT

Adler addressed ''feeblemindedness'' and its impact on lifestyle (Ansbacher & Ansbacher, 1956); however, it is difficult to know precisely what he meant by this term. He appears to believe that the ''feebleminded'' do not develop a lifestyle. In our work we have not found this to be true. We have seen a clear and observable lifestyle orientation. The behavior of the mentally retarded individual is goal directed, purposive, and predictable, as opposed to being random and reactive.

An important determiner of the mentally retarded individual's own perceptions seems to be the manner in which the family and society view the handicap. Frequently, for the mildly retarded individual, there is no indication of a problem until the child reaches school age, at which time his academic deficits are noted. Prior to this time, it is less likely that family perceptions would be colored by stigmas or stereotypical views of mental retardation. That is not to say that dependencies will not be fostered later. For example, a 30-year-old woman who is mildly retarded is living in a lovely apartment in the basement of her parents' home. This appears to be a great stride toward independence since she works to pay her rent and contributes toward her food bill; however, she is not allowed to use her stove (''she might get hurt'') and her phone is an extension (''we want to keep tabs on her'').

In cases of more immediately visible handicapping conditions (Down's Syndrome, cerebral palsy/mr) family and societal perceptions can have an immediate impact on the way the child perceives himself and the world. Families experience anger, disappointment, guilt, and sadness—strong emotions that are inevitably transmitted to the child. There may be faulty notions that the infant needs less loving and cuddling, which may result in the child's misbehavior as a means of gaining attention. Parents may also pamper or overprotect as a means of assuaging their guilt. This reaction could result in teaching dependence or the belief that "things (life) should always go my way."

The child's world may be limited by parental hesitancy to expose the child to outsiders; leaving the house is solely for visits to the clinic or doctor's office. Family and societal expectations become self-limiting or self-fulfilling as the mentally retarded individual is denied the opportunity to fail or succeed.

Wolfensberger poignantly outlines society's perceptions of the mentally retarded, including "subhuman organisms," "objects of pity," "menaces," and "eternal children" (Wolfensberger, 1972). It is highly likely that a child will incorporate the perceptions of his family and his society into his lifestyle.

The mentally retarded child with siblings appears to assume the role of the youngest, regardless of the chronology. When the younger siblings pass him in intellectual ability, maturation level, and social development, he slides down the chronological ladder as his siblings literally grow up around him.

Siblings may also view their mentally retarded brother or sister as a chore or as a source of embarrassment, or they may feel that their retarded sibling gets more attention. Indeed, the mentally retarded child may decide that attention, in general, can result only from extremes in behavior, good or bad.

STRATEGIES FOR INTERVENTION

If behavior is predictable, organized, and goal directed for the mentally retarded individual, then related strategies may be developed for use in a vocational, day activity, family, or school setting. As with the general population, these strategies and corresponding techniques may be used when specific problems occur.

In order to use lifestyle information in working with the mentally retarded individual, some insight must be obtained by the counselor into that individual's unique patterns of movement or goal orientation. Since functional skills are extremely varied within the mentally retarded population methods must be geared to the individual.

Observation of the individual is the most universally useful tool for gathering information. Observation most effectively takes place in the normal environment, which may include the school, home, job, workshop, or day activity program. The observer may look for such things as the following: (1) How does the individual respond to peers, siblings, neighbors—is this person sociable, antisocial, or nonsociable? (2) How does the individual respond to authority figures, parents, teachers, work supervisors, etc.? (3) How does the person react to stress, failure, challenge? (4) Are there any outstanding behavioral problems? (5) What is the overall impression this person creates?

After gathering observational impressions, it is helpful to obtain background data and information concerning the current problem. Background data may include previous testing, past program information, and case narratives. The presenting problem should be clearly stated, including information about where and when the problem occurs and what has been done in the past with respect to this problem.

Information about family constellation, family members' views of the mentally retarded individual, and how he fits into the family structure, is useful and important. Questions such as the following can provide insight into family perceptions and expectations: (1) What responsibilities does this person have in the home? (2) Who is this person closest to? (3) What does the family do for fun?

The nature of the face-to-face or interview situation will naturally vary with each individual, although it will serve as an important tool in all cases. For lower-functioning or for nonverbal individuals, the problem will need to be stated clearly and simply with frequent stops for verification from the client. Notations as to attending ability, body language, and general demeanor should be made. It may be necessary to request eye contact frequently.

For mildly or moderately retarded persons with good attending or verbal abilities, the counseling time may be used to determine the clients' perceptions of the problem. Questions regarding their ideas about themselves in the world, as relating to others, are useful. Creativity on the part of the counselor is helpful in finding ways to present questions that will evoke the desired information. One moderately retarded woman, in response to the question "How are your glasses?" solemnly replied, "My glasses are fine but my eyes ain't doing so good."

It is at this point that early recollections may be solicited, which will serve to verify patterns and goal orientations obtained from observations and other sources. Early recollections and dreams, in our experience with retarded individuals, occur with the same, or nearly the same, frequency and relevancy as in the general population.

Three approaches to applying lifestyle information include behavioral techniques, cognitive techniques, and family intervention.

Behavioral Techniques

Behavioral techniques or behavior modification is the most traditional approach, and it is used in virtually every mental retardation setting. With the additional knowledge of a person's lifestyle or mode of movement, behavioral approaches can be more appropriately tailored for each individual. Both traditional lifestyle counseling and behavior modification, it may be remembered, focus on the consequences or the usefulness of behavior. However, they differ in procedures for handling the consequences. Generally, encouragement (discussed below) is the preferred lifestyle technique, whereas rewards are favored by the behaviorists. Both appear to have their place in working with the mentally retarded.

By identifying, for example, that a particular person will go to great lengths to feel special, the counselor can develop a behavior plan that incorporates special counselor time or a special activity as a reward.

We have found it necessary and more effective to include the individual in the formulation of behavior plans. Thus, during the implementation we can refer to their agreement of the problem and their participation in choosing rewards, time frames, etc.

Cognitive Approaches

Cognitive approaches with mentally retarded individuals are less traditionally employed but have also been successful.

After the counselor has gathered adequate information to render an opinion of the individual's view of himself in the world, the impressions should be verified with him. Stating the counselor's observation as it relates to the problem may elicit an obvious recognition reaction such as a smile or a "knowing" look. For example, the statement "It seems to me, John, that you feel pretty special, and that others should treat you that way. Perhaps sometimes you refuse to work along with others to show just how special you are," may elicit definite agreement from John. We might then attempt to turn John's behavior around by encouraging him to be special by continuing to progress until he achieves competitive employment. Or, it may be that refusing to work won't be as effective a behavior for John since we have, to borrow an Adlerian phrase, "spit in his soup" (Allen, 1971). It is also possible that John may not agree that he feels special. He may offer different reasons for his behavior or the counselor may need to consider other options for use with him.

Another useful cognitive approach is helping the client "identify and solve the problem." Frequently, when a mentally retarded individual is "acting out," or exhibiting behaviors that are ineffective or unrelated to the cause, we take time to stop and identify the real problem. When the problem is identified we can work on a mutually satisfactory solution, and at the same time point out how ineffective the "acting out" behavior is. Too frequently the behaviors are viewed as the problem and the underlying issues are not addressed.

One nonverbal individual had been receiving counseling employing this approach and had made great strides toward decreasing ineffective behaviors. He was so good at it that he became quite innovative. One day when he was bothered by another worker grinding his teeth, he indicated the problem by gestures and proceeded to point to his ears and a box in the work area. The box contained ear plugs—an interesting solution!

Encouragement, another cognitive approach that is often employed by Adlerians, involves demonstrating to the client that he has the power to behave differently (Sweeney, 1980). With the mentally retarded individual, encouragement may involve stating clearly the counselor's observations of the person's strengths and accomplishments. For example, when an individual insists that he can't perform a certain task, it can be helpful for the counselor to point out the parts of the task he has done or to comment on previously mastered tasks.

Encouragement may involve challenging a particular client with a task, or it may mean not reacting to a client in ways that perpetuate his feelings about himself or the world. This may mean, for example, not becoming upset with the individual whose goal seems to be demonstrating how unlovable he is by continually antagonizing others.

The "helpless" and "dependent" individual who is guided and encouraged into a helping and giving role can begin to perceive himself in a new light. For example, a young moderately retarded woman, who expressed discouragement about her dependent life, was encouraged to volunteer at a local nursing home. As a result of her responsibility, she blossomed with a new usefulness and continues to delight the staff and residents as she moves from room to room spreading her cheery personality, even "reading" letters to residents.

Giving choices to mentally retarded individuals who have never felt in control of their lives serves as another method of encouragement. Although limits must sometimes be set, the use of choices gives power to the person to control his own behavior. One example would be an individual who frequently loses his temper in the work setting; he is given the choice of calming himself in a predetermined manner (such as taking a walk) or being clocked out and taken off the work floor. The difference between having the choice or being told "If you lose your temper, you will be clocked out," is important; the worker now feels in control of the situation.

Routine use of humor is a way of diffusing anger, gaining perspective on limitations, and changing self-perceptions. Not only can clients learn to express themselves in more traditional humorous situations, but they can learn to view their struggles and mistakes with less severity. The counselor must be willing to offer his own humanity as a model, exposing weaknesses or error, and sharing the humor with the client.

Family Intervention

Consideration of family influences and perceptions is necessary in working with any mentally retarded individuals since they are often firmly enmeshed in the family network, and may remain within the family structure for a long time.

The mentally retarded individual may be seen as the "bad one," "helpless one," or "protected one." We have found it helpful to share our observations with the family, encouraging them to alter their expectations and perceptions. With due respect to the tenacity of family dynamics, this is often a slow and gradual process. A first step might be as simple as encouraging the family to allow the adult individual to prepare his or her lunch each morning or to give more financial responsibility to their child.

In soliciting family assistance it is necessary for family members to agree with the need for change. This will involve checking their perceptions of the problem as well as recognizing patterns of behavior in and out of the home. Hopefully, they can supply consistency with respect to behavior plans developed in and out of the home.

The issue of dealing with the parents of an adult must be handled individually. The result of the intervention should always aim toward greater independence for the individual.

A Case Study

Debbie is a young woman who is moderately retarded in academic areas and only mildly retarded in self-care and social areas. She is an only child in a middle-class home. She is highly valued and somewhat pampered because she is not expected to participate in the day-to-day responsibilities at home. Debbie graduated from high school in a special education program and worked for six months as a housekeeper in a motel. She was referred to our sheltered workshop for work adjustment because she was slow on the job and sensitive to correction.

Upon observation in the workshop setting, Debbie appeared sociable, friendly, and usually willing to participate in the vocational and social aspects of the program. She responded to work supervisors' requests positively during instruction or correction, but would later be observed crying in the bathroom. Occasionally, she would "faint" on the floor or be found slumped in a chair having a "spell."

Work supervisors' comments and case narratives indicated that Debbie frequently appeared depressed and upset over specific incidents on the work floor or over stressful social encounters. Physical complaints varied from hyperventilation to self-inflicted nosebleeds, and occurred after Debbie was corrected or asked to perform a challenging task. Medical examination reports revealed no related physical problems.

In counseling sessions Debbie was highly verbal and sociable. She would refer to incidents with work supervisors from a strictly physical standpoint, "I felt faint," or "my stomach hurt." She also referred to various family events, such as a divorce of a cousin, as being highly upsetting to her, often reducing her to tears.

Debbie's earliest recollection was of going out of the house with her parents and discovering that her mother had forgotten to put on Debbie's underpants. She told her mother and reported feeling highly embarrassed.

Some assumptions about Debbie might be that she is highly aware of being vulnerable or that "making mistakes can be costly and embarrassing." One might also assume that Debbie does not feel responsible for her mistakes and that one way of not being responsible is to be physically ill. As a result of being the only child, a handicapped child, and a pampered child, Debbie never had to fight for a position in her family and appears to have remained highly dependent on, and unseparated from, her parents.

After a trusting relationship was established with Debbie, the above assumptions were presented for her consideration, i.e., "It seems that sometimes you get sick because the job is scary or things aren't going your way. I wonder if it's easier to cry and let others take care of you when life is tough?" Eventually, Debbie agreed with these observations and could begin to work on the tasks of facing stress, accepting criticism, and separating from her family. One of the first assignments was for Debbie to verbalize her fears and concerns about making mistakes. After a few months this resulted in a decrease in her physical complaints.

Through counselor modeling and role playing, Debbie began to use humor in viewing her actions. The high point occurred one day when she was crying and complaining and suddenly burst into laughter, saying, "I sound like I'm on 'Search for Tomorrow.' "

Communication with Debbie's family included suggestions for ways that Debbie might function more independently at home, by assuming household responsibilities such as laundry, cleaning, and food preparation. Future expectations for Debbie include competitive employment, a more independent living situation, and perhaps marriage.

SPECIAL CONSIDERATIONS AND LIMITATIONS

Limitations in working with the mentally retarded are primarily a function of counselor personality and needs. Progress will be slow with some individuals and gains may be small at times. Patience, creativity, and flexibility are important counselor attributes. A counselor must temper expectations with reality, but be cautious about setting limits on expectations.

Parental hesitancies to change ways of perceiving their sons and daughters can be limiting. However, families can learn to allow risk and movement toward more independent functioning through involvement, education, and support.

Societal perceptions represent limitations in working with the mentally retarded. This is particularly so when bias and judgments, based on stigmas and stereotypes, interfere with the individual's movement toward independence.

SUMMARY

In working with the mentally retarded individual, it is more important to consider functional abilities than intellectual performance scores. Lifestyle is, in part, determined by the individual's perceptions of his world, which may, in turn, be greatly influenced by familial and societal perceptions and stereotypes.

In addition to traditional behavioral techniques, lifestyle information may be used to address problems in a cognitive manner with the mentally retarded individual. This may include sharing observations, identifying and solving the problem, encouragement, choices, and humor.

There is no such thing as a "typical mentally retarded individual" any more than there is a "typical man." To the practitioner, individuality and uniqueness of the person should always be foremost, followed by consideration of how that person chooses to move through life.

REFERENCES

Allen, T.W. Adlerian interview strategies for behavior change. *The Counseling Psychologist*, 1971, *3*(1), 40–48.

American Association on Mental Deficiency. *Manual on terminology and classification in mental retardation*. Washington, D.C.: Grossman, 1973.

Ansbacher, H.L., & Ansbacher, R.R. (Eds.). *The individual psychology of Alfred Adler*. New York: Harper & Row, 1956.

Coleman, J.C., Butcher, J.N., & Carson, R.C. *Abnormal psychology and modern life*. Glenview, Ill.: Scott, Foresman, 1980.

James, W. *The principles of psychology*. Chicago: Benton, 1952.

Kirk, S.A. *Educating exceptional children*. Boston: Houghton Mifflin, 1972.

Sweeney, T.J. *Adlerian counseling*. Muncie, Ind.: Accelerated Development, 1980.

Wolfensberger, W. *The principle of normalization in human services*. Toronto, Canada: National Institute on Mental Retardation, 1972.

Chapter 16

Using a Lifestyle Counseling Approach with Visually Impaired Individuals

Stephen J. Aukward

In discussing a lifestyle counseling approach, this chapter presents practical suggestions and techniques for counselors in their work with adult individuals. It is not my intention to focus on deficits, losses, and disabilities but rather to emphasize assets and abilities and creative coping skills. Furthermore, it is assumed that clients are active participants in their rehabilitation and adjustment process. Lastly, this writer is speaking from a personal perspective as a blind individual as well as from a professional perspective with over ten years of experience in the field of rehabilitation.

It should be emphasized at the onset that individuals who are visually handicapped do not require a unique counseling approach. The Adlerian lifestyle approach, however, offers some practical techniques and ideas that may be of assistance in adjustment counseling for visually handicapped persons.

SOME BASIC CONSIDERATIONS

The following are some basic considerations underlying adjustment counseling with blind individuals. First of all, counselors need to have an awareness of their own attitudes toward blindness. Second, counselors have an obligation to safeguard the dignity of individuals, respect the integrity of their feelings, recognize the importance of the clients' own concepts of their needs and their rights to self-determination. Third, because the individuals seeking counseling happen to be blind, it does not necessarily follow that blindness or maladjustment thereto is the core of their problems or the major underlying cause of the need that they present. The counselor's efforts should be directed toward an understanding of the total constellation of needs and the place of the client's blindness in that constellation (Lowery, 1968a).

Even though some of the conditions imposed by blindness (impaired mobility, reduced control of environment, restriction of experiential field, etc.) constitute serious handicaps common to all blind persons, the adjustment of each person to these conditions will be different, reflecting the basic personality structure and the personal and social experiences of that person before and after blindness (Lowery, 1968a). These facts lead to a fourth point regarding adjustment counseling with blind persons: the counselor's focus is not primarily upon the problems presented by blindness, but—consistent with the lifestyle approach—upon the person who is blind. This safeguards counselors against the fallacy of attributing common problems, characteristics, and capacities to all blind persons; it also highlights the danger of counselors directing their helping activities with each blind client in relation to what they feel are the needs and capacities of "the blind."

Persons who are blind are more similar to than different from those who are sighted, despite popular misconceptions. The differences to which the counselor's helping activities are directed are not the physical differences of the blind client but the behavioral ones. This assumption leads the counselor to the recognition that the approach to helping blind persons (as well as sighted ones) who are in need must be directed toward understanding the nature of their need, the individual attitude and behavior, the causal factors that have contributed to the development of their needs, and their capacities and resources for dealing with them (Lowery, 1968a). The counselor should keep in mind that loss of vision does not result in total incapacitation and that there is nothing fixed in blindness that predisposes the client to disabling neuroses. With blind clients, as well as with those who are sighted, the counselor's activities are directed toward helping them make more productive use of their skills and capacities by freeing them from constricting fears and anxieties and by offering opportunities for the development and use of their strengths.

Blind persons have a right to strong and honest expectations from those in their environmental relationship—honest, not only in terms of their handicap but also in terms of broader social standards or norms. What one expects of a blind client (and the manner in which one conveys this) is important because of its influence as a motivating force. It may loom with greater importance if the expectations from others, such as the blind person's family and social group, are either too low or too high. It is important, therefore, to differentiate between individuals in terms of expectations, i.e., to gear the level of expectation to the individual's capacity to function. Expectation is thus seen not only as a force and motivation but also as an aspect of intervention that the counselor uses constructively only if its direction is based upon a differential diagnosis of each blind client's capacities.

NATURE OF DISABILITY

Since this chapter deals with adjustment to blindness, it is important to define each of these concepts. *Webster's Seventh New Collegiate Dictionary* (1963) defines the word "adjustment" as "a correction or modification to reflect actual conditions" (p. 12). In the context of this chapter, adjustment can be more operationally defined as the extent to which the self-concept agrees with the factual and actual self (Bauman, 1958). Lowenfield (1950) sees adjustment as "knowing and accepting what one can and cannot do" (p. 42). This definition may sound simplistic but it shows very succinctly just what adjustment to blindness involves. In addition, it introduces the important aspect of acceptance in adjustment to blindness.

Acceptance of Blindness

In this chapter I am concerned with the conditions facilitating acceptance of blindness as nondevaluating. Although blindness may be seen as inconvenient and limiting, the individual can still strive to improve the improvable where improvement will facilitate certain aspects of that person's life (Wright, 1960). It must be born in mind that there is a gap between accepting one's disability and accepting one's self in general. Scheerer (1954) defines self-accepting persons as those who:

1. rely on internalized values
2. have faith in their capacity to cope
3. assume responsibility for their behavior
4. accept praise or criticism objectively
5. accept things without self-condemnation
6. consider themselves persons of worth
7. do not expect others to reject them
8. do not regard themselves as different from others
9. are not shy or self-conscious.

Later in this chapter specific strategies for facilitating self-acceptance are discussed.

Most people look upon blindness as a state of sightlessness. This is not necessarily the case since most "blind" people can, in fact, see something. Perhaps citing the legal definition of blindness can clear up some of the confusion. In *Facts and Figures about Blindness* (1967), blindness is defined as:

Central visual acuity of 20/200 or less in the better eye, with correcting glasses; or central visual acuity of 20/200 if there is a field defect in which the peripheral field has contracted to such an extent that the widest diameter of visual field subtends an angular distance no greater than twenty degrees (p. 1).

This is the definition most often used for the purpose of determining eligibility for services to the blind in most rehabilitation agencies.

The Psychological Aspects of Blindness

The counselor needs to be aware of the psychological aspects of blindness. The mental health problems associated with blindness tend to reduce the coping capacities of individuals at a time when they most need emotional strength and stability. Rusalem (1972) pointed out that blind individuals will be learning new and unfamiliar techniques of living, developing relationships with professional personnel and peers, exposing themselves to possible frustration and defeat in undertaking assigned rehabilitation tasks, and abandoning the comfort of dependency. Anxious individuals with preexisting neurotic needs may experience blindness as a welcome respite from overwhelming guilt. For most others, however, blindness intensifies preexisting anxiety (Chevigny & Braverman, 1950).

It has been found that there are no identifiable psychological reactions that set the blindness experience apart from other crisis experiences. Rusalem (1972) indicated that both the initial and long-range problems of adjusting to blindness have much in common with the problems developing out of other significant encounters such as amputations, aging, or the sudden death of a loved one. When compared with other disabilities, blindness, at least in its early stages, does seem to have a cataclysmic effect upon those whom it strikes, often arousing feelings of extreme helplessness and despair. Literally, blind persons cannot "see" any way out of their difficulties. Many authors have reported that blindness is the most emotionally charged event that can occur to an individual.

It needs to be pointed out that emotional reactions to blindness are highly individual, suggesting that adjustment is an individual rather than a group matter. Bauman (1963) concluded that individual factors are the major determiners of emotional adjustment for blind persons. Much behavior is shaped by the stress of having to attend to nonvisual stimuli, which count for little in the life of the more relaxed sighted individual.

For some, new blindness may result in profound shock. This shock reaction may have functional value by providing a respite from other stressful interactions. Carroll (1961) and others have pointed out that during this shock reaction the individual may reorganize his life, gradually incorporating his altered physical and social status into a new self.

Blind individuals may feel the strain of social pressures to adopt the behaviors of sighted persons in such activities as eating, walking, and relating to others. However, behavior standards for those with sight can be inappropriate and even dangerous for those who are blind. Attempting to follow them may lead to inconvenience, deprivations, and frustrations that divert human energies and complicate emotional adjustment (Cutsforth, 1951). Gowman (1957) pointed out that the expectations of society play an important part in determining behavior. The blind person who is active and independent may violate well-established expectations, thereby inviting opposition and exclusion. This sense of isolation may complicate the blind person's ability to cope with blindness.

The blind individual is stripped of customary perceptual supports. When this happens withdrawal may be the first line of defense against the anxiety resulting from loss of visual perception. The sense of loss may be intensified by the sudden awareness of other dependencies. Fearing the loss of whatever social supports may be available to them, blind persons may adopt behaviors they believe will maximize the feelings of concern and responsibility others have for them (Cutsforth, 1950).

The role of personal strength in the rehabilitation of blind individuals is important in understanding the nature of this disability. The onset of blindness may precipitate shock. Numbed by the enormity of the catastrophe that has occurred, the individual withdraws from anxiety-producing stimuli in the environment. Rusalem (1972) pointed out that those with good ego strength use professional help constructively and move out of this stage and usually the depression that follows it. On the other hand, those individuals whose preblindness emotional adjustment was more tenuous tend to respond less favorably to professional intervention and endure more prolonged periods of shock and depression. Even those with good ego strength can succumb to numerous stresses in the environment.

Blindness may reactivate a variety of dependent feelings for an individual. Incidents in adult life that cast one in a dependent role may reawaken dependent conflicts. Unfortunately, the dependence of blindness may not provide for a free expression of aggression. Feelings of dissatisfaction, anger, irritability, and bitterness may develop as substitutes for more direct forms of hostility since many outlets of tension reduction may be closed to the blind, therefore limiting the externalizing of feelings and the draining off of emotional distress. A sound approach to adjustment counseling with blind individuals should offer a therapeutic environment that is rich in activities with tension reduction possibilities.

Most authors agree that blindness results in multiple losses almost unmatched in any other disabling condition. Carroll (1961) listed 20 major areas in which losses may occur as a result of blindness. These include loss of:

1. physical integrity
2. confidence in the remaining senses
3. reality contact with the environment
4. visual background
5. light security
6. mobility
7. techniques of daily living
8. ease of written communications
9. ease of spoken communications

10. informational progress
11. visual perception of the pleasurable
12. visual perception of the beautiful
13. recreation
14. career, vocational goal and job opportunity
15. financial security
16. personal independence
17. social adequacy
18. obscurity
19. self-esteem
20. total personality organization

Unless these losses are overcome, adjustment becomes precarious, since each loss represents a capacity to cope with aspects of the unseen environment (Rusalem. 1972). The greater the number of losses, the greater the need for professiona intervention.

Psychological constructs about all people sighted or blind often fail the test of universality. The individual nature of adjustment to blindness cannot be over-emphasized. All too often, as Rusalem (1972) pointed out, those who serve the blind succumb to the temptation to oversimplify, categorize, and rationalize behavior of clients. The heart of rehabilitation is the encounter between unique individuals. If the individuality of the client is short-changed, adequate adjustment and rehabilitation are not as likely.

IMPLICATIONS OF LIFESTYLE COUNSELING

Since it is very important to take an individualized approach when counseling visually handicapped persons, the Adlerian lifestyle method offers a unique and practical alternative. One of Adler's major contributions was the development of a means for understanding an individual by focusing on the goal-directed nature of one's behavior. Using variations of the lifestyle method will yield an increased understanding of the personal goals that are at work with the problems at hand. An increased understanding of a person's goals can be helpful in improving or understanding the behavior that is used to meet the goals (Rule, 1978). Adler noted that people frequently operate from a subjective framework and are not always aware of their goals. Understandably, people learn behaviors in keeping with the goals of the lifestyle that safeguard their sense of self-esteem. Thus the lifestyle is essentially an individual's unique mental framework for measuring self-worth as a function of interaction with others. The lifestyle method allows the person to understand, predict, and control experience (Mosak & Dreikurs, 1973), and particularly to evaluate whether the lifestyle is working as an advantage or disadvantage.

STRATEGIES FOR INTERVENTION

There are several strategies to assist the visually impaired individual in an emotional acceptance of disability. Cholden (1958) has emphasized the critical need to develop psychological acceptance of disability. The visually impaired person's aspirations, social relationships, body image, self-concept, and relationship to the physical world are strongly affected, if not completely changed. Cholden (1958) referred to the need for an "intra-psychic" change consisting of psychological acceptance of the new self that has a disability. Furthermore, he points out that rehabilitation efforts are wasted unless professional help is offered to deal with feelings, attitudes, interpersonal relationships, and inner life. Ideally, the goal of counseling is to help the client use his potentialities to the maximum and obtain satisfaction from life. I would like to emphasize here that the strategies discussed are meant to assist both counselor and client in the psychosocial aspects of adjustment to blindness. Many visually impaired individuals may also work with rehabilitation counselors or other related professionals in the field of rehabilitation of the blind.

Practical Suggestions

The counselor needs to be aware of some practical suggestions that may facilitate the counseling process with visually impaired persons. Lowery (1968b) emphasized that the counselor's tone of voice and choice of words carry full responsibility for communication with the visually impaired. In counseling the blind person, the counselor needs to use more direct verbal expression such as "yeses" and "uh-hums." When giving mobility assistance to the blind person the counselor should offer an arm to the client rather than taking the arm of the client. In offering a chair, it is helpful to lead the client to it and place his hand on it. In giving directions, use nonvisual cues. Also, if there are sounds or movements in the room, give the blind individual a casual explanation of what is happening. The counselor also needs to avoid making extraneous noises and other distracting sounds. Lastly, the counselor should look directly into the face of the client as if the client were sighted. If the counselor abides by the above suggestions the client will feel much more comfortable and less threatened during the counseling session. The above suggestions also allow the client the maximum level of self-reliance and independence in the counseling environment.

The Lifestyle Assessment

In a lifestyle approach to counseling, a first essential step is the completion of the lifestyle assessment, discussed previously in this book. The assessment is a valuable tool in determining a visually impaired individual's preblindness personality. Bauman (1972) emphasizes the importance of understanding the kind of person the visually impaired individual was before loss of vision. She further indicates that rehabilitation starts with an understanding of the effect of competition and the fear of failure upon the person prior to visual loss. Also, the lifestyle assessment would be invaluable in serving congenitally blind persons.

It is important to stress the positive information derived from the lifestyle assessment. Specifically, emphasis needs to be placed on personal strengths identified in the lifestyle. As with all lifestyle assessments it is important that the clients have an understanding as to how their lifestyle works to their advantage and disadvantage. In addition, the lifestyle enables the counselor and client to identify any mistaken notions that the client may have. It is important also to remember that the lifestyle process assists in the gaining of awareness or insight; however, this knowledge must be directed toward specific behavioral activities in order to benefit the client.

Information regarding the goal-directed nature of behavior derived from the lifestyle assessment can be very valuable to both counselor and client alike. For example, the individual who has been struggling as a sighted person may find, in blindness, a socially acceptable solution to all his struggles (Bauman, 1972). In some cases, the psychological effect of blindness may be very comforting. Some visually impaired individuals may use their blindness as a weapon to control the environment. On the other hand, Cholden (1958) described a number of reasons for the nonacceptance of blindness, including punishment for one's own or parents' sins, a sexual interpretation of blindness, an end to acceptance by society as a valid person, economic problems of the blind, and resentment of pity the sighted are thought to feel.

Encouraging Self-Direction

The counselor needs to be especially aware of the client's dependency needs and to avoid behaviors that undermine self-reliance. Self-direction in the counseling relationship is the most promising avenue for helping visually impaired persons to become self-reliant and independent. Most essential is the development of a genuine feeling that blindness is not devastating, that it can be overcome, that blind persons need not be treated as children, and that they have rights—one of which is self-determination. More than ever before, counselors need to be aware of their own attitudes as a critical variable in the rehabilitation process.

The development of self-esteem is a critical element in the psychological acceptance of disability. Self-esteem has been described as a warm and loving feeling toward yourself. It is the total acceptance of yourself and your disability as you are. Both the client and the counselor need to remember that improving self-esteem requires work. Norbom (1980) stated that there are three conditions for self-esteem: you have a basic need to feel good, you deserve to feel good, and you have to choose to feel good. Many individuals feel that they are not in control of their life when actually they are. The counselor's and client's strategies should be directed at reestablishing control of the environment by the client. To improve self-esteem many clients may need to challenge their previously mistaken notions about themselves. The lifestyle assessment can be a valuable tool in identifying these mistaken notions. The counselor and client may then choose to employ strategies advocated by Albert Ellis in rational-emotive therapy to challenge negative thinking patterns.

There are several behavioral activities the counselor can use to enhance the personal strength and self-esteem of visually impaired clients. It is important to emphasize here the active role that the client plays in achieving a psychological acceptance of disability.

Resources

It is essential for both counselor and client to learn more about blindness and adjustment to it. Many resources can be invaluable in this process. Perhaps the foremost work in the area of blindness is a book by Father Thomas Carroll entitled *Blindness: What It Is, What It Does, and How To Live With It* (1961). This book includes an exhaustive description of the losses caused by blindness; but, more important, it also describes strategies and activities for counteracting the effects of these losses. Father Carroll emphasizes the need to "die" as a sighted person and be reborn as a blind person. Another example of an excellent resource is an article by Hanan Selvin entitled "How to Succeed at Being Blind" in *The New Outlook*, December 1976. This article includes helpful information regarding aids and appliances the newly blinded person can benefit from. By consulting resource material, visually impaired persons can better deal with their feelings about blindness and gain helpful information on the practical coping skills they will need. The counselor and client should emphasize the practical application of the information.

The client will learn that there are many practical devices that will make life easier and relieve the person of many frustrations in the activities of daily living. State and private rehabilitation agencies serving the blind have professional persons who can familiarize the client with these aids and devices. In addition, the client can write for appropriate catalogs. By becoming proficient in the use of a variety of aids and appliances, the client can experience a sense of accomplishment and mastery that previously may not have seemed possible.

In addition, the counselor and client should be aware of the variety of organizations serving visually impaired persons. There are at least three national organizations serving the blind: The American Council for the Blind, The American Foundation for the Blind, and The National Federation for the Blind. Each can be a wealth of information and services for visually impaired persons. They offer resource information and, more important, an opportunity to share the blindness experience. Most of these national organizations have local chapters and affiliates that the blind person may want to join. These local organizations would provide a valuable social outlet as well as a source of support and information. It is very important for blind persons to realize that they are not alone in their quest to accept their disability and to deal with some of the practical aspects and inconveniences presented by it.

Mobility and Alternative Communication

For most blind individuals the first step to independence and self-reliance comes with mobility instruction. For many, however, learning mobility skills can be a very stressful and fearful process. The first use of the white cane can be a very trying experience. The counselor can be invaluable by providing emotional support and encouragement during this activity. Personally, I see mobility instruction as essential to reestablishing the blind person's feelings of self-esteem and control over the environment. Many clients, however, never seem to acquire this essential skill for independent functioning. The counselor may wish to coordinate efforts with the mobility instructor working with the client to assist in this activity.

Another important area for the visually impaired person is the development of alternative communication skills. Here again the client's ability to communicate can very positively effect feelings of self-esteem and an acceptance of disability. There is a variety of communication media available to visually impaired persons including braille, typing, handwriting, and electronic recording devices. It takes time and patience to acquire these new skills. Once again, the counselor's and client's ability to structure their learning activities is essential. Some clients may resist using braille since it seems to represent an admission by them that they are, indeed, blind. For this reason, the counselor may play an important role by helping clients express their feelings about the use of braille or other materials. The acquisition of these alternative communication skills will definitely enhance feelings of self-esteem as well as access to essential information, thus allowing for better control of the environment.

Recreational Activities

The visually impaired person can benefit from participation in a variety of recreational and physical activities. There is a tendency for visually impaired persons to pull back from many of the activities they formerly enjoyed as sighted individuals. Recreational activities can be a wonderful source of relaxation and can assist in reducing the ordinary stress of daily life. The sense of physical mastery and exercise can help the visually impaired person feel more self-confident and independent. Visually impaired individuals should avoid assuming that they cannot participate in a particular recreational activity. There are many possible adaptations. Examples of activities that may be explored include swimming, bowling, card playing, fishing, and a variety of others. Participation in such activities allows for social contact and more enjoyable usage of leisure time.

Vocational Planning

Another important area of intervention for the visually impaired person and counselor is vocational planning. Many vocationally related services are available from rehabilitation programs. For some it may be a reentry into the employment market or, for others, it may include preparation for that first job. A whole range of services is available through state vocational rehabilitation programs and should be explored if the visually impaired individual would like to pursue employment. Employment for visually impaired persons provides considerable economic independence, which obviously has beneficial effects on self-esteem and self-reliance. For some visually impaired individuals, participation in volunteer activities can also be very beneficial. Examples of volunteer activities may include advocating for improved services for the blind, lobbying for legislation affecting the blind, and a variety of other volunteer programs available within any community.

SUMMARY

As the reader can see, there is a vast range of activities in which a visually impaired individual can participate to foster increased personal strength and self-esteem. The activities described certainly are not all inclusive and are meant to serve only as examples of possible activities. The theme of the activities described is one of acting on the environment whereby the visually impaired person retains a sense of control and independence. The counselor can assist the visually impaired client in structuring some of these activities, by providing encouragement and support, and occasionally by challenging the visually impaired person to utilize his own and outside resources. In the final analysis, however, it is the visually impaired person who must choose to become involved and participate in the activities described.

REFERENCES

Bauman, M.K. *Adjustment to blindness: A study as reported by the Committee to Study Adjustment to Blindness.* Harrisburg, PA: Office for the Blind, 1963.

Bauman, M.K. *The initial psychological reaction to blindness.* Paper presented at the Seventeenth Biennial Convention of the Eastern Conference of Home Teachers, Richmond, 1958.

Bauman, M.K. Research on psychological factors associated with blindness. In R. Hardy & J. Cull (Eds.), *Social and rehabilitation services for the blind.* Springfield, Ill.: Charles C Thomas, 1972.

Carroll, T. *Blindness: What it is, what it does, and how to live with it.* Boston: Little, Brown, 1961.

Chevigny, H., & Braverman, S. *The adjustment of the blind.* New Haven: Yale University Press, 1950.

Cholden, L.S. *A psychiatrist works with blindness.* New York: American Foundation for the Blind, 1958.

Cutsforth, T.D. Personality and social adjustment among the blind. In P.A. Zahl (Ed.), *Blindness, modern approaches to the unseen environment.* Princeton: Princeton University Press, 1950.

Cutsforth, T.D. *The blind in school and society: A psychological study.* New York: American Foundation for the Blind, 1951.

Facts and figures about blindness, American Foundation for the Blind, New York, 1967.

Gowman, A.G. *The war blind in American social structure.* New York: American Foundation for the Blind, 1957.

Lowenfield, B. Mental hygiene of blindness. In W. Donahue & D. Dabelstein (Eds.), *Psychological diagnosis and counseling of the adult blind.* New York: American Foundation for the Blind, 1950.

Lowery, F. Basic assumptions underlying casework with blind persons. In S. Finestone (Ed.), *Social casework and blindness.* New York: American Foundation for the Blind, 1968. (a)

Lowery, F. The implications of blindness for the social caseworker in practice—implications in the treatment process. In S. Finestone (Ed.), *Social casework and blindness.* New York: American Foundation for the Blind, 1968. (b)

Mosak, H.H., & Dreikurs, R. Adlerian psychotherapy. In R. Corsini (Ed.), *Current psychotherapies,* Itasca, Ill.: Peacock, 1973.

Norbom, M.A. Steps to self esteem. *Accent on Living,* Summer 1980, 25(1), 68–70.

Rule, W.R. Rehabilitation uses of Adlerian life-style counseling. *Rehabilitation Counseling Bulletin,* 1978, 21(4), 306–316.

Rusalem, H. *Coping with the unseen environment.* New York: Teachers College Press, 1972.

Scheerer, M. Cognitive theory. In G. Lindzey (Ed.), *Handbook of social psychology.* Reading, Mass.: Addison-Wesley, 1954.

Selvin, H.C. How to succeed at being blind. *The New Outlook,* December 1976, pp. 420–428.

Webster's Seventh New Collegiate Dictionary. Springfield, Mass.: G. & C. Merriam, 1963.

Wright, B.A. *Physical disability: A psychological approach.* New York: Harper & Row, 1960.

Chapter 17

Lifestyle Approaches to Alcoholism

Susan Merl-Nachinson

During the past ten years alcoholism has emerged as a major public health problem. In the United States it ranks as the third leading cause of death behind cancer and heart disease. For the nation's youth, alcohol is involved in over 70 percent of teenage deaths due to suicide and accidents (*Chicago Tribune*, 1982). Over $25.37 billion is lost yearly to our nation's industry as a result of alcohol misuse and alcoholism (Kinney & Leaton, 1978). All these alarming facts together have generated a public interest that has only just begun.

Why do people drink? What constitutes alcohol abuse and alcoholism? We will try to answer these questions while considering alcoholism as a result of lifestyle adjustment. Some helpful intervention techniques for working with the alcoholic will be discussed and a framework for the treatment of alcoholism within the family will be described.

NATURE OF THE DISABILITY

Close your eyes and try to remember when you had your first drink of alcohol. Who gave it to you? What did it taste like? Most people are first introduced to alcohol at a young age by a family member, often during a special event or festivity. Often people report that they did not like its taste but that they felt "grown-up" drinking it.

Alcohol has played a special role in the American culture. Socially, it is used to celebrate a special occasion, to mourn a loss, to celebrate religious events, to ease social tension, or for medicinal purposes. Individually, alcohol may be used to forget problems, to relax, to help express feelings, to get high, or to feel sexy. It can help the drinker seem glamorous, tough, or grown-up. In one year, the average American drinks 2.6 gallons of liquor, 2.16 gallons of wine, and 26.6 gallons of beer (Kinney & Leaton, 1978). Multiply this by the 68 percent of the adult population that drinks alcohol and the result indicates that a great deal of alcohol is being consumed.

It is estimated that at least 10 percent of the U.S. adult population becomes alcoholic, that is, becomes addicted to alcohol. According to the California Medical Association, there are an estimated 3.5 million teenage alcoholics. However, there are no precise figures on those who occasionally get into trouble with alcohol—the alcohol abuser or misuser.

During the past decade, more questions have been raised about what constitutes alcoholism and who becomes alcoholic. Until recently, alcoholism (or drunkenness, as it used to be called) was considered a moral sin deserving of strict punishment to ensure that the inebriated person mend his ways. Our own temperance movement was a key example of this.

Today, alcoholism is defined by many professionals as a disease, with signs, symptoms, and a progression similar to other diseases. However, this concept is not universally accepted. For instance, the New Hampshire Christian Civic League in 1974 devoted an entire issue of its publication to a criticism of the disease concept. The assertion was made that the disease concept gives sanction to the "odious alcohol sinner" (Kinney & Leaton, 1978).

Jellinek (1960), considered the father of alcohol studies, delineated five species of alcoholism—alpha, beta, gamma, delta, and epsilon. He indicated that the gamma species is the most prevalent form of alcoholism in the United States. The gamma species differs from the others in that it is marked by a progression from psychological to physical dependence. In this species, he explained, there are four phases of alcoholism: prealcoholic, prodromal (warning sign), crucial, and chronic. It is during the last two phases that one loses control over the amount of alcohol consumed. The National Council on Alcoholism published guidelines to aid the physician, counselor, or helper in determining the diagnosis of alcoholism (National Council on Alcoholism, 1972).

It is important to note here that "alcohol abusers" and "problem drinkers" are terms having different meaning in the sense that these individuals have not yet experienced a loss of control over their drinking. They do experience a host of other problems related to their drinking. Quite often this type of drinking is a response to situational stress and may be repeated only occasionally.

IMPLICATIONS FOR LIFESTYLE ADJUSTMENT

Why is it that some people become alcoholic and others do not? There have been many theories postulated that elaborate on the genetic, psychological, and environmental/cultural factors that lead to alcoholism. It is likely that these all act in combination to produce the alcoholic individual.

Adler's approach to understanding human behavior asserts that man (in the generic sense) creates his own personality from his heredity and his environment. Each individual draws his own conclusions about how he sees himself, others, and his own unique view of the world. These views make up what Adlerians call the lifestyle. The basic feeling common to virtually every individual is a sense of inferiority. This feeling of not-enoughness sets into motion behaviors that attempt to elevate the person to a feeling of superiority or mastery over his environment. How individuals choose to do this is decided, although not always consciously, by their private logic, which directs all of their behavior (Ansbacher & Ansbacher, 1956). The lifestyle is mostly developed by approximately age five or six and is reflected in all spheres of the individual's psyche and personality (Lombardi, 1973).

In this view, the alcoholic can be conceptualized as an individual, like all others, striving for mastery and a place of significance. One way in which this person chooses to do this is through the use of alcohol, a decision that, as will be discussed later, can backfire. Alcohol is a means of adaptation that reflects a person's own private logic about himself, others, and the world.

Adler states that alcoholics "have built up their original character in a situation of great pampering, in which they were dependent on others. Usually this involved exploiting the mother" (Ansbacher & Ansbacher, 1956, p. 423). Although this conclusion may be somewhat oversimplified, it can be useful when related to Adler's overall conception of human development. Thus, for example, an individual struggling from a felt minus position and with a goal to be dependent and taken care of might turn to alcohol to feel better about himself. At first alcohol may help this person to experience feelings of competency, increased self-esteem, and enhanced self-image, thereby counteracting his feelings of vulnerability, inadequacy, and dependency.

Oftentimes the alcoholic views himself through his own private logic as incapable of coping with life's demands and, although he wants to be protected and taken care of, he cannot tolerate the intimacy of such a relationship (Schwartzman, 1977/78). Rather than decreasing these feelings of vulnerability, this fear of intimacy serves to increase it. Perhaps these dynamics are most apparent with what may be called the "inadequate" lifestyle (Mosak, 1971). It is important to mention that not every individual with an inadequate lifestyle turns to alcohol and not every alcoholic will have an inadequate lifestyle.

Once alcohol has been used in this maladaptive way, as Johnson (1980) points out, the drinker learns the effect alcohol has on his mood and purposely starts drinking to seek it out. At the onset of use, by altering the dose, the person can control the effect it has. However, as alcohol continues to be used, the drinker begins to experience problems that are due to its chemically addicting properties: blackouts, hangovers, embarrassments, etc. In this prodromal (warning sign) phase the person continues to experience increased feelings of adequacy and competency through alcohol use. Yet the individual begins to suppress distress about the problems it also causes and to rationalize his behaviors. As physical tolerance builds, more and more alcohol is required to achieve the desired effect.

In the crucial and chronic phases, the individual loses control over the amount of alcohol consumed and many problems ensue, e.g., physical illness, loss of friends and family, and increased withdrawal signs when he is not drinking. This process can take as long as 15 years or as few as 2 years for the teenage alcoholic. Now the drinker needs to drink, if only to alleviate withdrawal symptoms!

At this point the cruel paradox takes hold; the more the alcoholic drinks in an effort to increase self-esteem, the lower his self-esteem plunges. The alcoholic continues drinking with the hope that it will make him feel better. But it doesn't. Ironically, according to Johnson (1980), the alcoholic now has to drink simply in order to feel "normal." The way this person has attempted to implement his lifestyle, which, for example, may be something like, "I am inadequate, others are more adequate and must take care of me, the world is a scary place," has become harmful and restrictive. Although it is maladaptive, it is still used to protect the self and its mistaken goals. This is reminiscent of the old joke about the man who always tore up his newspaper and threw it out the train window. When his friend asked him what he was doing, he replied, "I'm keeping elephants off the tracks." His friend replied that there were no elephants on the tracks, to which he retorted, "See how effective it is."

The following is a brief example of how a person might use alcohol as a function of one's lifestyle:

Brief Example

A bright, pretty, 17-year-old high school junior was referred to counseling by her guidance counselor because of the "dramatic change" in her personality. She is the second youngest child in a family of six children and there are six years between her and her youngest brother. Her drinking history indicates occasional alcohol use beginning at age 10, with increased use thereafter, so that by age 13 she was drinking almost daily.

She identified the onset of use with her mother's return to work, her feelings of not fitting in at school, not making good enough grades, and confusion around her budding sexuality. Alcohol, she said, gave her a feeling that she was O.K., that she could handle herself with her peers, and that she could actually kiss a boy. By age 13, however, she began to do poorly in school and have violent arguments at home. At the time of referral her parents and the school had labeled her incorrigible.

Her earliest recollections indicated that she had been babied and taken care of by the entire family for 6 years until her youngest sibling was born. She recalled events when her older siblings would do things for her and then brag to her parents that she had accomplished them herself. She stated she wanted other people to help her, but she didn't feel she could trust anyone.

This young woman has never had a personal sense of accomplishment. She was plagued by a feeling that others have to do things for her because she would fail on her own. As she matured and more was expected of her, she became riddled with insecurities. When her mother left home to go to work, this girl felt she could not make it, so she turned to alcohol to increase self-esteem. Unfortunately, as with most teenagers, the addiction process took hold in a very short period of time.

STRATEGIES FOR INTERVENTION

Shulman (1973) notes that successful therapy helps the individual consider new patterns of moving from an inferior to a superior position. He states one must break free of the restraints of the current lifestyle. When alcohol has been used as the tool to adjust to a particular lifestyle, it is first necessary to eliminate alcohol use from the individual's diet altogether. This may or may not require hospitalization, depending on the physical complications surrounding withdrawal. Once this has been accomplished, it is now necessary to look at the context within which the individual used alcohol—both intrapsychically and interpersonally.

It is the counselor's job to educate the client about the nature and extent of the illness. The counselor will also try to understand the reasons why the individual used alcohol initially and how he has magnified the scope of his problems through its use. Through counseling, the alcoholic can learn and practice new and appropriate ways of coping with his problems.

As the counselor helps the client to understand the biased goals of the client's characteristic patterns of psychological movement in life, the client is more inclined to move in a less limiting manner and more in keeping with the reality of the situation. First the alcoholic must be helped to understand his lifestyle. Then through counseling, this client must learn how and why alcohol is no longer a productive way of coping with his lifestyle. With increased awareness, he is in a better position to exercise a greater range of decision making. For most alcoholics, this includes a decision about abstinence and a plan for maintaining lifelong sobriety. For the alcohol abuser, this might include decisions about when and how much he will drink at any given time. The therapist can aid the client in discovering and utilizing already existing personal strengths while developing new ones. An example of this is discussed below:

Brief Example

A 34-year-old female alcoholic entered treatment complaining of a general state of anxiety and depression. An in-depth case history revealed that Mrs. X had been drinking regularly for the past five years and that any attempt at controlled drinking resulted in loss of control within one to two weeks. Mrs. X agreed to an abstinence program and it did not appear that hospitalization was necessary at this time.

Mrs. X was having many problems in her marriage and with her children because of her alcoholism. However, it emerged in counseling that she was respected on her job because of her skills at organization and office management. Helping Mrs. X transfer these office skills to her home enabled her to find a temporary solution. Her already existing skills could be applied to help her in an area where she felt "overwhelmed" with responsibilities she didn't know how to take care of. Counseling continued to work on the reasons for her feeling overwhelmed and she later learned how to express herself more effectively to her family as well as redistribute home responsibilities.

Considering the Family System

Present alcohol literature (Hafen, 1977) and research (Steinglass, 1979) indicate that treating the whole family system when one individual is symptomatic (in this case, the alcoholic) is essential. What happens is that the family of the alcoholic comes to both expect the alcoholic behavior and reinforce the symptoms. Therefore, if the alcoholic is treated only individually, no real change is likely to take place. Once back within the family system the alcoholic will be influenced by the same set of communication stimuli and reinforcers that motivated and supported the alcoholic's behavior in the first place. Often when the alcoholic spouse gets better outside of the family system and then returns to it, the nonalcoholic spouse may start to show symptoms. (This is called the seesaw phenomenon.)

This process indicates that the alcoholism acts as a homeostat (regulator) for other family problems (Swartzman, 1977). Feldman and Pinsof (1982) have described a model to help the counselor assess how an individual's symptoms may be acting as a homeostat for other family problems. This approach does not mean that the alcoholism should not be treated as such. However, if the alcoholic is simply treated for this disease, without examining and changing the larger context in which he lives, there is not likely to be any long-term desired change.

A family can be compared to the beads of a necklace; if one bead breaks away the remaining beads must shift positions to compensate for the missing piece. Thus, as the alcoholic draws further away from the family, the rest of the family members frequently shift positions to fill the void. Alcoholism affects all members of the family in some way. Black (e.g., 1981) has lectured and written extensively about the effects of alcoholism on the alcoholic's children. In many instances the children's response to the alcoholism is an attempt to stabilize the family system, as illustrated in the following case example.

CASE EXAMPLE

Bob, a 39-year-old veterinarian, and Rita, a 38-year-old college student, and their two teenage daughters were referred to counseling because of their 14-year-old daughter's promiscuous behavior. Counseling revealed that Bob was in the chronic stage of alcoholism and felt isolated and ridiculed by the family. Rita felt she had too much responsibility for managing the home, the children, and her schoolwork. It became apparent that the 16-year-old daughter was Rita's chief confidante and supporter and was later titled "mini-mommy" in the counseling sessions. The identified patient, the 14-year-old daughter, attempted to stabilize her family system through her acting out behavior. When she saw Rita and her sister ally together and Bob's drinking increase—which resulted in his being quite distant from the family—she swung into action. Her behavior was an attempt to bring Bob back into the family as a parent who had to discipline her. As her previous attempts failed and Bob's drinking increased, her behavior became worse, which eventually brought the family into counseling.

Mozdzierz and Friedman (1978) point out that Adler's approach is compatible with a general family systems theory. They say:

> The nature and characteristic of any system in which an individual interacts is in part a reflection of each individual's movement. The particular characteristics of an interactional system, then, would be a reflection of both individual striving toward personal goals . . . and mutual striving toward mutually defined goals (which requires application of common sense). (p. 232)

One form of marital interaction that may use alcoholism as a homeostatic mechanism is what Mozdzierz and Friedman (1978) call the Superiority-Inferiority System. This is comparable to Bowen's (1978) identification of the overadequate/underadequate marital system. It is important to note that inferiority, or a feeling of not-enoughness, characterizes everyone to varying degrees, including those in a "superiority" position.

Perhaps one of the more obvious examples is the previously discussed alcoholic with an inadequate lifestyle, who is heavily invested in displays of inadequacy. Such a person would most likely be found in the Inferiority (or underadequate) Role. The Inferiority Role (I.R.) spouse demonstrates incompetency, hyper-dependency, acts more immature, less intelligent, and more "out of control." Often the I.R. partner idolizes the Superiority Role (S.R.) spouse. The Superiority Role (overadequate) spouse acts more intelligent, organized, and controlled, and often complains about the I.R. spouse's negative behavior. This interaction is a manifestation of each spouse's individual lifestyle (Mozdzierz & Friedman, 1978). As long as the S.R. spouse stays focused on the I.R. spouse's symptoms (in this case, alcoholism), the S.R. spouse does not have to face his or her own feelings of inferiority and inadequacy. The I.R. spouse may seem to be an easy target—but there is a secret agenda. The tacit message from the spouse is something like "Prove your competence and try to solve my symptoms." Of course, the S.R. spouse cannot control the alcoholic's drinking, so the alcoholic gains momentary feelings of superiority (adequacy), as in the case of Bob and Rita.

Rita presented the family problems as being all Bob's fault. She complained that he purposely avoided her and the kids, he drank too much, he did not discipline the children, he did not participate in any household responsibilities, and that he had no sexual desire. She described him as lazy, inept, out of control with his drinking, and physically unkempt. Bob agreed with all his wife's complaints and described Rita as a hard-working, responsible, and controlling person. As counseling progressed Rita described her feelings of frustration and inadequacy at being unable to control Bob's drinking. She blamed herself for not being able to "make him stop." Bob expressed the feeling that his drinking was one area in which Rita could not tell him what to do, and this felt somewhat satisfying to him.

Family counseling for the alcoholic's family begins with educating the family about alcoholism—its signs, symptoms, and progression. The family members must also be made aware of how the alcoholism has affected each of them and what role each played in maintaining or enabling the symptom to continue. As with most family counseling, it is necessary to expose the nonproductive family rules (spoken and unspoken). In the preceding example, this family apparently had a rule that said one spouse must be inferior and one spouse must be superior. Such a relationship simply cannot operate if it suddenly contains two equally effective adults. Either new rules have to be made—usually with the help of the therapist— or one spouse may revert to inferior (underadequate) behavior. Again, it is not always the alcoholic who displays the symptoms.

In the alcoholic family, the roles and boundaries usually become confused. One child may assume a parental role with respect to the other children, or even a grandparent role, acting as the parents' parent. This grandparent role not only interferes with the natural consequences of the alcoholic's drinking, it also has permanent effects on the child.

It is necessary to redefine more appropriate family roles, so that each member can assume a rightful place within the family. When faced with the superiority/ inferiority spouse system, the counselor must help broaden the fixed role descriptions, adding flexibility to the family's interactions, and allowing for some role reversals when necessary. Thus, the alcoholic spouse can find a way to be competent and give direction to the family, while the nonalcoholic spouse can find a way to be taken care of.

Another goal of family counseling for the alcoholic's family is improving communication. According to Satir (1967), communication should become more clear, congruent, noncontradictory, direct, and honest as a result of counseling. For the alcoholic who has most likely been suppressing his feelings for a long time, rationalizing and making excuses for his behavior, and feeling quite guilty, open and direct expression may be difficult. The spouse who has been expressing exclusively negative feelings for a while, receiving little or no verbal response from the alcoholic, may also find it uncomfortable to explore this new, more vulnerable form of communication. That was the case with Bob and Rita.

After five months of weekly marital or family counseling, Bob still found it difficult to tell Rita what he would like to see change about her and about their relationship. He was inclined to insist she is "fine, just the way she is." However, Rita complained that Bob got angry at her, but he didn't tell her the reasons why. Bob confirmed this and related that he was afraid of Rita's verbal attacks. He indicated that when he became closemouthed, Rita whipped into a sarcastic tirade. Both spouses ended up very angry at each other, yet neither knew quite why it all happened.

The counselor assigned Bob the task of telling Rita when he was angry at her; he was not to withdraw. Rita made an agreement to refrain from sarcasm when Bob explained his angry feelings; she agreed instead to respond in a way that would indicate she understood why Bob was angry. Also, if she sensed Bob's anger, she was not to become hostile but was to ask, "Are you angry?" and accept a simple answer. After two weeks of practice, both spouses reported that they felt closer to each other and better understood.

The preceding represents only a few of the goals and techniques of family counseling for the alcoholic. No counselor should consider the job complete, however, until the alcoholic and the family are introduced to an appropriate self-help group. These groups include, but are not limited to, Alcoholics Anonymous for the alcoholic, Al-anon for the spouse, Al-ateen for the children over 12, Al-atot for children under 12, and Families Anonymous for parents of teenaged alcoholics. These groups are often helpful in bridging the gap from professional treatment to community support. Most alcoholics and their families find sobriety to be a process, which must continue long after professional therapy has ended; indeed, for many the process lasts their entire life.

SPECIAL CONSIDERATIONS

Family counseling as previously described would *not* be indicated under two conditions: when there is no family or when the family refuses treatment.

Regarding the first condition, the assumption is that the alcoholic had been removed for a long period of time from the family system. For example, John was a chronic alcoholic for the past 25 years. The past six years he has been living on skid row. His wife divorced him over eight years ago and his three children are grown and only one of them lives in the same town as John.

Under the second condition, the family consistently and adamantly refuses treatment. For example, Melissa was a teenaged alcoholic and the daughter of two alcoholic parents. While Melissa was in an adolescent alcoholism in-patient program, her parents steadfastly refused to be interviewed and visited Melissa only once to bring her clothes and money. Melissa was referred to a halfway house where she remained for 18 months. At the end of that time she moved in with friends she had made from A.A.

CONCLUDING REMARKS

The change in emphasis from treating the alcoholic individually to treating the alcoholic and the family is receiving widespread recognition. Family treatment can also be viewed as a form of prevention, since statistics indicate that children of alcoholics have a 50 percent greater chance of becoming alcoholic than the general population. Once in treatment, these children have an opportunity to learn about alcoholism and to explore the ways they have adapted to it that may be harmful to them in the future. Counseling provides children and their parents with a framework for understanding their own individual behavior and the way they have interacted with each other to maintain unhealthy rules, roles, boundaries, communication, dependency, and symptoms.

REFERENCES

Ansbacher, H.L., & Ansbacher, R.R. *The individual psychology of Alfred Adler*. New York: Basic Books, 1956.

Black, C. Innocent bystanders at risk; The children of alcoholics. *Alcoholism*, 1981 *1*(3), 22–26.

Bowen, M. *Family therapy in clinical practice*. New York: Jason Aronson, 1978.

Deadly Alcoholism. *Chicago Tribune*. March 25, 1982, p. 6.

Feldman, L., & Pinsof, W. Problem maintenance in family systems: An integrative model. *Journal of Marital and Family Therapy*, 1982, *8*(3), 295–308.

Hafen, B.Q. *Alcohol: The crutch that cripples*. St. Paul, Minn.: West Publishing, 1977.

Jellinek, E. *The disease concept of alcoholism*. New Haven: College & University Press, 1960.

Johnson, V.E. *I'll quit tomorrow*. San Francisco: Harper & Row, 1980.

Kinney, J., & Leaton, G. *Loosening the grip*. St. Louis: C.V. Mosby, 1978.

Lombardi, D.N. Eight avenues of lifestyle consistency. *The Individual Psychologist*, 1973, *10*(2), 5–9.

Mosak, H.H. Lifestyle. In A.G. Nikelly (Ed.), *Techniques for behavior change*. Springfield, Ill., Charles C Thomas, 1971.

Mozdzierz, G.J., & Friedman, K. The superiority-inferiority spouses syndrome: Diagnostic and therapeutic considerations. *Journal of Individual Psychology*, 1978, *34*(2), 232–43.

National Council on Alcoholism. Criteria for the diagnosis of alcoholism. *American Journal of Psychiatry*, August 1972, *129*(2), 41–49.

Satir, V. *Conjoint family therapy*. Palo Alto, Calif.: Science & Behavior Books, 1967.

Schwartzman, J. Under the influence: The alcoholic at risk. *Drug Forum,* 1977/78, *26,* 177–185.

Shulman, B.H. *Contributions to individual psychology.* Chicago: Alfred Adler Institute, 1973.

Steinglass, P. An experimental treatment program for alcoholic couples. *Journal of Studies on Alcohol,* 1979, *40*(3), 159–182.

Chapter 18

A Systematic and Interdisciplinary Use of Lifestyle Counseling with the Public Offender

James Michael Gould

Scene 1

Excerpts from a central classification committee receiving inmate requests for a custody reduction.

Committee Member 1 (transportation administrator with security background): "The problem with you bleeding-heart liberals is that you've never had to clean up after one of these guys has blown someone to pieces on the kitchen wall."

Committee Member 2 (counselor): "We are talking about a property offender."

Committee Member 3 (chief of classification): "It's all academic, gentlemen, we have no 'B custody' (medium) beds available. Next docket."

Scene 2

Excerpts from an informal conversation following a discussion between a superintendent and a counselor who proposed to initiate a new institution's first treatment program. The proposal has been turned down.

Superintendent: "Off the record, I really don't think any of these programs really work. The more you give these inmates, the more they want, until you can't give any more. Then you've got a real problem on your hands. Don't quote me because I'll deny I've said this."

The conversation continues and the superintendent acknowledges the success of A.A. Six months later the counselor sponsors the first meeting in the institution. Three months later the superintendent is promoted. Three months later still, the counselor begins to screen candidates for a problem-solving course he initially proposed twelve months earlier.

Scene 3

A Sunday afternoon in suburbia. A counselor receives a phone call from the maximum security prison informing him that an inmate on his case list has been seriously injured by another inmate while he was being transferred from the institution for security reasons. During the week the inmate had requested protective custody in the prison jail because of an alleged homosexual attack by three other inmates. As a result of this incident in which the inmate received serious head wounds, information had been obtained indicating that the injured inmate was involved in drug traffic and that the most recent attack was retributional in nature and probably contracted through the inmate lines of communication. The incident occurred early Sunday. The original transfer had been postponed from Friday because of a disturbance in another major institution, which diverted the transportation priorities until the major instigators could be removed and transported to separate institutions. The counselor was informed so that he would be prepared to meet with the injured inmate's family the next day.

Scene 4

Sunrise. A crisp autumn Monday. The alarm, a struggle to the shower, a bite to eat, a cup of coffee, and a breath of fresh air. Into the car. Twenty-five miles west on a country road a shining cyclone megalith on top of a hill lies on 700 acres of the most beautiful farmland this city slicker has ever known. The institution grows larger. The parking lot of red clay, the superintendent's office. The double gates. Hundreds of inmates waiting for the trucks to take them to the jobs on the farm, on the roads, etc. I expect the usual jibes, the onslaught of requests, demands, improprieties. I've learned to walk the gauntlet like a dancer through fire. My stomach rates a six on the Richter scale. Perhaps by Wednesday I will be able to breathe again.

These experiences are presented as a way of introducing some of the fundamental problems that exist with regard to public offenders. The systematic-contextual and multidisciplinary concerns that must be faced in dealing with the public offender have been neglected and left ununified. One result is the failure to adequately prepare prospective counselors to deal with the complexity of issues and this could potentially nullify the effects of any treatment approach.

Lifestyle counseling as a therapeutic individual or group approach to public offenders applied as if they existed within a vacuum is not enough. Counselors, psychologists, social workers, recreational therapists, etc., need to develop a philosophical framework that can be utilized in dealing with the system that employs them (the state, the correctional system, the institution, their department), their role within it, and the context in which the public offender is encountered (American society, race, class, and the inmate society). This may be done by drawing from the disciplines not only of psychology but also of sociology and criminology, in order to help clarify the problem of crime in America and the plight of the public offender.

In this article I will begin the process of applying an Adlerian philosophy of "social interest" as a means of assessing and responding to the needs of the clinician and the public offender that arise from these systematic, contextual, and multidisciplinary considerations. I hope to provide a theoretical experiential model, which goes beyond lifestyle and holistic counseling, that the counselor can use in dealing with the client. This may also be used in defining their roles within the prison system and the contexts in which the criminal is encountered. In this process I will highlight the benefits of Adlerian psychology and caution practitioners on its limitations as seen from other than psychological perspectives.

THE PUBLIC OFFENDER VERSUS THE AMERICAN CRIMINAL

For the purpose of this article, "public offender" refers to any individual who is apprehended, tried, and found guilty. Although I will focus later on interventions with public offenders in the correctional setting, public offenders will also be encountered on probation, parole, and in halfway houses. They are to be distinguished from other criminals who are not labeled as such despite regular involvement in illegal activities. It is important to distinguish between these groups in order to have a realistic approach to the former.

The major difference between these two groups is that the public offender is involved in more obvious criminal behaviors and has been a failure even as a criminal. Public offenders are aware that they represent a class of criminals that have been designated for punishment within a larger class of criminals who are not designated for punishment. This is due to the peculiarities of enforcement and the hidden nature and tacit acceptance of other types of crime. It is important to realize that the crimes of the public offender are often behaviors performed within the context of the ghetto and defined as criminal within another context, i.e., the courts (Burglass & Duffy, 1974). It is also important to note that the public offender may be a pampered person, a getter, a victim, an inadequate person, or a fighter, but that these types of individuals may be found equally represented in the general population.

The public offender can be said to have life problems merely because he is presented within the context of the criminal justice system. Saying this avoids the classical analytic dilemma of diagnosing and labeling, as well as the resistances that arise with these value judgments especially within a society in which crime has historically been firmly entrenched as a way of life, a means of upward mobility in business, closely allied with political interests, organized labor, and economic opportunity (Bell, 1969).

How is it that there is so much crime in America? It seems to be a product of a lawless frontier society, with a high degree of cultural diversity within the context of an opportunistic, materialistic, and highly competitive society (Durkheim,

1927) in the throes of "anomie" (Merton, 1969). This analysis, made decades ago, still seems to hold true.

There is empirical evidence, based on a review of 113 studies, that 42 percent of the public offenders do not differ psychologically from the normal population (Schuessler & Cressey, 1950). Although genetic and chemical research may ultimately provide more information, the likelihood seems to be that a sizable psychological overlap exists between the criminal and normal populations. Thus, the relevance of some of the Adlerian-related concepts may be increased; i.e., some criminals as well as some normal persons may have a superiority complex in regard to their ability to achieve, sexual callousness, and professional loyalties (Worchel & Hillson, 1958; Foulds, 1960). Incidentally, these same terms could be descriptive of the American businessman from a feminist perspective.

IMPLICATIONS FOR LIFESTYLE ADJUSTMENT

The history of the American approach to the public offender has been a progression of treatment from retribution as a deterrent to further crime on to rehabilitation of the offender's personality and then on to the correctional approach of today. With the advent of modern psychology, the use of punishment has been brought into question. The failure of rehabilitation has resulted in a realization that there is a great difficulty involved in rehabilitating the personality and this has led to a reeducational focus of correction. This has been a "de jure" progression within a "de facto" state of punishment that persists and arises from the conditions of incarceration and has cast a shadow over all facilitative efforts. It is indicative of a need to correct our system as well as the public offender. This will be discussed below within the context of social interest and professional advocacy.

Adler (Ansbacher & Ansbacher, 1956) indicated the counterproductive nature of punishment and public focus on the alleged proliferation of crime waves. He also acknowledged the importance of recognizing the basic attitudes of public offenders that deter them from success in the areas of work, sexuality, love, and family. Thus, according to Adler, it would be desirable to avoid all approaches that will lead to challenging and further isolating public offenders, who already perceive society as against them. These considerations have significant implications for a correctional system that removes the offenders from their communities, places them in isolation, denies conjugal visitation rights and meaningful work, and restricts visitation in general.

It seems logical to approach the criminal, not from a perspective of theoreticians but the public offenders' conception of themselves as "victims." By approaching them from an educational perspective as opposed to a therapeutic cure, we place responsibility for their lives on the public offenders. Frankl (1955), in referring to neurotics, stated that "such people want to create alibis for their weaknesses. They accept them as something given instead of recognizing in them a task for reeducation or, better, self-education" (p. 99). With a reeducational approach, we avoid coercion to our conception of the world and respect the autonomy of the individual. This opens the door to exploring with clients how they violated their own autonomy by claiming that they have developed along lines other than what they have chosen, believing themselves to have been forced in a particular direction by society (Burglass, 1974).

This approach is consistent with examining the lifestyle of an individual's development along nonproductive lines. In working with the decision-making, problem-solving model and an understanding of lifestyle counseling, I believe I have, in keeping with Burglass's (1974) goals, been able to educate clients in the origin and purpose of their attitudes and beliefs, to help them free themselves of the myths and fictions foisted on them by themselves and others, and finally, to approach life as a journey and a struggle to find the truth within themselves, a process, not a treatment, on the road to truth. By examining the surrender of autonomy through the use of reaction versus decision, the process of individual liberation that would lead to cultural or class liberation where needed is begun.

If anything has impressed me in working with public offenders, it is their apparent sharing, for the most part, of the same problems and concerns as the general population. The only difference seems to be their expression of their frustrations and discouragement in a criminal manner, which seems more related to the environmental and sociological conditions already discussed.

However, before the client is able to develop and progress along this journey, in which we are relying on the Socratic belief that an individual has the capacity to find the truth within himself when the information is provided, there are more basic needs that must be met. These are related to Maslow's (1968) needs hierarchy. In order to meet these, we as counselors and educators can utilize the Adlerian concept of social interest to extend beyond our relationship with the client to the systematic, contextual environment in which we encounter the public offender.

Maslow, Adler, Frankl, and Malcolm X

An obvious dilemma in working with the public offender, who often comes from a deprived environment or who is at least living in the deprivation of incarceration, is the realization brought into focus by Maslow's concept of hierarchy of needs. Maslow postulated that individuals have a need for food, safety, shelter, love, beauty, and actualization that can only be fulfilled progressively if the preceding needs have been met. Sometimes, priorities do get out of order: Baruth and Eckstein (1978) talk about two counselors who spent their first two weeks of working in a prison setting rat traps.

The correctional system can be viewed as a system with the same basic needs of feeding, housing, and security. Therefore, it is important for the counselor to realize how these needs are going to impact on his exposure to the client and definition of his job. This is apparent in the counselor's classification duties. The counselor needs to be aware of the role of the particular institution within a larger system and its relationship to the concerns of the community, especially in terms of the issues of security with violent and sexual offenders.

The broad political situation is often one in which the existence of a correctional facility in one's district is viewed as a deficit. If one is located there it can only hurt a politician and can never be an attribute, particularly if a mass disturbance occurs. This unfavorable assessment of a correctional facility is most likely to occur when the community is largely unconcerned with the internal conditions of the correctional system and is primarily concerned with it as a form of protection from the public offender. This narrow perspective, therefore, is further justification for advocating a greater social interest on the part of the community members.

In the meantime, the counselor will need to be able to function within the existing conditions. This can occur through a metaphysical realization that questions relating to purpose and meaning in life can aid the inmate in transcending the bitter conditions of incarceration. I have always urged clients and counselors to read and utilize Frankl's *Man's Search For Meaning* (1963) as well as *The Autobiography of Malcolm X* (1966) as an attempt to rise above the situation.

The inmate who is functioning from either a pampered or victim image will look at his surroundings and try to utilize the circumstances in which he finds himself as an excuse for not trying to progress. Since the counselor is within the criminal's field, the inmate will try to win the counselor's support for his view of himself as a victim of society's cruel and unusual punishment.

It is important for the counselor to be aware that these conditions exist; but, on the other hand, he should be able to return responsibility to the inmate population for its nonproductive activities, e.g., creating within itself a climate that tolerates violence and sexual abuse by silent consent. The public offender should not be pitied, but recruited in efforts to improve the conditions of his situation, the institution, and the system.

The goal is the realization by the offender of the meaning of Frankl's statement (1967) that the essential question in life is "not what I demand of life, but what life demands of me" (p. 122). From a broader, yet related, perspective, it behooves us also who are interested in this problem to become involved in the political arena, thereby modeling "social interest" for public offenders and the reality of their concern.

The recognition of the many needs of the public offender and the system is consistent with the use of lifestyle counseling in an eclectic approach advocated by Rule (1982). However, we need to expand the holistic psychology to a holistic multidisciplinary approach. One of the major assumptions of Adler's individual psychology is that man is a social being whose behavior can only be fully understood in a social context. In fact, Adler regarded personal problems as social problems. We need to expand the conception of the individual's problems as problems the society must share.

ROLE OF THE CORRECTIONAL COUNSELOR

It is not sufficient to talk about the modality of lifestyle counseling within the correctional setting as if, in and of itself, it will produce a major impact. This would distort the nature of correctional counseling by ignoring the employer, that is, the correctional system, the context in which the client is encountered, and the majority of tasks the counselor will be required to perform.

Regarding the counselor's tasks, they can be utilized as alternative means of gathering information related to lifestyle counseling, instead of being looked upon as necessary evils that the counselor must endure. They are a function of a competitive environment created by scarce resources and have generated a call for greater social activism. The tasks have to do with administrative matters, casework, systems integration, social advocacy, the counselor-psychologist relationship, and the treatment team.

Administrative Aspects

The counselor needs to understand the administrative juggling required in managing security, housing, industry, education, and treatment and how these will define and influence his institution, his caseload, and the participants in any treatment or educational activity. Also, the counselor needs to understand the mission of his institution within the local, state, or federal system, on both a long- and a short-term basis. This understanding can include politically hot issues, e.g., fluctuating security versus treatment priorities with violent and sexual offenders.

Thus, the administrative task of the counselor is knowing the system in which he works. It involves the use and maintenance of records, court and legal procedures related to sentencing, parole eligibility, and sentence reductions. Additional concerns are classification involving job, custody, and institutional status as related to productivity, safety, and community ties.

An understanding of these factors can influence the treatment or an assessment of the potential of the individuals. It can facilitate matching them with available resources in various institutions and increase the accessibility of particular programs to the target inmate.

Casework

The casework of a counselor is usually voluminous and is assigned on a basis unrelated to counseling, e.g., dormitory residence. These duties entail much paperwork and consume quite a bit of time. Files can be utilized for the purpose of increasing awareness of lifestyle consistency in identifying participants and for the wealth of accumulated information involved.

The eight avenues of lifestyle counseling identified by Lombardi (1973) (case history, interviewing, expressive behavior, psychological testing, family constellation, early recollection, grouping, and systematic behavior) can be explored in presentence investigations, mandatory monthly interviews, observation on the yard, in recreation, diagnostic-reception data, visiting day, and informal interaction that arises as a result of the residential nature of the correctional setting. The areas of early recollection and family constellation interpretation are often better handled by the psychologist for reasons that will be discussed below.

Systems Integration

Another important area is systems integration, which Wein (1982) describes as a major focus of present-oriented crisis intervention within this setting. The counselor is often the middleman in a correctional setting and a prison society. Sykes and Sheldon (1973), in talking about the prison society, stated "there is a striking pervasive value system. This value system commonly takes the form of a prison code in which brief normative imperatives are taken as imperative guides for the inmate's behavior, in relation with fellow prisoners and custodians" (p. 129). This is an important aspect for the counselor to realize and look for in the perception of the inmate. The counselor should note whether the public offender considers the counselor to be a custodian as opposed to one who integrates the inmate and the correctional system by providing the public offenders with guidance in utilizing the system to their maximum benefit. Treatment outcomes will be directly proportional to the extent the offender buys into the value system. Those values are the basis of dialogue and can be reframed into the concept of "Social Interest" (see Chapter 2).

Cressey & Irwin (1962) present a view of the "thief," "convict," and "legitimate" culture, which seems more realistic and consistent with Adler's view of the criminal attitude. This framework is most helpful in identifying the reeducation potential of the public offender and can be utilized to identify many inmates who are the most amenable to nonrecidivism. In addition, Sykes and Sheldon (1969) identify the factors of concern for advocacy and the prevention of a school for crime.

Advocacy

The need for advocacy stems from the environmental conditions that add fuel to the public offender's discouragement in the form of rejection, impoverishment, figurative castration, extensive social control, and a loss of physical security. In addition, there may be organic and nutritional issues that seem to be related to the criminal's activity levels, both prior to and while being incarcerated. Adler pointed out that the criminal has one of the highest levels of activity on the negative side of life (Ansbacher & Ansbacher, 1956).

Hippchen (1980) noted six areas that may be correlated with violent forms of behavior: vitamin-mineral deficiency, hypoglycemia, cerebral allergies and addictions, environmental contaminants, minimal brain dysfunction, and neural receptor imbalances that are also related to hyperactivity. The counselor needs to be vigilant for these possibilities and advocate institutional dietary changes that could ameliorate the first three.

The issue of potential safety will be greatest for the unincarcerated culture offender. The counselor can have an effect on this with classification changes. Advocacy is both an institutional and a societal consideration that could lead to the decriminalization of drug abuse or more creative treatment of alcoholic habitual offenders (e.g., taking their cars rather than their licenses and not expecting them to drive illegally). The presence in the prison of individuals such as these only compounds violence and security problems related to contraband materials.

The legal and economic disenfranchisement of the inmate and the prison system from the free market is directly related to the individual and the correctional system's impoverishment. This results in overcrowding, ineffective vocational training, and a drain on the taxpayer. The loss of autonomy, social rejection, and isolation could be reduced by a free flow of traffic into the institution via family and community visitation, which could also function as an aid to internal security by a dilution of the "convict culture." Conjugal visits could lead to couple and family counseling.

To advocate these changes almost presumes a political stance by the counselor. Stevich (1980), in talking about social interests in relation to locus of control, quotes Teng (1970), who reported that "internals" in the Rotter (1972) scale were significantly more cooperative, i.e., higher in social interest, than "externals." Along the same vein, Majumder, McDonald, and Greever (1977) found internally oriented rehabilitation counselors had more positive attitudes toward the poor. To the extent that the inmate is impoverished by the environment, that we are approaching the public offender and the system from a perspective of social interest, those findings give a clear direction for the need for "internals" as models for the public offender and as advocates for basic human rights. This is in contrast to the use of punitive "externals," which has been the general practice.

Counselor-Psychologist Relationship

Since many of the tasks that the counselor will be dealing with are very time consuming, it is beneficial to form an alliance with the psychologist. The psychologist may have more training in working with the therapeutic techniques related to

Lombardi's (1973) eight avenues, especially early recollections, family constellation, and grouping.

Close cooperation is the optimal approach to lifestyle counseling in the correctional setting. The counselor has much to do, e.g., caseloads, classification,
administrative, casework and advocacy, in addition to contending with other
disruptive factors that are time consuming and interfere with regular individual
and group techniques.

In terms of group counseling, Rule (1982) has noted seven goals for holistic,
lifestyle group formation; these are very similar to those discussed in Chapter 3 of
this book. His citation of Hare's (1962) six characteristics of group interaction
supports this division of labor. The counselor-psychologist alliance is the beginning of the creation of a network, which will be discussed later.

The Treatment Team

To team or not to team has been the question. By this time it is obvious that the
counselor's duties will bring him into regular interaction with administrators,
industrial staff, educators, recreational staff, classification officers, and security.
It is only natural to try to coordinate these activities so that the often competing
interests within the institutional setting can be best manipulated.

The creation of a treatment team can be a process by which the counselor and
other staff can become more educated about various institutional needs as well as
how they are related to the needs of the public offender. It also provides the
counselor with half a dozen other perspectives on particular offenders as well as
daily material for the counselor in the use of crisis intervention techniques,
rational-emotive techniques, and problem-solving approaches. In helping the
inmate to adjust to the demands of the prison "world," it becomes the dress
rehearsal for the outside world.

A STRATEGY FOR INTERVENTION AND EXPANDING THE NETWORK

Once correctional counselors are able to mobilize and manage the multitude of
responsibilities involved in a systematic, contextual, and multidisciplinary
approach, they somehow often manage to instigate specific group therapies or
approaches. By recruiting interested inmates into these programs and by providing
additional training to those who have demonstrated growth, mastered new skills,
and expressed an interest to continue the process, counselors can develop the next
link of the network, the indigenous inmate peer teacher or counselor.

I have found the use of a problem-solving skill model, active listening skills
training, and supervision of the inmate peer teacher an effective means of provid-

ing further training for both new members and old members. This is also an ensurance of continuity of the program despite high staff turnover, a chronic problem in the field. An added bonus is that this is a means of freeing the counselor to attend to the development of community programs like A.A. and other needed services.

By working closely with the staff psychologist in the training of the peer teachers and the general development of an educational approach to problem solving, I have been able to evolve a continuum of reeducation leading from basic problem-solving skills to group therapy, which the psychologist can facilitate.

This process also can be viewed as a technique for observing the movement of the public offender along the hierarchy of social interest, as elaborated by Nystul (1976), from the egocentric to the altruistic level of social responsibility and commitment. In addition, the opportunity to work shoulder-to-shoulder with staff members helps break down social isolation and break through the defensive superiority complex noted by Worchel and Hillson (1958) and Foulds (1960). If the progress continues, the public offender may be able to reach a sense of completion that is analogous to the concept of social interest or a feeling of oneness with the community of man. This development can be stimulated with the use of music, poetry, leisure counseling (Rule & Stewart, 1977), and recreational counseling (Gould & Ansbacher, 1975); in addition, meditation, art forms, and spiritual development groups can be utilized.

The decision-making model (Burglass, 1972), that I have utilized, contains a seven-step process of problem solving, examining (1) the situation, both external and internal, (2) the possibilities, (3) evaluating the possibilities, (4) applying the decisional criterion, (5) decision, (6) action, and (7) ratification. The model was originally designed for volunteer counselors and has an Adlerianlike emphasis on principles of self-determination and community responsibility and the ethics of autonomy and individual commitment.

This approach was based on a political, social, and psychological perspective of criminality. It circumvents the disadvantages of label and value judgment and deals with the public offender as an individual who was unable to solve major life problems. The progression through the phases of the decisional criteria is equivalent to moving through the three levels of social interest. It addresses the issues of private logic by dealing with the processes that contribute to the formation of perceived or consenting victim images, reaction (impulsivity) versus decision, and the lack of the fundamental skills of problem solving. These skills were taught within a classroom format requiring the reading of Frankl's *Man's Search for Meaning* (1963). Rituals, art forms, and symbols were utilized to reframe experience from deficit to gift and self-images, from victims to creators. My research has indicated that the short-range approach was statistically significant in improving decision-making skills as measured by *The Means and Problem Solving Scale* (Platt & Spivak, 1971); however, there was no significant difference on the Rotter scale as a measure of victimage (external) versus creator (internal), although this is not surprising in view of the short-term nature of this study (Gould, 1979).

PROBLEMS AND FUTURE DIRECTIONS

In my efforts to present a realistic approach to lifestyle counseling in a correctional format, I have attempted to approach the life problems of the public offender from a historical, system-conscious, contextual, and multidisciplinary perspective. I have been able to identify a number of problems and, unfortunately, too few solutions; however, I hope to have given a direction in which to proceed. I have tried to reframe lifestyle counseling as more than a format but an essential element of Adlerian philosophy of social interest. This philosophy holds the seed to the solutions of the problems cited and the myriad, yet to be isolated, that flow from the history, the systems, the context and limitations of the social sciences to which we look for solutions. I have proposed a situation-specific approach that has both inherent strength and weakness due to this specificity. There are also problems with some of the basic assumptions, e.g., the concept that self-actualization is always on the positive side of life (Jahoda, 1958).

We are at ground zero after a century of efforts to return the public offender to society in a better condition than when he comes to us. We need to reevaluate the situation to discover how we managed to arrive at this point. To the extent that we have not "de facto" progressed beyond punishment, rehabilitation and corrections have not failed, but rather have never really been tried. We need to move from a fear of the public offender and our own failure to a more courageous, creative, and innovative effort to bring about change. As practitioners, we need to look within ourselves for our own unique approach to these problems. There are indications (Garfield & Bergen, 1978) that positive outcomes are related to the use of a conceptual framework in which we have faith and competency.

REFERENCES

Ansbacher, H.L., & Ansbacher, R.R. (Eds.). *The individual psychology of Alfred Adler*. New York: Basic Books, 1956.

Baruth, L.G., & Eckstein, D.C. *Lifestyle theory, practice and research*. Dubuque, Iowa: Kendall-Hunt, 1978.

Bell, W. Crime as an American way of life. In W.A. Rushing (Ed.), *Deviant behavior & social process*. Chicago: Randy McNally, 1969.

Burglass, M.E. *Thresholds manual for correctional counselors*. Bucks County, Pa.: Correctional Solutions Foundation, Inc., Department of Corrections, 1972.

Burglass, M.E., & Duffy, M.G. *Thresholds teachers manual*. Cambridge, Mass.: Correctional Solutions Foundation, Inc., 1974.

Cressey, D.F., & Irwin, J. Thieves, convicts and the inmate culture. In W.A. Rushing (Ed.), *Deviant behavior and social process*. Chicago: Rand McNally, 1969.

Durkheim, E. *Les Regles de la Methode Sociologique*. Paris, 1927.

Foulds, G.A. Attitudes towards self and others in psychopaths. *Journal of Individual Psychology*, 1960, *16*, 81–83.

Frankl, V. *The doctor and the soul*. New York: Knopf, 1955.

Frankl, V. *Man's search for meaning, an introduction to logotherapy*. Boston: Beacon Press, 1963.

Frankl, V. *Psychotherapy and existentialism*. New York: Washington Press, 1967.

Garfield, S.L., & Bergen, A.E. The evaluation of therapeutic outcomes. In S.L. Garfield & A.E. Bergen (Eds.), *Handbook of psychotherapy and behavior change* (2nd ed.). New York: Wiley, 1978.

Gould, J.M. The short-range effects of a modified thresholds decision-making model on the problem-solving skills of adult male offenders. Unpublished paper, 1979.

Gould, J., & Ansbacher, H.L. Function pleasure in Adlerian psychotherapy. *Journal of Individual Psychology*, 1975, *31*, 150–157.

Hare, A.P. *Handbook of small group research*. New York: Free Press, 1962.

Hippchen, L.C. *Some possible biochemical aspects of criminal behavior*. Paper presented at the annual meeting of the Academy of Criminal Sciences, Philadelphia, March 20, 1980.

Jahoda, M. *Current concepts of positive mental health*. New York: Basic Books, 1958.

Lombardi, D.N. Eight avenues of lifestyle consistency. *The Individual Psychologist*, 1973, *10*(2), 5–9.

Majumder, R.K., McDonald, A.D., & Greever, K.B. A study of rehabilitation counselors locus of control and attitudes towards the poor. *Journal of Counseling Psychology*, 1977, *24*(21), 137–141.

Malcolm X, *Autobiography of Malcolm X*. New York: Grove Press, 1966.

Maslow, A.H. *Towards a psychology of being* (2nd ed.). Princeton: Van Nostrand, 1968.

Merton, R.K. Social structure and anomie. In W.A. Rushing (Ed.), *Deviant behavior & social process*. Chicago: Rand McNally, 1973.

Nystul, M.S. Identification and movement within the three levels of Social Interest. *Journal of Individual Psychology*, 1976, *32*, 55–61.

Platt, J.J., & Spivak, G. *Manual for the Means-End Problem Solving Procedure* (MEPS). Philadelphia: Hahnemann Medical College, 1971.

Rotter, J.B. *Application of a social learning theory of personality*. New York: Holt, Rinehart & Winston, 1972.

Rule, W.R. Holistic approaches to offender rehabilitation. In Hippchen, L.C. (Ed.), *Holistic approaches to offender rehabilitation*. Springfield, Ill.: Charles C Thomas, 1982.

Rule, W.R., & Stewart, M.W. Enhancing leisure counseling using an Adlerian technique. *Therapeutic Recreational Journal*, 1977, *11*, 87–93.

Schuessler, R., & Cressey, D.F. Personality and characteristics of criminals. *American Journal of Sociology*, 1950, *55*, 476–484.

Stevich, R.A., Devon, P.N., & Willingham, W.K. Locus of control and behavioral versus self-responses measure of social interest. *Journal of Individual Psychology*, 1980, *36*, 183–190.

Sykes, G.M., & Sheldon, N.L. The remote social system. In W.A. Rushing (Ed.), *Deviant behavior and social process*. Chicago: Rand McNally, 1973.

Teng, M.S. Locus of control as a determinant of job proficiency employability and training satisfaction of vocational rehabilitation clients. *Journal of Counseling Psychology*, 1970, *17*(6), 487–491.

Wein, M.L. Personal communication, October 1, 1982.

Worchel, P., & Hillson, J.S. The self-concept in the criminal—an exploration of Adlerian theory. *Journal of Individual Psychology*, 1958, *14*, 173, 181.

Part V

The Counselor as a Person

Chapter 19

Ethical Issues in Lifestyle Counseling for Adjustment to Disability

Rochelle V. Habeck

Many practitioners believe lifestyle counseling to be particularly applicable for facilitating the adjustment of persons with disability. In order to protect the welfare of clients, the ethical counselor would carefully evaluate alternative counseling approaches and techniques before adopting any specific orientation in practice. This evaluation might prompt such questions as: How well does this approach facilitate my efforts to meet the counseling needs of my clients? How appropriate are the philosophical tenets and methods of this approach for the setting, role, and administrative constraints within which I have agreed to work? What evidence exists that supports the assumptions of this approach and/or argues for the use of this approach over others available to me? How consistent are the skills required to appropriately use this approach with my own competencies and training? How conducive is the approach for enabling me to function according to the ethical standards I espouse?

REVIEW OF CONCEPTS

The purpose of this chapter is to stimulate the reader to weigh these and other ethical considerations in regard to lifestyle counseling and rehabilitation. Potential pitfalls and possible advantages to assist the counselor in evaluating this approach are discussed. In order to consider these issues more carefully, it may be useful to review and define the concepts of ethics in counseling, adjustment to disability, and lifestyle counseling.

Ethics in Counseling

One of the characteristics of a profession is responsibility for maintaining high standards for autonomous function among the group members. This, in part, is achieved through a written code of ethics (Wright, 1980). To function as an ethical counselor implies that one behaves in accordance with the rules of conduct or standards of the profession. Counselors working with disabled persons can find applicable standards in the codes of various professional organizations.

These codes cover many aspects of counselor functions, including relationships with clients and families, relationships with other agencies and professionals, administration, research, evaluation, and training. Ethical behavior is delineated with regard to confidentiality, competent service, conflicts of interest, assessment methods, moral and legal issues, and other matters. All proclaim the counselor's primary obligation to respect the dignity and worth of the individual and the commitment to promote fundamental human rights and full functioning of the individual (American Psychological Association, 1981; National Rehabilitation Counselor Association Ethics Subcommittee, 1972; American Personnel and Guidance Association, 1981).

Although written standards for counselors are readily available, ethical issues are often not easy to identify and ethical solutions are not always easy to attain. An effective counseling relationship requires a measure of objectivity to achieve respect for the client as an individual, yet the counseling process involves making judgments and choosing modes of action that necessarily entail choosing between values (Golightly, 1971). Regardless of the counselor's theoretical orientation or the counseling methods employed, these unavoidable value judgments, along with limitations in the art and science of counseling and human imperfection, make ethical issues an important consideration in the application of any counseling approach.

Adjustment to Disability

In rehabilitation, the concept of adjustment to disability is widely used yet poorly operationalized and variably defined. Often the term is applied to psychological functioning, although the outcome criteria for adjustment in rehabilitation are typically physical/functional and social and vocational/economic. Most authors recognize the contribution of a variety of factors for influencing the adjustment of persons with disability (e.g., environment, family, social attitudes). Nevertheless, rehabilitation practitioners often continue to focus their counseling efforts only at the psychological level of the individual, ignoring the impact these other factors may have. Likewise, practitioners often assume the need for counseling in the adjustment to disability, despite research findings (e.g., Wright, 1960) that show no necessary association between particular disabilities (e.g., missing limb) and particular personality characteristics (e.g., depression), nor that severity of disability is correlated with level of adjustment.

Despite findings to the contrary, perhaps the most persistent bias that interferes with "objective" counseling in rehabilitation is the notion that disability is a necessary source of maladjustment. To date, there is no evidence that specific type or degree of severity of disability constitutes sufficient cause for psychological maladjustment (Shontz, 1977). On the contrary, even with severe somatic change the basic personality structure of most individuals appears to be stable. Although it may become temporarily disorganized, personality is characterized as malleable, yet stable, and able to reestablish equilibrium by drawing on preexisting resources for integrating the crisis into the self (Shontz, 1977). Some disabled persons would add that the experience of disability can have positive effects (e.g., personal growth, career development) along with the inconveniences and hardships.

Disability seems to have a greater impact on the external (e.g., income, leisure activities) characteristics of the lifestyle than on the holistic personality. Research indicates that stability of personality extends from the formative years while the sociological, or external, characteristics of the lifestyle are tenuous realities subject to change by major life events such as disability (English, 1977). Some research suggests that the best predictor of favorable response to certain traumatic disabilities is a history of previously successful adjustment in coping with life stresses (Shontz, 1977). These findings lend support for the use of lifestyle as a relevant basis to assist persons who want help in integrating the impact of disability.

Theoretical concepts that have been used to explain psychological effects of disability are varied and there is little empirical basis for choosing one model over another. As reviewed by English (1977), these theories range from those based on psychological theory to those based on sociological theory, and differentially emphasize the impact of body image, social role, motivation, early childhood, social attitudes, behavioral skills, cultural conditions, interpersonal interactions, and social learning on subsequent psychological response.

Roessler and Bolton (1978) add two important considerations to the concept of adjustment in disability. They conceptualize adjustment in rehabilitation as a process characteristic rather than a status to be achieved. The focus is shifted to the particular way in which the individual deals with problems and how effective these methods are for resolving problems, rather than on whether the individual has achieved some desirable state of adjustment (e.g., freedom from anxiety). The authors also discuss the issue of frame of reference as a factor in determining adjustment. Differences in the self-reported views of clients versus the views of professionals analyzing client data have been noted (Roessler & Bolton, 1978). In such cases, whose view is to be considered valid?

Similarly, Cobb (1962) emphasizes the significant impact of the personal meaning of disability to each individual and argues that counseling must therefore be directed toward individual situations and reactions rather than psychological processes that are assumed to be constant across groups of persons.

One's values and assumptions regarding the nature of adjustment and one's beliefs about the factors that promote or impede its development will have a bearing on the method one views as being most facilitative for the client and on the choices one makes within the counseling process. These influences are subjective and subtle. Counselors have different levels of self-awareness of their existence and varying ability to recognize or control their influence in counseling.

In summary, adjustment can be defined according to a variety of theoretical views. These views are important as they will influence the nature of the counseling intervention offered. For example, in rehabilitation, adjustment is often described in functional terms as the ability to manage one's environment (Roessler & Bolton, 1978). Intervention in this case emphasizes training in skills and behaviors to generate rewards and avoid punishments. Or as Trieschmann (1974) has simply stated the issue, the key to coping with disability is having the ability or resources to receive enough satisfaction and rewards to make life worthwhile.

Lifestyle Counseling

For purposes of this chapter, lifestyle is considered to encompass two assumptions; first, that the behavior of individuals is holistic, such that people develop styles or patterns of living; and second, that the behavior of individuals is goal oriented, such that a person's major goals in life influence much of his or her thoughts, feelings, and actions. As a result of adopting these assumptions in counseling persons with disability, the practitioner is influenced in terms of the focus of counseling and how the impact of the disability is viewed. The implications of these assumptions will be considered in more depth below.

A summary of conclusions related to the key concepts may be helpful at this point. It is assumed that as professionals, all counselors ascribe to some set of ethical standards that uphold certain principles for appropriate conduct and client welfare. Bearing these general ethical standards in mind, one must recognize that situational variables and individual counselor differences in values, understanding, and beliefs will influence their interpretation in practice. Consequently, ethical issues are often complex. Weighing the ethical merits of a particular counseling approach challenges us to reexamine our beliefs and assumptions that form the value framework from which we operate. Some important areas for awareness might include one's assumptions about counseling and human values in rehabilitation, one's perceptions about disability and its consequences, and one's values and beliefs regarding what constitutes adjustment—for the individual and for society. It is important to bear these general professional and personal issues in mind as we examine some specific ethical issues for lifestyle counseling in rehabilitation.

POTENTIAL PITFALLS

Interpreting Lifestyle

One important issue to consider relates to the accuracy of the lifestyle assessment. In lifestyle counseling, the counselor discusses strategies for change with the client based on inferences made from some combinations of early recollection, family constellation, and other interview data. However, the reliability or validity of these assessment techniques has not been fully substantiated. Although the techniques for gathering the information are fairly well delineated, there are very few specific guidelines on how the counselor is to put the information together to interpret the lifestyle assessment and form strategies (Gushurst, 1971). Consequently, the client might conceivably provide the same information to different counselors and receive different assessments of their lifestyle with different views about the client's basic mistakes and appropriate strategies for change. Without clear guidelines for accurate interpretation of assessment data, counselors are subject to errors in the interpretation of lifestyle data and, consequently, in the strategies they offer. In this sense, lifestyle assessment is more of an art than a science.

Prescribing Strategies

Another ethical problem in lifestyle counseling is the moral bind that faces a counselor in using this somewhat prescriptive counseling approach. Following assessment, it is the counselor's function to identify the mistaken notions in the client's lifestyle. Other counseling approaches share this dilemma, particularly those that share recognition of the effect of cognition on emotion (e.g., rational-emotive therapy, cognitive behavioral therapy). The problem, simply stated, is that there are no objective standards to use in deciding what constitutes "mistakes." The counselor is in the position of imposing his or her values in identifying mistakes and prescribing strategies for change. This may be softened by a negotiating or sharing approach with the client; however, it is important to remember that the prescriptive approach assumes that the counselor's values are superior to those of the client.

According to Lowe (1959), Adler intended that therapists should remove themselves from cases where the client's values run counter to those held by the therapist, thereby avoiding a situation that could create emotional conflicts for the therapist. He recommended that in situations of conflicting values, only those therapists who are democratic and have sufficiently flexible values to accept those of persons different from themselves should continue the counseling relationship (Lowe, 1959).

Counselor Competence

In both these areas, assessing lifestyle and prescribing strategies, considerable responsibility rests with the counselor. This leads to the related issue of counselor competence. Typically, personality assessment, diagnosis, and interpretation to facilitate client insight are considered sophisticated skills that require extensive training and supervision. The step-by-step approaches that have been written as guides to lifestyle assessment appear deceptively simple, as do the cookbook and computer-generated interpretations for tests like the MMPI. Although these handy tools assist the counselor in collecting and compiling client data, they also afford access to persons who lack necessary background about their limitations and appropriate use. In the application of lifestyle counseling in rehabilitation, the counselor should be mindful of using this method in accordance with one's level of skill. Ethical standards require that counselors function within the parameters of their training and competence (American Psychological Association, 1981).

Angers (1958) points out the dangers of superficial, evaluative labeling that, while applicable at the time, leads to errors because of partial descriptions of the client rather than assessment based on the whole style of life. For example, a hospital environment may provide a very limited and perhaps distorted view of behavior. Patients are often labeled by staff as uncooperative, unmotivated, noncompliant, and other pejorative terms when their behavior conflicts with the needs of the staff or interferes with institutional functioning. These pigeonholes can not only severely limit the effectiveness of rehabilitation but are also passed on verbally or in reports that influence future interactions with the client. Effective use of lifestyle assessment can combat this problem by providing a more holistic view of the individual and a broader framework for understanding the client's goals and interpreting behavior.

In a related vein it is important that the counselor consider the appropriateness of lifestyle counseling for the setting in which the practitioner functions and the context in which the person is being seen. Many counselors in rehabilitation function as part of a team where there is some delineation, formal or informal, regarding each professional's role. Some counselors function in a specific role, such as job placement or work evaluation. Other counselors are part of a medical treatment setting, where clients have come seeking physical restoration. Before determining an appropriate intervention strategy it is important for the counselor to weigh carefully the role he or she has in relation to other professionals as well as the client's understanding of the purpose of counseling.

Informed Consent

Informed consent is a critical component of ethical counseling practice. Clients have a right to be informed of the purpose of counseling, the specific approach used by the counselor, the limitations of the approach, and the alternatives available (American Personnel and Guidance Association, 1981). Clients have the right to choose whether they will participate in counseling. When clients seek out counseling, these rights are somewhat easier to safeguard. In rehabilitation, counseling is often offered as "part of what we do here" and these rights are easily overlooked. For clients who are not self-referred, counselors must carefully examine their assumptions regarding client needs before providing unsolicited lifestyle counseling. While it is reasonable to expect that disability may create inconveniences that interfere with a realization of an individual's major goals, it is neither reasonable nor ethical to assume individuals with disability necessarily need or want the benefit of lifestyle counseling to assist them.

In addition, the insight orientation of lifestyle counseling may not be appropriate for persons with limited cognitive ability or those without verbal skills. Psychotherapy research offers inconclusive evidence to support one counseling technique over another (Garfield & Bergin, 1978). However, for some specific problems or situations, certain techniques have been demonstrated to be more effective than others; for example, the use of behavior modification for operant pain. The counselor has an ethical responsibility to know and to make available the most effective means of treatment available, regardless of personal preference.

Psychological Orientation

Perhaps the most severe theoretical shortcoming in the application of Adlerian principles and lifestyle counseling in adjustment to disability is its almost exclusive psychological orientation. As Ford and Urban (1964) point out, not all overt behavior is determined by an individual's view. Some behavior is determined by situational stimuli. In Adlerian theory the emphasis is on the individual's subjective perspective (the "fictions" that direct one's behavior) in order to reorganize dynamic factors and create insight as a sufficient precondition to change. It is important to note that these assumptions were developed with a population having psychiatric difficulties, where the focus on individual psychology may be sufficient. In rehabilitation, the problem of lifestyle counseling is that psychological distress or maladjustment implies an error in the client's view, attributing crisis to the individual's lifestyle. As Mosak (1979) points out, not all suffering stems from a person's lifestyle. Many people with adequate lifestyles (i.e., satisfactory relationship to the basic life tasks of work, relationships, sex, etc.) "develop problems or (psychological) symptoms in the face of intolerable or extreme situations from which they cannot extricate themselves" (Mosak, 1979, p. 66). In regard to disability, then, one must use caution to avoid an overly psychological orientation to the assessment and interpretation of current difficulties, and consider the impact of very real external stressors such as societal attitudes, genetic factors, environmental constraints, and physical discomfort.

THEORETICAL ADVANTAGES

In previous chapters, many of the assets associated with lifestyle counseling have been discussed. In this section, some major characteristics of Adlerian theory that form the basis for lifestyle counseling are reviewed in regard to their contribution to the ethical functioning of the counselor in rehabilitation settings.

Holism and Human Worth

The concept of holism, or the unity of personality, is a central focus in viewing the lifestyle. In rehabilitation, this orientation can assist the client and the counselor to see the effects of the disability within the totality of his or her identity and may help to integrate this characteristic as only one part of the whole person. Understanding the subjective schema of the individual's lifestyle can allow the counselor to help the client see unnecessary restrictions imposed by the lifestyle and thus facilitate the development of new patterns of thinking and behavior that incorporate the functional limitations of the disability (Rule, 1978). Redefining the self to emphasize the assets associated with the whole lifestyle can serve to expand the behavioral options and thus increase the individual's chances for satisfaction in pursuing his or her overriding goals.

Associated with this concept of holism is the emphasis on human worth and dignity in Adlerian theory. Ansbacher (1971) compares Adlerian concepts with those of humanistic psychology, recognizing the creative power of the individual versus deterministic models in which behavior results from genetics and/or environment alone. Sahakian (1978) describes the personalistic psychotherapies as having high regard for persons. Human beings, unlike objects, are placed beyond value and therefore possess dignity. He viewed Adler and other cognitive theorists as being grounded in personalism. Dowd and Kelly (1980) describe individual psychology as featuring the capacity of man to transcend the limits of heredity, environment, and immediate experience. According to these authors, individuals are viewed as creative, unified, dynamic organisms, whose lives move in a consistent pattern toward subjectively developed goals. From this perspective, individuals with disabilities are not viewed as necessarily defined or determined by the disability characteristic, but as goal-oriented persons capable of transcending specific limitations and integrating these characteristics into a unified identity.

There is similarity in many of the assumptions and values that underlie individual psychology and those associated with the general philosophy of rehabilitation. In addition to the high regard for persons, both philosophies emphasize the importance of dignity and self-esteem. The individual is valued, in both systems, although the idiographic techniques of lifestyle counseling may be better suited to the recognition and enhancement of the individual than are the institutionalized systems of rehabilitation services. Nevertheless, in individual psychology and rehabilitation, the individual is viewed as an active agent in the helping process, not as a passive victim (O'Connell, 1976). Both processes can be participatory, with the client actively involved in setting goals.

Preparation for independent activity is the major focus of the rehabilitation process. This process is described in Adlerian terms by Sonstegard, Hagerman, and Bitter (1975) and demonstrates the comparability of these helping systems. The individual is prepared and motivated best not by doing for the client what he or she can do for himself or herself, but by providing experiences of life in an orderly and progressive manner. Those learning "to meet and face the obstacles of life . . . will not be lacking" (Sonstegard, Hagerman, & Bitter, 1975, p. 22). The lifestyle can be used to enhance the client's awareness of his or her subjective goals to facilitate the client's participation.

In rehabilitation therapy as in Adler's concept of psychotherapy, the focus is on education and development. The process-oriented concept of adaptation as opposed to the static concept of adjustment has been used in both models (Mosak, 1979; Roessler & Bolton, 1978) as consistent with their change-oriented approaches. Ansbacher (1971) describes the view of man in individual psychology as active, self-determined, striving "in-spite-of" to overcome difficulties and inferiorities. The values on which individual psychology is based are generally compatible with the goals and philosophy of rehabilitation and are capable of enhancing the rehabilitation process from a counseling point of view.

Social Interest

Another major assumption of individual psychology that has implications for the counselor in rehabilitation settings is the notion of social interest, or *Gemeinshaftsgefühl*. This concept has been described in detail elsewhere (Chapters 2 and 9). In brief, social interest is considered to be a trainable cognitive process—an innate aptitude to be developed—and the ultimate criterion of mental health. Ansbacher (1978) considers the process as incorporating the basic drive for superiority along with training and socialization for social interest. Successful integration of these two components, according to Ansbacher (1978), results in optimistic activity within the parameters of the useful side of life.

The emphasis on social interest as the criterion of mental health has resulted in the consideration of individual psychology as a value psychology. This is not unlike the ethical criticisms levied against rehabilitation, with its emphasis on productive activity as the determinant of success. These socially determined goals can create an ethical problem in the counselor's obligation to respect the individual and facilitate his or her own goal. Nevertheless, the notion of social interest may have some applicability in rehabilitation, based on preliminary research with a group of severely disabled persons identified as effective copers. In this study, the individuals judged as having achieved the most successful adaptation to their

disability were all found to have a high level of community involvement, productive activity, and a prominent role in advocacy efforts for the disabled (Blom, Ek,
Irwin, Kulkarni, Miller, & Frey, 1982). These findings lend empirical support for
social interest as an important component in the mental health and effective coping
of persons with disability. In Adlerian terms, social interest remains undeveloped
in the failures of life or those who are unable to cope effectively. Correspondingly,
interdependence and cooperation, considered essential ingredients to achieving
mental health, are also applicable skills necessary to the achievement of successful
independent living in rehabilitation as well.

Optimism

According to Brown (1976), Adlerian principles parallel many Afro-American
values, and can be viewed as more applicable to the needs and concerns of
minority clients. She views the theoretical assumptions—that things can indeed
change—as forming an optimistic psychology for oppressed people.

Like other cognitive theories of psychotherapy, this approach can be seen as one
that empowers the individual; although recognizing the limitations of an environment, it assists the client to identify ways in which he or she can exercise some
choice in response. The use of lifestyle counseling for counselor self-awareness
may be one means for counselors to identify and to understand the role their values
play in their own lifestyle in order to clearly identify conflicts that arise in
counseling relationships with clients. Lowe (1959) emphasizes the importance of
ethical standards for the therapist. He notes that the goal of reshaping the client's
perception is to promote the emergence of moral values as social interest; therefore, therapists who lack a system of moral values would be unable to evoke them
in a client.

SUMMARY AND CONCLUDING REMARKS

An ethical problem confronting any counseling approach in disability stems
from unsupported assumptions about the psychological consequences of disability. Some specific ethical pitfalls in the use of lifestyle counseling for persons
with disabilities were discussed. The major problems include (1) incomplete
empirical support for the techniques of lifestyle assessment, (2) lack of specific
guidelines for interpreting lifestyle information and forming prescriptive strategies, (3) the moral bind of imposing the counselor's values as superior to the
client's in determining mistakes and goals, and (4) the psychological orientation
of lifestyle counseling, which may overlook problems that result from the environment, from social attitudes, and from physical factors such as heredity and genetic

abnormality, all of which cause difficulties for disabled persons who have otherwise adequate lifestyles.

Aspects of lifestyle counseling and Adlerian theory that promote ethical functioning of the counselor with disabled persons were also discussed. The major
assets are (1) the emphasis on a holistic view of the person, which incorporates the
disability as only one characteristic in a unified personality; (2) regard for the
dignity and creative power of the individual; (3) compatibility of the philosophy
and methods of lifestyle counseling and rehabilitation; (4) congruence in their
respective goals of increasing capability for productive and independent functioning as well as the promotion of social interest; and (5) the role of the counselor in
this approach vis-à-vis professional standards for ethical counseling.

According to the ethical standards of the National Rehabilitation Counselor
Association (1972), counselors "have a commitment to the effective functioning
of all human beings; to facilitate the function or refunction of persons at some
disadvantage to achieve viable goals" (p. 218). In doing so, the counselor must
maintain an objective relationship with the client and "refrain from urging the
client's acceptance of values, lifestyles, . . . that represent . . . the counselor's
personal judgment of values" (p. 219). Counselors must function "within the
limits of his (her) defined role, training and technical competency" (p. 220). In
regard to an unconventional or offensive lifestyle of the client that may jeopardize
reaching a vocational goal, the counselor should "explore with the client the
possible effects of his (her) lifestyle on rehabilitation. But . . . the client should be
permitted to make his/her own decision . . . without undue influence from the
counselor," unless it is known to be illegal or definitely destructive to the client or
others (p. 219).

In the ethical standards of the American Personnel and Guidance Association
(1981), the counselor must "inform the client of the purposes, goals, techniques,
rules of procedure and limitations . . . at or before the time the counseling
relationship is entered . . . Counselors must recognize the need for client freedom
of choice" (p. A). Since lifestyle assessment is used as the appraisal technique to
provide prescriptive and interpretive data about the client, counselors are obli-
gated to follow the same guidelines delineated for the appropriate use of other
psychological tests and assessment methods. This would include the selection of
methods based on their measurement properties and appropriateness as well as the
cautious use and interpretation of unvalidated data.

Maintenance of these and other ethical standards is a difficult, but intrinsic,
aspect of the provision of counseling services. No counseling approach will free
the counselor from the ethical conflicts of value judgments inherent in counseling
relationships. The lifestyle approach has its own particular pitfalls as well as other
ethical problems common to other methods. At the same time, lifestyle counseling
has some unique aspects that make it particularly well suited to the needs of
persons with disabilities and for the ethical functioning of the counselor. Coun-

selors who have a realistic awareness of their own lifestyle as well as their professional competence and who use caution in the interpretation of lifestyle data in the application of lifestyle counseling would seem to be well prepared to strive for ethical counseling of persons with disabilities.

REFERENCES

American Personnel and Guidance Association. Ethical standards. *The Guidepost*, 1981, Supplement A–D.

American Psychological Association. Ethical principles of psychologists. *American Psychologist*, 1981, *36*, 633–638.

Angers, W.P. The dangers of evaluative labeling. *Vocational Guidance Quarterly*, 1958, *7*, 26–30.

Ansbacher, H.L. Alfred Adler and humanistic psychology. *Journal of Humanistic Psychology*, 1971, *11*(1), 53–63.

Ansbacher, H.L. The development of Adler's concept of social interest: A critical study. *Journal of Individual Psychology*, 1978, *34*, 118–152.

Blom, G., Ek, K., Irwin, S., Kulkarni, M., Miller, K., and Frey, B. *Coping with handicaps: Implications for adults with physical disabilities.* Paper presented at the meeting of the National Rehabilitation Association, Anaheim, Calif., September 1982.

Brown, J.F. Parallels between Adlerian psychology and Afro-American value system. *The Individual Psychologist*, 1976, *13*(1), 29–33.

Cobb, B. Cancer. In J.F. Garrett and E.S. Levine (Eds.), *Psychological practices with the physically handicapped.* New York: Columbia University Press, 1962.

Dowd, E.T., & Kelly, F.D. Adlerian psychology and cognitive-behavior therapy: Convergences. *Journal of Individual Psychology*, 1980, *36*, 119–135.

English, R.W. The application of personality theory to explain psychological reactions to physical disability. In R. Marinelli & A. Dell Orto (Eds.), *The psychological and social impact of physical disability.* New York: Springer, 1977.

Ford, D., & Urban, H. *Systems of psychotherapy.* New York: Hawthorn Books, 1964.

Garfield, S., & Bergin, A. (Eds.), *Handbook of psychotherapy and behavior change: An empirical analysis* (2nd ed.). New York: Wiley, 1978.

Golightly, C. The philosopher's view of values and ethics. *Personnel and Guidance Journal*, 1971, *50*(4), 289-294.

Gushurst, R.S. The technique, utility and validity of life style analysis. *The Counseling Psychologist*, 1971, *3*(1), 30–40.

Lowe, W.L. Value systems in the psychotherapeutic process. In K. Adler & D. Deutsch (Eds.), *Essays in Individual Psychology.* New York: Grove Press, 1959.

Mosak, H.H. Adlerian psychotherapy. In R. Corsini (Ed.), *Current psychotherapies* (2nd ed.). Itasca, Ill.: Peacock, 1979.

National Rehabilitation Counselor Association Ethics Sub-Committee. Ethical standards for rehabilitation counselors. *Journal of Applied Rehabilitation Counseling*, 1972, *3*, 218–228.

O'Connell, W.E. Adlerian aphorisms. *The Individual Psychologist*, 1976, *13*(1), 18–28.

Roessler, R., & Bolton, B. *Psychosocial adjustment to disability.* Baltimore: University Park Press, 1978.

Rule, W. Rehabilitation uses of Adlerian life-style counseling. *Rehabilitation Counseling Bulletin,* 1978, *21,* 306–316.

Sahakian, W.S. Personalism and Adlerian psychology. *Journal of Individual Psychology,* 1978, *34,* 191–200.

Shontz, F.C. Physical disability and personality: Theory and recent research. In J. Stubbins (Ed.), *Social and psychological aspects of disability.* Baltimore: University Park Press, 1977.

Sonstegard, M., Hagerman, H., & Bitter, J. Motivation modification: An Adlerian approach. *The Individual Psychologist,* 1975, November, 17–22.

Trieschmann, R. Coping with disability: A sliding scale of goals. *Archives of Physical Medicine and Rehabilitation,* 1974, *55,* 556–560.

Wright, G.N. *Total rehabilitation.* Boston: Little, Brown, 1980.

Chapter 20

Lifestyle Self-Awareness and the Practitioner

Warren R. Rule

> For even saintly folks
> act like sinners
> Unless they have their
> customary dinners.

Many practitioners in the helping professions would like to believe that the above quotation, from Bertolt Brecht, does not pertain to them. In fact, some seem to believe, either consciously or dimly consciously, that functioning as a helping practitioner somehow cleanses the lifestyle into saintly purity.

A great deal has been written in the lifestyle literature about the usefulness of lifestyle methods for helping clients. Extremely little has been written on how the practitioner can help himself using the lifestyle method, and, in doing so, become a more effective counselor. This dearth of literature makes one wonder if the fact has been too often overlooked that the client and the counselor are both human beings whose lifestyles work at times to the disadvantage of self and others. The purpose of this chapter is first to highlight the importance of overall practitioner self-awareness, second, to discuss lifestyle implications for the counseling role, and, finally, to explore action considerations.

PRACTITIONER SELF-AWARENESS

The benefits of increased practitioner self-understanding appear to be considerable. Appell (1963) asserted that the most important dimension in the counseling relationship is counselor self-understanding. Passons (1975) concluded that:

> . . . it is recognized that the person of the counselor is the essential instrument in his work. Stripped of all professional accouterments and

rhetoric, who the counselor is remains the primary factor in his functioning. His values, beliefs, needs and other personal characteristics permeate everything he does in his many functions as a counselor. (p. 4)

Shoben (1962) stated that the counselor is well-served if he has insight into
himself and his counselor frame of reference because the choice of any given
counseling perspective is a reflection of one's own personality. Lister (1964)
concluded that one's personal theory of counseling is heavily influenced by one's
hypotheses regarding effective and satisfying human relationship in general. He
noted that :

Each beginning counselor has already spent years formulating hypotheses about himself and others and the nature of the world in which he
lives. In the broadest sense, the counselor's personal theory refers to the
hypotheses he has come to view as reliable guides to satisfying human
relations. Although many such hypotheses are largely implicit and
inarticulate, they nevertheless constitute patterns for counseling behavior or personality theory. For example, the student whose experience
has led him to believe that his effectiveness in human relations requires
that he prevent others from getting the upper hand is apt to maintain tight
control of topics covered in the counseling interview. . . . If a student
believes that people are basically trustworthy and capable of responsible
behavior, he will probably have a higher threshold for the perception of
"clear and imminent danger" than the student who has found others
untrustworthy and irresponsible. (p. 209)

Passons (1975) contends that a congruence must exist between the counselor as
a person and his theory of counseling. Moreover, attempts by others or by himself
to impose theory that does not fit will result in a state of dissonance. Thus, Passons
(1975) recommends that the first step in formulating a personal theory is for the
practitioner to attain a high level of awareness of his philosophical beliefs, values,
needs, etc. Without this awareness, the base of his personal theory may be shaky.
In addition, as the counselor becomes more aware of himself, he endangers his
ability to evaluate other theories of counseling in terms of their appropriateness to
him. As Shoben (1962) has concluded, if there were a theory that was "right" for
every counselor, there would not be so many of them.

LIFESTYLE IMPLICATIONS FOR THE COUNSELING ROLE

Aside from the issue of how the lifestyle works to an individual's advantage and
disadvantage in one's personal life, which will be touched on below, the issue of
how a person's lifestyle relates to his work as a counselor is an intriguing, and

hopefully beneficial, concern. It may be remembered that, according to Adlerian theory, the lifestyle that one has formed as being useful for coping with life in general will also be the same lifestyle used for coping with the life task of work. This area of "work" includes one's activities and thoughts on matters such as relating to clients, colleagues, and supervisors. Also included are eagerness to experiment with different counseling approaches, reaction to client noncooperation, telephone conversations, organization of daily activities, internal evaluation of job success, etc.

From the perspective of counselor-client interaction, counselor lifestyle notions, attitudes, and goals can both enhance and detract from the counseling relationship. For instance, the counselor who has concluded at a dimly conscious level that intellectual superiority is the way to go in life may well alienate clients (by abstractions, big words, oratories, etc.) who aren't on an intellectual wave length for solving problems. Yet he may help those clients who are very similar or who rely too heavily on other methods in coping with difficulties. Similarly, a counselor whose style is heavily laden with mandates of self-control may be able to keep a level head during a client's nonproductive emotional outbursts yet fail to provide a spontaneous, emotionally warm model for clients who may profit immensely from such a counselor. Related to this is the counselor who treats himself as if he should control others. He can help clients who need structure in the counseling process but may antagonize those clients who are also like this or who simply want to make their own decisions. Furthermore, the counselor who is heavily invested in being right and avoiding being wrong may well have the tendency to be overly stubborn, or even engage in seemingly irrelevant behaviors such as repeating himself frequently (to make sure his ideas are fully understood)—thereby impressing some clients with his rightness, but annoying others.

In addition, the counselor who has learned at a vague level of consciousness that he only feels OK when he is getting constant approval can possibly help some of those clients who profit from his extra efforts to please them. Yet this notion can work to his disadvantage if he avoids confrontation when appropriate or if he is too hard on himself for not getting the desired amount of approval-assurance from certain clients. The counselor who displays moral superiority or goodness-togetherness may be encouraging as a well-intentioned person to some clients. But he might create an image of saintliness to some other clients and, in doing so, inadvertently create discouragement. In addition, the counselor who has concluded at a vague level of apprehension that OK-ness means driving and striving for a place of special importance can find many of his clients "unmotivated" who do not share this intense conviction. But, on the other hand, he may be able to spur on successfully some other clients who need a shot in the arm or who relate well to the counselor's projection on them. Additional examples abound.

An important point is that counselors are both people and counselors. They therefore have broad notions about self, others, and life that can and do creep into the counseling role by thought, word (as well as silence), and deed. Obviously, the same holds true for clients—they are both people and clients. In terms of compatibility between counselor and client, some research studies, e.g., Gerler (1958), Carson and Heine (1962), Mendelsohn and Geller (1965), have indicated that counselors and clients who are either very similar or very dissimilar on personality variables are generally less apt to do as well together as are counselors and clients who are neither too similar nor too dissimilar. Possibly too much reinforcing empathy is going on at one extreme and not enough at the other. Although these findings do not warrant the status of an ironclad rule, the practicing counselor may want to keep an eye on this variable when compatibility difficulties seem to be occurring.

Because all behavior—including "helping" behavior—is regarded as being goal directed, a lifestyle question that may be worth exploring for the practitioner is "What does 'helping' do for me?" Related to lifestyle notions regarding self and others, a host of purposive, self-serving possibilities may exist, such as increasing rightness, fostering praise, encouraging redemption, nurturing control, guaranteeing an audience, ensuring importance, granting goodness, recharging batteries, bestowing specialness, heightening self-elevation, and so on.

ACTION CONSIDERATIONS

Many believe that characteristics of the lifestyle become most apparent when the individual is experiencing some stress or when life is not going his way. A thought that may be worth pursuing, based on one's lifestyle notions, is: "What do I keep telling myself about myself when things have not worked out for me?" Similar to Ellis's (1971) rational-emotive approach, the task is to pinpoint and to challenge the self-message that has a "should" or a "must" attached to it.

A practitioner could also make a concerted effort to work into his everyday thinking the Adlerian belief in the goal-directed nature of behavior. This might be particularly helpful as this phenomenon relates to characteristics the counselor does not quite understand about his manner of approaching some of his work activities. By stretching the imagination a little, the counselor may be able to make the connection between a lifestyle notion and a hard-to-understand behavior or behavior pattern that is in the service of that notion. Examples of this are the constant apologies and expressions of good intentions for one whose lifestyle notions dictate pleasing and winning approval, or possibly the power and/or recognition demands that underlie a quick temper, or the avoidance-of-failure purpose beneath the feeling of being unable to concentrate when beginning a task. Sometimes much can be learned by viewing an "unwanted" behavior or feeling as a safeguard for self-esteem.

During the helping process, the counselor may profit by becoming more aware of his initial experience of a negative thought or feeling (e.g., frustration, anger, anxiety, boredom, etc.) or visceral reaction and using this awareness as a "triggering device" for self-exploration. By attempting to match up the initial negative experience with what one suspects are some of his lifestyle notions, the counselor is better equipped to take a more accurate look at what is going on and then to act accordingly—ideally for the ultimate benefit of both the client and the counselor.

The counselor may want to consider his guesses as to some of his lifestyle notions from the perspective of how this awareness can be used to build upon strengths. By guessing in which direction one's energy is inclined to flow, the counselor may choose to capitalize upon and enhance those aspects that work to his advantage and minimize those that work to his disadvantage. For example, if control over the environment is a strong dimension in one's lifestyle notions, a consideration is to sharpen one's organizational skills some more or even concentrate on administrative efforts. If intellectual mastery is prominent, one could explore those counseling approaches that emphasize cognitive problem solving. If putting others in one's service is a dominant theme, maybe the counselor can increase his skills in areas that could be naturally self-fulfilling, such as public relations or employer development.

The mental act of encouraging oneself can often lead to gratifying results. By subvocalizing something like "You're still OK even when you are not . . . e.g., perfect, Number One, pleasing everyone, in control, right," can help move oneself off the vertical plane of comparisons and onto a more satisfying horizontal plane of accepting the various parts of the self that one continually keeps on trial.

Having identified what one suspects is a lifestyle notion or goal underlying a problem area, one is then able to take a stand on one or several of the following actions: (1) to accept how the lifestyle notion or goal is working, yet want to learn different, more effective ways of behaving in order to implement the goal more satisfactorily; (2) to desire to reduce the felt intensity of a lifestyle notion or goal by attempting to change one's thoughts, e.g., mental self-discipline, self-encouragement, internal challenging, self-rewards and punishments, etc.; (3) to desire to reduce the felt intensity of a lifestyle notion or goal by attempting to behave in ways that are counter to the goal, e.g., learning new behavior, doing more or doing less of already learned behavior; (4) to decide not to decide to do anything. It's worth emphasizing that individual lifestyle goals are dimensions that a person takes a sensitive position on. Both the behavior that is a function of this sensitivity as well as the sensitivity itself can be altered. People—including counselors—can change!

Many types of action steps exist for those willing to take the necessary risks. For example, telling a client about one's own lifestyle notions can be risky, e.g., "I've got a tendency to want . . . (to be right about, to control, approval for, etc.) things, so let me step back from this so my bias doesn't get in your way," yet it can yield surprising dividends. Or an individual can even try taking a small creative risk when things are not going so well when it is suspected that one's own lifestyle is contributing to the difficulty. One way to do this is to laugh fully at oneself by vividly imagining a ridiculously exaggerated version of a lifestyle notion. Examples are: for a counselor who treats himself as righteously perfect—a white robe, halo, angel wings, surrounded by a dazzled, yet humble, congregation; for one who demands of himself that he be a number-one achiever—a king's crown, a battleax, ribbons and medals, perched atop a throne while competitors and servants bow and do homage from below.

Additional homework considerations can be found in an excellent book by Lazarus and Fay (1975) entitled *I Can if I Want To*. Although not written from a direct lifestyle point of view, it provides many helpful strategies for changing thoughts and behaviors.

The process of using the lifestyle approach, either in part or totally, can be further enhanced by sharing in a group setting with fellow practitioners. In this manner, the group members can provide additional validity checks as well as vicariously learn from their fellow group members.

Overall Stress Management

Stress is a key factor in everyone's life. Here, too, the counseling practitioner is no exception, because stress is a significant part of the individual's professional *and* personal life. As discussed previously, the lifestyle, with all its advantages and disadvantages, is at work in all areas of living.

Schafer (1978) has provided a useful concept of stress management that is consistent with lifestyle self-awareness: "Managing stress wisely means knowing what amount of stress is right for you and keeping control of the pace of your life so you neither stagnate nor are overwhelmed with too much to do" (p. 20).

Stress has been viewed as a bodily response and as a perception. Selye (1974) defines stress as "the nonspecific response of the body to any demand made on it" (p. 14). Woolfolk and Richardson (1978) regard stress as "a perception of threat or expectation of future discomfort that arouses, alerts, or otherwise activates the organism" (p. 9). Both views are helpful in understanding the broad range of ways in which stress operates.

In the physical realm the innate fight or flight response, which we inherited from our primitive ancestors, results in many bodily changes when stimuli coming in are interpreted as threatening. The pupils enlarge so that we can see better, hearing becomes acute, blood pulsates through the head to stimulate thought processes, heart and respiratory rates increase to energize the system, and so forth. Most contemporary threats, however, cannot be dealt with in a fight or flight manner, as could ancient threats of fierce animals or savage competitors. Thus, this programmed response to stress can take a bodily toll over the years and is said to contribute to symptoms including heart attacks, headaches, colitis, and allergies.

Other realms are closely connected to the physical realm. The emotional realm and the behavioral realm are descriptive types that can be related to the physical and to the cognitive realms. The emphasis in this chapter is on the cognitive realm. It is this realm that, for the individual, seems to assess the degree of "awfulness" of the perceived threatening stimuli; this assessment, in turn, appears to contribute to the nature of response in the physical, emotional, and behavioral realms. In addition, the cognitive realm seems to lend itself best to self-awareness and self-management strategies that are consistent with the lifestyle conceptual framework.

Not all stress is negative. As discussed in the chapter on avocational counseling for lifestyle adjustment, stress can be both pleasant and unpleasant. Selye (1974) defines unpleasant, negative, or intense stress as *distress*. Prolonged distress can result in damaging wear and tear on the mind or body, destructive behavior toward others, or interference with everyday living. Individuals vary in their comfort zones of stress and degree of desired stimulation from stress.

Thus, awareness of individual lifestyle vulnerability, along with the accompanying awareness of personal sensitivity to various types of stressors, can be particularly beneficial. This may be especially helpful when one is confronted with personally threatening experiences. For example, some of the major experiences that can lead to distress, according to Schafer (1978), are overload; understimulation; absence of meaning; role conflict, including personal desires conflicting with the expectations of others, expectations associated with one role conflicting with expectations associated with another role, and different expectations of a single role conflicting with each other; role ambiguity; transitions; loss; unfinished business; "negative" life scripts; and a perceived gap between ideals and reality.

Schafer (1978) organizes the main personal approaches to managing stress into three areas:

1. Managing your stressors—controlling the pace of your life.
2. Managing your stress filter—taking care of yourself so that stressful events will have minimal harmful effect on mind and body and developing personal qualities that will soften the impact.
3. Managing your coping response—coping with distress constructively so it will be reduced rather than increased; i.e., live with the distress, withdraw from the stressor, relate to the stressor differently, change the stressor, or accept the situation and thereby lower the stress.

In one of his most famous essays, "A House Divided," Abraham Lincoln (Sandburg, 1960), master of the metaphor, concisely expressed a potent concept that speaks to the heart of lifestyle self-awareness, action considerations, and stress management: "If we could first know where we are, and whither we are tending, we could better judge what to do, and how to do it" (p. 33).

Related to this, Shoben (1962) has observed that the counselor who "knows himself" and can use his theoretical tools flexibly is indeed fortunate. He further concludes that the "counselor who achieves this kind of honesty in dealing with his cognitive self is likely to enjoy a sense of personal growth that is denied to others" (p. 621).

So, in response to the question "Why should I concern myself with an increased awareness of biased lifestyle notions? After all, I am completely free to choose what I want to think and do," the Adlerian suggestion might be to look for a common attitude or pattern of movement that ties together those features of your working style that you want to change. For in doing so, you may well be really exploring the hidden notions influencing "where you are" in relation to "where you want to be." Aided by this self-insight, you now have an increased opportunity to plot a straighter course or even to change the destination.

SUMMARY

Very little has been written in the counseling literature on the disadvantages of the counselor's lifestyle. The benefits of increased practitioner self-awareness seem to be useful in human interaction as well as in developing one's personal approach to counseling.

The counselor's lifestyle is likely to operate at a dimly conscious level in ways that are both advantageous and disadvantageous to the client. Exploring the question of "What does helping do for me?" may yield worthwhile results for the practitioner.

Action considerations that result from practitioner self-awareness may take many directions: self-disputing, identifying blind spots, focusing on triggering cues, building upon strengths, challenging vertical comparisons, creating goals and behavioral strategies for change, humorous self-confrontation, peer feedback in a group setting. In addition, the practitioner may profit by incorporating into his self-awareness a place for overall stress management.

REFERENCES

Appell, M.L. Self understanding for the guidance counselor. *Personnel and Guidance Journal,* 1963, *43*, 143–148.

Carson, R.C., & Heine, R.W. Similarity and success in therapeutic dyads. *Journal of Consulting Psychology,* 1962 26(1), 38–43.

Ellis, A. *Growth through reason.* Palo Alto, Calif.: Science & Behavior Books, 1971.

Gerler, W. Outcome of psychotherapy as a function of client-counselor similarity. *Dissertation Abstracts,* 1958, *18*, 1864.

Lazarus, A., & Fay, A. *I can if I want to.* New York: Morrow, 1975.

Lister, J. The counselor's personal theory. *Counselor Education and Supervision,* 1964, *3,* 207–213.

Mendelsohn, G.A., & Geller, M.H. Effects of counselor-client similarity on the outcome of counseling, *Journal of Counseling Psychology,* 1965, *10*(1), 71–77.

Passons, W. *Gestalt approaches in counseling.* New York: Holt, Rinehart, & Winston, 1975.

Sandburg, C. The most enduring memorial to Lincoln. In R. Newman (Ed.), *Lincoln for the ages.* New York: Doubleday, 1960.

Schafer, W. *Stress, distress and growth.* Davis, Calif.: International Dialogue Press, 1978.

Selye, H. *Stress without distress.* New York: Signet, 1974.

Shoben, E.J., Jr. The counselor's theory as a personality trait. *Personnel and Guidance Journal,* 1962, *40,* 617–621.

Woolfolk, R., & Richardson, F. *Stress, sanity, and survival.* New York: Sovereign, 1978.

Appendix A

Suggested Readings

Adler, A. *Understanding human nature.* New York: Fawcett, 1969. (Originally published, 1927).

Adler, A. *Problems of neurosis.* (P. Mairet, Ed.) New York: Harper & Row, 1964. (Originally published, 1929).

Adler, A. *The science of living.* (H. Ansbacher, Ed.) Garden City, N.Y.: Doubleday, 1969. (Originally published, 1929).

Allen. T.W. The individual psychology of Alfred Adler: An item of history and a promise of a revolution. *The Counseling Psychologist,* 1971, *3*(1), 3–24.

Ansbacher, H.L., & Ansbacher, R.R. (Eds.). *Superiority and social interest* (2nd ed.). Evanston, Ill.: Northwestern University Press, 1970.

Ansbacher, H.L., & Ansbacher, R.R. (Eds.). *The individual psychology of Alfred Adler.* New York: Basic Books, 1956.

Dreikurs, R. *Psychodynamics, psychotherapy, and counseling.* Chicago: Alfred Adler Institute, 1967.

Dreikurs, R., & Soltz, V. *Children: The challenge.* New York: Hawthorn, 1964.

Eckstein, D., Baruth, L., and Mahrer, D. *Life style: What it is and how to do it* (2nd ed.). Dubuque, Iowa: Kendall-Hunt, 1982.

Ford, D.H., & Urban, H.B. *Systems of psychotherapy.* New York: Wiley, 1963.

Mosak, H.H. *On purpose.* Chicago: Alfred Adler Institute, 1977.

Mosak, H.H. Adlerian psychotherapy. In R. Corsini (Ed.), *Current Psychotherapies* (2nd ed.). Itasca, Ill.: Peacock, 1979.

Mosak, H.H., & Mosak, B. *A bibliography for Adlerian psychology.* Washington, D.C.: Hemisphere, 1975.

Nikelly, A.G. *Techniques for behavior change.* Springfield, Ill.: Charles C Thomas, 1971.

Rule, W. Rehabilitation uses of Adlerian life-style counseling. *Rehabilitation Counseling Bulletin*, 1978, *21*, 306–316.

Shulman, B.H. *Contributions to individual psychology*. Chicago: Alfred Adler Institute, 1973.

Sweeney, T.J. *Adlerian concepts: Proven concepts and strategies* (2nd ed.). Muncie, Ind.: Accelerated Development Press, 1981.

Walton, F.X., & Powers, R.L. *Winning children over*. Chicago: Practical Psychology Associates, 1974.

Resources and Training Opportunities

Information on resources and ongoing training opportunities throughout the world may be obtained from:

North American Society of Adlerian Psychology
159 North Dearborn Street
Chicago, IL 60601

Some of the major Adlerian training institutes in North America are:

Alfred Adler Institute
159 North Dearborn Street
Chicago, IL 60601

Alfred Adler Institute
37 W. 65th Street
New York, NY 10023

Alfred Adler Institute
5501 Green Valley Drive
Bloomington, MN 55436

Alfred Adler Institute
4 Finch Avenue, West
Suite 10
Willowdale, Ontario
Canada

Adler-Dreikurs Institute of Human Relations
Bowie State College
Room 1110—Robinson Hall
Bowie, MD 20715

Lifestyle Form
(Variation of Dreikurs' Form)

Warren R. Rule

I. *Family Constellation:* List all siblings in descending order (including client). Give sibling's age in terms of + or − the number of years age difference from client. Include siblings that died as well as step-siblings in the home. Age six is the approximate age cut off for this entire lifestyle section.

A. *Description of Siblings* (Only children are compared with significant playmates)
1. Who was most different from the client? _____
In what ways different?

2. Who was most like the client? _____
In what ways like?

3. What kind of kid was the client? (Expand on "personality" characteristics)

4. Describe other siblings:

B. *Ratings and Descriptions*
List highest and lowest sibling for each attribute and, if the client was at neither extreme, draw an arrow in the middle space toward the sibling to which he leans. Only children compare with significant playmates. Sometimes general impressions must be used. Try to limit client responses of "I don't know."

	HIGHEST		LOWEST
1. Intelligence			
2. Hard-working			
3. Grades in school			
4. Helping around house			
5. Conforming			
6. Rebellious—overtly			
7. Rebellious—covertly			
8. Trying to please			
9. Actually pleasing			
10. Critical of others			
11. Critical of self			
12. Considerateness			
13. Selfishness			
14. Wanting to have own way			
15. Getting own way			
16. Sensitive feelings easily hurt			
17. Temper tantrums			
18. Stubbornness			

	HIGHEST		LOWEST
19. High standards of:			
achievement	_____	_____	_____
behavior	_____	_____	_____
morals (right and wrong)	_____	_____	_____
20. Athletic	_____	_____	_____
21. Strong (physically)	_____	_____	_____
22. Strong (emotionally)	_____	_____	_____
23. Tall	_____	_____	_____
24. Pretty or handsome	_____	_____	_____
25. Masculine	_____	_____	_____
26. Feminine	_____	_____	_____
27. Sense of humor	_____	_____	_____
28. Methodical, neat	_____	_____	_____
29. Charming	_____	_____	_____
30. Sociable	_____	_____	_____
31. Mischievous	_____	_____	_____
32. Withdrawn	_____	_____	_____
33. Excitement seeker	_____	_____	_____
34. Daring	_____	_____	_____
35. Chip on shoulder	_____	_____	_____
36. Obedient	_____	_____	_____
37. Bossy	_____	_____	_____
38. Sulky	_____	_____	_____
39. Fighter	_____	_____	_____
40. Cheerful	_____	_____	_____

41. Who was the most spoiled? _____

    By whom? _____

    How? _____

    _____

    For what? _____

42. Who was the most punished? _____

    By whom? _____

    For what? _____

43. Who had the most friends? _____

    What kind of relationship existed with friends for client? (e.g., leader, follower, observer, etc.)

44. What would usually happen after client threw a temper tantrum?

After he pouted when he didn't get his way?

45. What fears does client remember having?

46. What did client do during his leisure time?

47. What kind of imaginary playmates did client have?

48. What kind of day dreams or childhood fantasies did client have?

49. What was client's favorite story as a child?

50. Did the client have a nickname?

51. What kind of idols (from TV, radio, stories, Bible, movies, songs, fairy tales, nursery rhymes, etc.) did the client remember having?

52. Did client have any disabilities or prolonged illnesses?

53. Were there any exceptional talents, achievements, or ambitions of the client?

54. Does the client recall any childhood habits?

55. Religion?
    Approximate size of town or city lived in before age 6?
    Socioeconomic class?
56. What strong family values existed?

C. *Siblings' Interrelationships*
   1. Who took care of whom? _____
   2. Who played with whom? _____
   3. Who got along best with whom? _____
   4. Which two fought and argued the most? _____
       _____
   5. Who was father's favorite? _____
   6. Who was mother's favorite? _____

D. *Description of Parents*
   1. How old was father when you were born? _____;
       mother? _____
   2. What kind of person was father?

       Father's birth order?
       What kind of job?
   3. What kind of person was mother?

       Mother's birth order?
       What kind of job?
   4. Which of the children was most like father? _____
       In what way?

5. Which of the children was most like mother? _____
   In what way?

6. Which parent did you like more? _____
   For what reasons?

7. If father could have really molded you exactly to suit his notion of an ideal child, how would you have been?

8. If mother could have really molded you exactly to suit her notion of an ideal child, how would you have been?

9. What could you have done to make father the maddest at you?

   The happiest?

10. What could you have done to make mother the maddest at you?

    The happiest?

11. What kind of relationship existed between father and mother?

    a. Who was dominant, made decisions, etc.? _____
    b. Did they agree or disagree on methods of raising children?
    c. Did they quarrel openly?
       How did the quarrels end?

       How did you feel about these quarrels?

       Whose side did you take? _____

12. Who was more ambitious for the children? _____
    In what ways?

13. What kind of family atmosphere existed in the home?

14. Did any other person (grandparent, uncle, aunt, family friend, boarder, etc.) live with the family? Were there any other significant figures in your childhood? Describe them and your relationship to them.

15. Can client recall any childhood uniqueness or unique situations not covered in previous questions?

16. Are there any significant events from later childhood or early adolescence that the client would like to indicate?

II. Next, the client is asked to describe his six (6) earliest childhood memories (or dreams). Please keep the following points in mind.

- The early memory (recollection) must be a specific incident, event, occurrence, or happening that you can remember. Early memories of incidents that occurred over and over again (example: "We *used to* do such and such," or "I did this *many* times") are not true early recollections and consequently should not be written down. However, a remembered childhood dream that occurred over and over *is* to be written down.
- Write down any early recollection that comes to the client's mind, even if he is not sure the incident actually occurred.
- Report any specific recollection that he thinks of regardless of how insignificant it may seem to him.
- Write down the recollections in the order that the client remembers them, even if you are not sure which ones really occurred earlier. It is not important that the recollections be reported in their true chronological order; rather, in the order that they are remembered.
- Write down only those recollections which occurred approximately before age eight (8).

Description of Early Recollection (or Dream) No. _____, and age _____ of occurrence.

1. How were you feeling (i.e., your emotions) during this incident? (Keep in mind that sometimes we have mixed feelings about events.)

2. Were any *other people* there?

3. What is the clearest, *most vivid* part of the recollection for you?

4. If you can remember, what happened *right before*? How were you feeling?

5. If you can remember, what happened *right afterward*? How were you feeling?

6. (If appropriate) What was your *purpose* for behaving like that?

7. What was the most important thing you learned from that incident?

Abbreviated Lifestyle Form
(Variation of Dreikurs' Form)

Warren R. Rule

Please respond to all of the questions *as you remember yourself and your family before approximately age six.*

I. Family Constellation: List all siblings in descending order, from oldest to youngest (including yourself). Give sibling's age in terms of + or − the number of years age difference from you. Include siblings that died as well as step-siblings in the home.

A. *Siblings* (Only children are compared with significant playmates; clients with only one sibling describe different and similar characteristics)

1. Who was most different from you? _____
In what respects?

2. Who was most like you? _____
   In what respects?

3. What kind of kid were you? (Expand on "personality" characteristics)

B. *Parents*
   1. If father could have really molded you exactly to suit his notion of an ideal child, how would you have been?

   2. If mother could have really molded you exactly to suit her notion of an ideal child, how would you have been?

3. What kind of person was father?

4. What kind of person was mother?

5. What kind of family atmosphere existed in the home?

II. On the following pages, you are asked to describe your three earliest childhood memories. Please keep the following points in mind.

- The early memory (recollection) must be a *specific* incident, event, occurrence, or happening that you can remember. Early memories which describe incidents that occurred over and over again (example: "We *used to* do such and such," or "I did this *many* times") are not true early recollections and consequently should not be written down.
- Write down any early recollection that comes to your mind, even if you are not sure the incident actually occurred.
- Report any specific recollection that you think of regardless of how insignificant it may seem to you.
- Write down the recollections *in the order that you remember them,* even if you are not sure which ones really occurred earlier. It is not important that the recollections be reported in their true chronological order; rather, in the order that you remember them.
- Write down only those recollections which you think occurred approximately before age eight (8).

III. Description of recollection (or dream) No. ____, and age ____ of occurrence.

   1. How were you feeling (i.e., your emotions) during this incident? (Keep in mind that sometimes we have mixed feelings about events.)

   2. Where any *other people* there?

   3. What is the clearest, *most vivid* part of the recollection for you?

   4. What happened *right before*?

      How were you feeling *right before*?

   5 What happened *right afterward*?

      How were you feeling *right afterward*?

   6. (If appropriate) What was your purpose for behaving like that?

   7. What was the most important thing you learned from this incident?

Index

A

Ackerman, J.M., 47
Acting out
  alcoholism case study and, 283
  mentally retarded and, 259
  psychiatric disabilities and, 243-45
Activities, leisure counseling and,
  179-82
Adjustment. *See* Disability adjustment;
  Work adjustment
Adler, Alfred, 26, 121, 150, 151, 153,
  156, 164, 169, 208, 209, 227, 238,
  292, 309, 312, 313
  alcoholism and, 279
  child's environment and, 81-82
  concept of lifestyle and, 4-5, 6-7,
    15-21, 122, 158-61
  death of sibling and, 93
  "feeblemindedness" and, 256
  goal-directed behavior and, 270
  misunderstanding of, 8
  motivation and, 97
  older brother attitude and, 154
  problems of living and, 158
  resistance and, 120
  RET and, 161
  social problems and, 294-95
Administrative duties (correctional
  counselor), 295

Adult development
  adulthood stages and, 106-107
  aging and, 112
  basic assumptions concerning, 106
  continuous nature of, 105-106
  counseling and, 113-14
  the couple (marriage and career) and,
    108-109
  early parenthood and, 109-110
  goals and strategies and, 114
  individual autonomy and, 107-108
  late parenting and, 111
  middle parenting and, 110-11
  stage transitions and, 112-13
Adults
  adjustment to disability and, 68-70
  symptoms and, 63
Advocacy
  correctional counselor and, 296-97
  defined, 197
Afro-American values, 314
Aging, 112
Al-Anon, 295. *See also* Alcoholism
Alcoholism, 62
  Asthma symptoms exacerbation
    study and, 66
  defining, 277-78
  intervention strategies and, 281-86
  lifestyle adjustment and, 278-80
    example of, 280-81

Johnson, V.E., 279, 280
Joining (therapeutic process)
  asthma example and, 76
  counseling and, 72-73, 74
  psychiatric counseling and, 235-39
Joswiak, K., 175

K

Kanfer, F.H., 181
Keeney, B.P., 124, 127, 128
Kelly, F.D., 312
Kern, R.M., 25
Kerr, M.E., 62
Kirschenbaum, H., 176
Kir-Stimon, W., 51, 55
Kubler-Ross, E., 30
Kuder Preference Record-Vocational,
  175

L

Labeling, 225
Lakein, A., 180
Lankton, S., 190
Lassiter, R.A., 199
Lazarus, Arnold, 47, 161, 176, 324
Leaffer, T., 130
Le Fevre, C., 131-32
Leg amputation (physical therapists
  case study), 222-23
Leisure. *See* Avocational counseling
Leisure Activities Blank (LAB), 174
*Leisure Counseling Assessment
  Instruments*, 175
Leisure Interest Inventory, 175
Levinson, D., 106
Lewinsohn, P.M., 176
Liebman, R., 75
Lifestyle
  Adler and, 4-5, 6-7, 15-21, 122,
    158-61
  alcoholism and adjustment in, 278-80
  counselors and, 320-22, 323

defining, 3-4, 15-16, 61
ethics and interpreting, 309
goal-directed behavior and, 18-19
heredity and environment and, 17-18
holistic approach and, 16
mentally retarded and development
  of, 256-57
public offender and adjustment in,
  292-95
resistance to change and, 120-22
social context and, 18
subjective determination and, 20-21
Lifestyle assessment
  the blind man, 271-72
  childhood memories and, 22-23, 24
  as ethical problem, 309
  family constellation and, 23-24
  information sources for, 22
  interview for, 24-25
  physical therapy and, 207, 225
Lifestyle counseling. *See also*
  Counselors;
  Relationship stage of counseling;
  Strategies for intervention;
  specific condition or disability
  adult development and, 113-14
  alcoholism and, 278-81
    case study of, 283-85
  alternatives to, 26, 29-30, 46-48, 305
  analysis of disabled individuals and,
    51-55
  disability adjustment and, 10
  ethics in, 305-306, 308, 314-16
  group setting and, 11-12
  independent living and, 198-99
  lifestyle interpretation and, 38-40
  medical information and, 139
  mentally retarded and, 256-57
  physical therapy and
    adjustment in, 208-212
    case study of, 222-25
    in intervention, 212-22
  psychiatric disabilities and, 227-28,
    248-51
  public offenders and, 295-98
  resistance to change and, 119-20, 130-33

mentally retarded and, 257-63
N.L.P., 186-93
paradoxical approach to, 77-78, 126, 242
physical therapy and, 212-22
psychiatric disability and, 240-48
pragmatic approach and, 248-51
public offenders and, 298-300
resistance to change and, 119-20, 130-33
specific goal considerations and, 45-46
structural approach to, 77-78
supplemental techniques and, 46-48
visually impaired and, 271-75
work adjustment, 150-57
Stress, 208, 209, 322
aging and, 112
cancer case history and, 140, 142
counselor and, 97
counselor and management of, 324-26
disability and individual autonomy and, 108
family system intervention and, 78
leisure and management of, 181-82
marriage and preschool children and, 109
mentally retarded work adjustment case study and, 262
reliance on lifestyle and, 39
sequence of responses to, 31
Stroke (physical therapist case study), 223-25
Strong-Campbell Interest Inventory, 175
Stubbins, J., 11
Stuck state, 189, 192
Subjective determinations, 20-21
Subjective experience, studying structure of. *See* Neuro-Linguistic Programming (N.L.P.)
Sullivan, H.S., 50
Superior and inferior spouse system, 283-84
Sutton-Smith, B., 25

Sweeney, T.H., 48
Sykes, G.M., 296
Symptoms
adult family members and, 63
aggravation (asthma) example and, 65-67
alcoholism case study and, 284
client's sense of loss of control and, 143
dramatic presenting, 113
onset and maintenance (anorexia nervosa) example and, 67-68
physical therapist and, 216
prescription (resistance to change), 124-26
significance of, 54
Systemic lifestyle
adult disability adjustment and, 68-70
exacerbation of symptoms (asthma example) and, 65-67
family adjustment (epilepsy example) and, 63-65
intervention and, 70-78
onset and maintenance (anorexia nervosa example) of physical symptoms, 67-68

T

Takata, N., 175
Targ, D., 111
Tavormino, J.B., 83, 94
Taylor, J., 25
Teamwork (public offender client), 298
Teenagers, alcohol and, 277, 278, 280, 286
Teng, M.S., 297
Tharp, R.G., 181
Theory. *See also* Lifestyle *entries*
coherence, 120, 121, 122, 133
familial patterns of interaction and, 81-82
other approaches to disability adjustment and, 26, 29-30

About the Editor

Warren R. Rule is an associate professor in the rehabilitation counseling department at Virginia Commonwealth University. He received a Ph.D. from the University of South Carolina and has been a rehabilitation counselor and a counselor in higher educational institutions. Dr. Rule is a Fellow in the Society for Personality Assessment and has published in the areas of rehabilitation, counseling, and psychology. He has served in different editorial capacities for Adlerian and rehabilitation journals and publications.

About the Contributors

Stephen J. Aukward holds a master of science degree in rehabilitation counseling from Virginia Commonwealth University. He has been employed by the Virginia Department of Rehabilitative Services for over nine years in a variety of rehabilitation facilities throughout Virginia. Currently, he is a rehabilitation counselor at the Community Rehabilitation Center in Norfolk, Virginia. He is recognized as a certified rehabilitation counselor (C.R.C.) by the Commission on Rehabilitation Counselor Certification. Legally blind since the age of 16, he has been both a consumer and provider of rehabilitation services.

Martha Stover Barlow is a licensed professional counselor in Virginia and is employed as a child and family specialist at Valley Community Mental Health Services in Staunton, Virginia. She has her B.A. from Bridgewater College, Bridgewater, Virginia, and an M.S. in rehabilitation counseling from Virginia Commonwealth University. Ms. Barlow has trained in the family systems theory and psychotherapy at Georgetown University. She has also participated in extensive training and supervision in family communications and structural family therapies. Ms. Barlow is married and the mother of two sons.

Joe Bauserman completed his master's degree in rehabilitation counseling in 1975 at Virginia Commonwealth University and is completing his Ph.D. in counseling at the University of Virginia. He has nine years' experience in community mental health and is presently supervisor of clinical services at Hanover Family Counseling Center in Ashland, Virginia. In addition, he is on the adjunct faculty at Virginia Commonwealth University, where he teaches individual and family counseling, and is a licensed professional counselor with a practice in individual, marital, and family counseling.

Patricia C. Franco has a master's degree in rehabilitation counseling from Virginia Commonwealth University. She holds national certification in her field and is a licensed professional counselor in Virginia. Ms. Franco is currently coordinator of the Cancer Rehabilitation and Continuing Care Program, Medical College of Virginia, and is engaged in various activities including direct patient care, teaching, and research.

James Michael Gould is a Philadelphian who began working in the criminal justice field in 1973. He received a B.A. from LaSalle College where he studied criminal justice. He obtained an M.S. in rehabilitation counseling at Virginia Commonwealth University, while working in the Virginia state correctional system as a counselor and part-time program treatment supervisor. Currently he is pursuing a doctoral degree in counseling psychology at Temple University, where he also works as the assistant to the director of the doctoral program.

Rochelle V. Habeck received her Ph.D. in rehabilitation counseling psychology from the University of Wisconsin-Madison and her master's degree in rehabilitation counseling from Virginia Commonwealth University. She has worked as a counselor and program coordinator in cancer rehabilitation at the Medical College of Virginia and the Wisconsin Clinical Cancer Center. She is currently working as an assistant professor in the counseling program at Michigan State University, where she is also affiliated with the University Center for International Rehabilitation.

Larry Katz received an M.S. in rehabilitation counseling from Virginia Commonwealth University in 1980 and earned certification as a neuro-linguistic programming practitioner in 1982. He lives in Takoma Park, Maryland and is employed by a vocational adjustment program in Fairfax, Virginia.

Martha Hughes Lassiter is an educational specialist for the Virginia Department for the Visually Handicapped. She received her doctorate from the University of Virginia. Dr. Lassiter is on the adjunct faculty of the rehabilitation counseling department at Virginia Commonwealth University.

Robert A. Lassiter is professor of rehabilitation counseling at Virginia Commonwealth University and coordinator of vocational evaluation, work adjustment, and independent living in rehabilitation. He received a Ph.D. from the University of North Carolina, where he was chairman of the rehabilitation counseling program. Dr. Lassiter has had varied experiences in rehabilitation at the executive, supervisory, and practitioner levels and has made numerous contributions to the professional literature.

Susan Merl-Nachinson received her M.S. degree in rehabilitation counseling from Virginia Commonwealth University in 1975. She has worked both as a clinician and an administrator in a variety of alcoholism treatment settings. She currently resides in Chicago, Illinois, where she has a private family counseling practice and works as an educator in the alcoholism sciences for various institutes of higher education. She is an Illinois state certified senior alcoholism counselor. She is married and has one child.

Beverly Marie Momsen is a licensed professional counselor in private practice and is the training officer for Henrico County in Richmond, Virginia. Originating from Minnesota, she has taught at Virginia Commonwealth University and worked in student affairs at the University of Minnesota and Virginia Commonwealth University. She earned a doctorate in counseling from the University of Virginia.

Rita M. Riani received a bachelor of science degree in physical therapy in 1973 at Russell Sage College in Troy, New York, and is a registered physical therapist. She received a master of science degree in rehabilitation counseling at Virginia Commonwealth University in Richmond, Virginia, in 1983. She is presently supervisor of the rehabilitation section of the physical therapy department at the Medical College of Virginia Hospitals.

Kathleen Phayer Sadler received her B.S. in social welfare in 1971 and her M.S. in rehabilitation counseling in 1974, both from Virginia Commonwealth University in Richmond, Virginia. She has been employed as a rehabilitation counselor and presently works for Chesterfield County Mental Retardation Services in Virginia as a program director.

Gail Fitzpatrick Scott is currently employed at the Henrico Area Mental Health and Mental Rehabilitation Center in Richmond, Virginia, in the adult outpatient unit. She has worked there since her graduation from the Virginia Commonwealth University in 1975, where she earned an M.S. in rehabilitation counseling. She is the mother of three children, a daughter and two sons. Ms. Scott is a licensed professional counselor.

Michael D. Traver received his M.S. in rehabilitation counseling at Virginia Commonwealth University and his Ed.D. at the College of William and Mary. His experience has included both outpatient and inpatient psychiatric consultation. Presently Dr. Traver is employed by the Behavioral Services Unit of the State of Virginia, an agency that provides mental health services to juveniles committed to the Department of Corrections.

J.I. Wainwright completed his master's in rehabilitation counseling in 1976 at Virginia Commonwealth University. He is a licensed professional counselor with eight year's experience in community mental health and presently works as director of outpatient services at Chesterfield Community Mental Health Center in Chesterfield, Virginia. In addition, he is on the adjunct faculty at Virginia Commonwealth University, where he teaches group counseling, and has a certificate of training in divorce mediation.

Patricia Muller Weiss received her B.S. in psychology from Bethany College, Bethany, West Virginia, in 1967, and her M.S. in rehabilitation counseling from Virginia Commonwealth University, Richmond, Virginia, in 1981. She presently works as rehabilitation services supervisor for Chesterfield Vocational Services, a Chesterfield County (Virginia) Mental Retardation Services vocational training facility for mentally retarded adults.